Language in the Brain

Language in the Brain

Critical Assessments

Fred C. C. Peng

continuum
LONDON • NEW YORK

Continuum
The Tower Building
11 York Road
London SE1 7NX

15 East 26th Street
New York
NY 10010

British Library Cataloguing-in-Publication Data
A catalogue record for this book is available from the British Library.

ISBN 0–8264–8701–7 (hardback)
ISBN 978082638843 (paperback)

Acknowledgements
The publishers would like to thank the following copyright holders for permission to reprint their material:

Poznan Society for the Advancement of the Arts and Sciences for permission to reprint Fred C. C. Peng's 'A Brief History of Linguistics: What Went Wrong?' from *Lingua Posnaniensis* 46, 2004, pp. 45–72.

Typeset by YHT Ltd, London
Printed and bound in Great Britain by MPG Biddles, Norfolk.

Contents

Preface

As one linguist friend told me recently, 'Much of linguistics has condemned itself to irrelevance and the pursuit of intellectually trivial questions out of an incapacity to understand where the real questions lie.' I concurred because I had told him that linguistics is losing steam everywhere. He continued to lament that, 'This is due to the domination of mechanistic and computer models in the past few decades. But I don't think that is the whole story. It is amazing how a discipline can so ably shoot itself in both feet! There is also a lot of reinventing the wheel and a dearth of new questions and lines of inquiry being developed. Further, it remains very tribalistic and cult-driven.'

He then solicited what I might have in mind, hoping to hear the expansion of what I had said to him about 'losing steam everywhere'. I replied that my feeling of linguistics was summarized quite well by him and that there were two things I could add: (1) the lack of knowledge in the biological and social foundations of language among linguists who are too eager to speculate by argumentation but not willing to present facts on how the brain works *vis-à-vis* human behaviour; the computer can never replace the human brain; (2) the mixed up illusion by linguists in thinking that the mechanistic rules they 'invent' about language represent the brain functions of language, as may be evidenced by the claims of *Agrammatic Aphasia* (see Peng 1992c for more details) and *Pathways of the Brain* (Lamb, 1999). I added that using medical terminology does not make their works fit to represent how the brain functions *vis-à-vis* language as behaviour; nor does it indicate that they know how complex the brain functions are in respect to human behaviour, language behaviour included.

The aforementioned are general remarks which may be taken as an assessment of the current situation in linguistics. These general remarks have become the major concern of my pursuit of the solution to a seemingly simple, but in reality a highly complex, question: 'What is language?' Although there is not a single grain of pretence on my part, nor is there any illusion to think that the question can be answered satisfactorily by a stroke of magic in one piece of research, at least I can begin to undertake this first step to head off the current crisis in linguistics and, by extension, show a new direction in semiotics and behavioural neurology.

This book is therefore a monograph, the first one of a series which I have begun to undertake, in the hope that the quest for the answer to the question 'What is language?' will be the central theme of the series. By extension, it is also hoped that the series will stimulate and encourage thousands of like minds to join forces with me in the exploration of the answer to this fascinating question that is bound to give rise to a new realm of investigation regarding the brain functions of memory which govern language in the brain as behaviour.

As a monograph, it is not a textbook, because many of the new ideas have yet to enjoy consensus. However, it can be used as a reference book. Thus, I have adopted the tone in keeping with the register and style of arguments, critical statements and theoretical constructs.

The series is mentioned in the Preamble, in anticipation of some kind of consensus which, it is hoped, will be reached when the series is completed. It is hoped that the series will become a hallmark in neurolinguistics, or behavioural neurology, and consequently in the basic sciences; this monograph is but the first step to set the pace of the series.

To those colleagues with whom I have expressed strong disagreement I extend a cordial invitation for their public responses, if any, so as to help salvage the sinking discipline, called linguistics, and to prevent the same fate from happening to semiotics. To those colleagues who have voiced their opinions in the past, publicly or privately, regarding the current situation in both linguistics and semiotics, I express admiration and, by taking this opportunity, salute their courage. At one and the same time, I also encourage intellectual interaction, through more open debates, among practitioners in different disciplines, especially among social scientists and neuroscientists, in order to avoid premature sensationalism, errors in imitation and reinventing of the wheel.

If this monograph can become a milestone for the new direction of the study of human language and, by extension, to explore and theorize its origin, the objective of this monograph will have been met. However, it is hoped that the exploration and theorizing should not be through subjective human-centredness by looking down upon non-human primates or other animals; rather, such endeavours should be undertaken through objective observation and investigation, from within, of the central and the peripheral nervous systems in terms of both neuroanatomy and neurophysiology and, more importantly, from without, of the nervous systems control of behaviour in varying social contexts of situation – human or non-human.

Fred C. C. Peng

Acknowledgements

This monograph could not have been undertaken without the intellectual benefits I received from the following people: the late Dr William A. Smalley, who was the first teacher to initiate me to linguistics; Dr Eugene A. Nida and his late wife, Althea Nida, from whom I received financial aid during the first year as a graduate student at the University of Buffalo; the late Professor George L. Trager and the late Professor Henry Lee Smith, Jr. from whom I benefited in training of structural linguistics during my academic years at the State University of New York at Buffalo (1960–64); and the late Professor Charles F. Hockett from whom I received further training in structural linguistics at Cornell University (1962–63).

I am also indebted to the anthropology faculty at SUNY Buffalo, where I benefited from training in cultural anthropology, physical anthropology and archaeology, and the faculty of the School of Medicine at SUNY Buffalo, where I benefited from medical training in the basic sciences.

My realm of specialization also owes its debts to the various training hospitals in Taiwan. Specifically, I should mention Taipei Veterans General Hospital, Taichung Veterans General Hospital and the Tri-Service General Hospital in Taipei, Taiwan, where I gained most of my clinical experiences. Through their sponsorships I obtained several research grants from the Executive Yuan of the Government of Taiwan to conduct research on language disorders in various kinds of patients – notably, patients with aphasia, epilepsy, Parkinson's disease, Alzheimer's disease, Fischer's disease, Huntington's disease, Pick's disease and spino-cerebellar ataxia (SCA).

In the course of writing this monograph, I had the privilege of obtaining agreement from several friends/colleagues and my daughter to review an earlier version of the manuscript before it was submitted to the publisher. Their encouragements are herewith acknowledged: Dr Eugene A. Nida, a staunch structural linguist and a pioneer in the theory of translating, was also instrumental in getting a job for me in Japan when structuralists were having a hard time finding employment in the late 1960s in North America. Professor Roger Matthews, a teacher of English literature, whom I have known since 1966, was a colleague for many years and some of his suggestions as points of subject matter and presentation have been incorporated into the text. Professor J. Peter Maher, a close linguist friend since 1976, made suggestions on terminology and the change of organization. His suggestions on terminology were well taken, which led to some precautious modifications. His work is quoted several times in the monograph. Professor Joseph Decchichis is a linguist of the younger generation. Though first trained in the transformational-generative tradition, he abandoned it in 1980, before turning to ethnographic studies which eventually took him to Japan. Professor Stuart Picken is a philosopher and a theologian. Although he could provide only limited assistance regarding improvement of the manuscript, he has been very helpful to me personally. And my daughter, Professor Virginia M. Peng, is always a very constructive critic of my academic works. Trained as a systemicist, she now leads with other systemicists in Japan an association called the Japan Association of Systemic and Functional Linguistics.

Last but not least, I would like to express my appreciation for the administrative and logistic support I have received from the Department of Neurosurgery and the Neurological Institute of Taipei Veterans Hospital, with which I am affiliated as a consultant. Thanks also go to Ms Jennifer Lovel of Continuum, whose help in obtaining the various permissions to include the figures employed in the monograph was very much appreciated.

Preamble

This book is the first of a series of monographs, plus a textbook, I have planned to finish as a result of the research that has been going on for quite some time at the Neurological Institute, Department of Neurosurgery, Taipei Veterans General Hospital. The series will take several years to complete, hopefully at a rate of one volume per year. The tentative titles of the monographs and the textbook are as follows:

1. Language in the Brain: Critical Assessments;
2. Language Disorders: A Critical Perspective;
3. A Critical Introduction to Neurolinguistics;
4. Language and the Brain Functions of Memory, and
5. Central and Peripheral Nervous Systems Control of Language.

The reason for completing this series is my conviction that language has been mystified and misunderstood to an outrageous proportion, so much so that even geneticists have begun to tap the human genome purporting to have identified 'a gene that controls the development of speech and language'. In *The Times* (London, 10 April 2001), its science correspondent reported, under the heading 'Speech gene discovery proves Darwin's instinct was right', that the gene 'has been identified for the first time in a breakthrough that will transform understanding of a uniquely human ability'.

The science correspondent must have been struck by 'the discovery'. As will be shown throughout this book, the 'gene' so discovered is nothing but one of the many genes affecting human behaviour that result in language disorder when altered, a cause that is absolutely unrelated to the phylogeny or ontogeny of language. However, I should hasten to add that the language disorders so observed may arise from environmental factors, such as some children in a family picking up the 'bad habits' from their elders in the same family.

The many genes which affect human behaviour as a new phenotype, language behaviour in particular, are the genes underlying mitochondrial disorders (or encephalopathy), Pick's disease, Alzheimer's disease, Parkinson's disease, spino-cerebellar ataxia, Huntington's disease, to mention just a few. Thus, associating disordered language behaviour with any defect of a gene as a phenotype in the human genome proves nothing about the original role of the defective gene. Put differently, any gene for the outcome of abnormal behaviour, i.e., a new phenotype, as in the case reported by *The Times*' science correspondent, who along with the 'geneticist(s)' make no distinction between language and speech by lumping them together, on the one hand, but separating language from speech, on the other, is no proof at all for the origin and/or development of language in the brain as normal behaviour. Speech is a part of language, as will be shown throughout this book.

The statement made by the 'discoverers' is no better than saying that 'a gene has been identified that causes cleft palate and, therefore, controls the development of speech and language'. Language in the brain as behaviour is not controlled by any gene any more than it is a thing which can be used; nor is it an organism, as was so believed by some linguists in the past, when it changes.

A gene is a functional concept which directs cell development to form an organ or alters it, as in baldness and/or grey hair, and not a structural one, such as a substance or a molecule in the cell. In contrast, language is behaviour reflecting what the individual's brain does collectively when engaged in interactions with other individuals. Consequently, there is no language gene in the brain, any more than language in the brain can be claimed to be innate.

Note that the report of a mutated form of the gene, linked in 2001 to a speech disorder that impairs movement of the mouth, lips and tongue, also claimed that the gene caused grammatical problems, such as use of the wrong word tense in English. Hence, it has found the language gene. If this gene is believed to be the language gene in humans, does it imply that people who speak a language without any inflections for word tenses do not have that gene? Todd Disotell, associate professor of anthropology at New York University, is critical of the view: 'The best analogy I can give is that we know of a gene responsible for muscular dystrophy and that affects how you walk. Because some people have that mutation, does that make it the gene for walking? No.' (quoted from *The Daily Yomiuri*, 20 August 2002).

As if the claim of the language gene is not enough, German researchers at the Max Planck Institute for Evolutionary Anthropology in Leipzig, Germany, now claim that 'a gene linked to language became widely established in the human population within the last 200,000 years, perhaps because it helped people communicate better and survive' (quoted from *The Daily Yomiuri*, 20 August 2002). The gene is identified as FOXP2, but one of the researchers, Svante Paabo, cautioned that 'While the FOXP2 gene is not believed to have caused speech to emerge, it probably allowed humans to speak much more clearly.' Note that these German researchers make no distinction between language and communication, on the one hand, and between language and speech, on the other.

If that gene became widely established in the human population because it helped people communicate better and survive, or, as Paabo put it, if 'those who first had the gene may have had a survival advantage because their improved communication abilities may have allowed them to hunt better', why have so many languages already disappeared or why are so many more languages fast disappearing today? Paabo added that it enabled the boys to 'tell nice stories to the girls. Or sing beautifully, maybe.' It has possibly not occurred to him that the Japanese deaf people can tell nice stories in Japanese Sign Language and can use it to 'sing' even more beautifully. Is there a separate gene that can be linked to sign language in general, since sign language is also language? These geneticists do not understand what language is and are recommended to read 'The misunderstood geneticist', which is a book review by Pollack (2001) of *The Misunderstood Gene* (Morange, 2001).

Any such claim cannot lend credence to the ups and downs of the philosophy (or 'theology') of the innateness of language which has plagued linguistics for many centuries. Unless the claimer takes into account 'the full interplay of all genes for all relevant cells, tissues, and/or organs of a developing whole organism', to quote, adapt, and otherwise modify a passage from Pollack's review, their claims will go down as a farce in the history of science; so will the claim of innateness of language in the history of linguistics. This book is to repudiate any claim of this sort for the good of linguistics and semiotics and, by extension, of behavioural neurology in particular and neuroscience in general.

Introduction

I have arranged the contents of this book into six parts. Each part pertains to the question 'What is language?' in the hope that some clues to the answer can be thought to have been provided. If we are lucky, the answer may be within our reach before the end of the twenty-first century.

Part I 'What Is Language?' presents three historical perspectives to illustrate the prevalent conceptions of what most people think of language. It consists of three chapters: Chapter 1 'A Brief History of Linguistcs: What Went Wrong?', Chapter 2 'Historical Perspective from the Semiotic Point of View', and Chapter 3 'Historical Perspective from the Medical Point of View'.

1. Since in linguistics, which has a history of more than two millennia, language is the object of study, the linguistic point of view takes a brief look at what language was thought to be in the past by linguists and their predecessors, philologists, and what it is thought of currently by practising language scientists. It is accompanied by a section on the rationale of having neuroanatomy as a must in the analysis of language, if it remains to be called 'linguistics'. Otherwise, as things are going every which way, it may end up being a separate discipline of its own, quite apart from the study of language, with probably a different name: pseudo-theology.
2. The semiotic point of view, as semiotics does not go as far back in history as linguistics, illustrates its original roots in the medical science, on the one hand, and the merging with linguistics in the realm of general semantics, on the other (Pula, 2001). It is also accompanied by a chapter on the importance of neuroanatomy for the brain functions in the interpretation of signs, that is, the reconstructions of meaning in varying social and cultural contexts of situation, which is what semioticians do without being aware of or knowing the brain functions underlying such reconstructions.
3. The medical point of view demonstrates the vast difference which exists between linguistics and other disciplines in the medical and paramedical sciences. It also incorporates what most lay people, that is, non-linguists, would think of language. For the most part, it embraces three domains: (1) language and speech are two separate entities;

(2) language and speech are indistinguishable; and (3) language is made up of ordinary words in the brain. Since this point of view is already equipped with the knowledge of neuroanatomy, what is needed for this point of view is to remedy the deviation, so as to come to terms with reality.

Given the brief literature review and the explanation of what language is currently thought of by people in varying disciplines, Part II 'What Can Be Done about the Current Situations?' proposes some ideas to remedy the current situations in linguistics and semiotics. There is only one chapter in Part II.

'A Mild Proposal' is, therefore, presented as Chapter 4 in order to prepare for the answer to the question 'What is language?' That is, language is not a thing, nor is it an organ, let alone an organism. Rather, language is behaviour which utilizes body parts: the vocal apparatus and the auditory system for oral language; the brachial apparatus and the visual system for sign language. Other non-language behaviours utilize these and other body parts, too. Such body parts are controlled by none other than the brain for their functions.

However, for some peculiar reason, language has been mystified by linguists and non-linguists alike; worse still, it is grossly misunderstood by linguists, as if language is some kind of unknown cognitive ability, a set of rules, dubbed 'competence' by most, thereby referring arbitrarily its manifestation to a mere theatrical notion called 'performance', all because language has two aspects – which have been mixed up and taken for granted interchangeably by linguists and semioticians. The two aspects of language are actually like the two faces of Janus: one looking inward to the individual's nervous system and the other looking outward to society where each individual interacts with other individuals. It is this fact that has been ignored and/or left out in linguistics and semiotics. I have, therefore, introduced the new core distinction of Individual vs. Social to add to the Saussurean traditional core distinction of *langue* and *parole*, which has been known to linguists for quite some time. Through the combinations of these two core distinctions, it is hoped that definitive clues for the answer to the question can be found.

To facilitate the understanding of these combinations of the two core distinctions, I have devoted one chapter to elaborate the importance of the individual aspect of language. It is intended to pave the way for facilitating the introduction and explanation of new ideas which will occupy Part III and Part IV.

Since linguistics has been influenced by other disciplines in the past, I have added a chapter to encourage the interdisciplinary interactions between social scientists and neuroscientists. The reason is that the answer to the question 'What is language?' cannot be undertaken by people with just one discipline in mind. However, as each discipline has its own territoriality, it is often guarded against 'outsiders'. To penetrate this invisible barrier for a constructive two-way intellectual interaction will be a formidable task that awaits conscientious linguists, semioticians and neuroscientists to accomplish for the sake of advances in the language sciences.

Part III is then designed to introduce what is new to most linguists and semioticians, namely, functional neuroanatomy. Many of the ideas expressed may even be new to the medical and paramedical people, for these ideas were cultivated over the past two decades or so by me through the painstaking endeavours of clinical practice and academic research in both linguistics and neuroscience.

There are seven chapters in Part III 'The Individual Aspect of *Parole*'; however, I have omitted the introduction of the vascular system in the brain, which is reserved for the next monograph, *Language Disorders: A Critical Perspective*. The chapters are: Chapter 5 'Language Behaviour and Body Movements', Chapter 6 'The Physical Basis of Life', Chapter 7 'Embryonic Development of the Nervous System', Chapter 8 'Fetal Development of the Nervous System', Chapter 9 'Phylogenic and Ontogenic Origin of the Complexity of Neuronal Circuitry', Chapter 10 'Species-Specific Formation of the Human Vocal Apparatus' and Chapter 11 'Structural Divisions of the Nervous System'.

Part IV 'The Individual Aspect of *Langue*' consists of six chapters: Chapter 12 'Language in the Brain is Memory-Governed', Chapter 13 'Language in the Brain is Meaning-Centred', Chapter 14 'Language in the Brain is Multi-faceted', Chapter 15 'Language in the Brain is also Stratified', Chapter 16 'Evolution of Language: What Evolved?' and Chapter 17 'Cerebral Dominance and Cerebral Laterality: Fact or Fiction?'.

Such new ideas, because they reflect the factual phenomena of life itself in phylogenic and ontogenic terms and come closer to actual human language behaviour, are likely to 'shock' or even 'irritate' many traditionally minded linguists, semioticians and neuroscientists.

Part V 'Production and Reception' literally marks the beginning of the long quest for the answer to the question posited initially. It shows the results of such painstaking endeavours, containing mostly new ideas related to language in the brain; in so doing, I have departed from the long-held tradition that has been cherished by linguists, semioticians and neuroscientists. It has two chapters: Chapter 18 'The Construction of Meaning: Mapping of Content onto Expression' and Chapter 19 'The Reconstruction of Meaning: Coupling of Expression and Content'. They illustrate how the two planes, Content and Expression, function in the brain, from the point of view of production and reception. It is hoped that it will also inspire other like minds to start paying attention to language as behaviour, rather than beating around the bush.

Part VI 'Summary and Conclusion' offers a summary of the distinction between language in the brain and the individual aspect of language on the basis of the fundamentals of what I think language as behaviour requires. This Part has one chapter, Chapter 20, which depicts my realization. It draws many conclusions regarding the scientific contributions of this monograph, and where and how the individual and the social aspect of language can meet. The social institutions seem to be an ideal realm for the union of these two aspects of language. But first and foremost is the conclusion of including people with language disorders of any kind in the study of language by linguists, semioticians and neuroscentists who have thus far ignored them.

Although some linguists have begun to pay attention to aphasic patients, as if their abnormal language behaviours are simply a result of the distortion of the 'rules' these linguists have invented, the fact remains that there are no such things as nouns, verbs, adjectives, or subject and predicate, in the brain; these notions are the artifacts of the theory of grammar (or grammatics) linguists have created for their own purpose of discourse. Thus, ten points are drawn in the conclusion, the key issue of which lies in how to unravel the mystery (or enigma) surrounding the brain functions of memory and cognition, so as to bridge the two aspects of language.

In remembrance of

My Parents

彭清良 MD

彭林芳

PART I WHAT IS LANGUAGE?

General Remarks

In this first part, I shall raise the fundamental question of 'What is language?' by examining three areas of investigation from their historical perspectives. The aim is to explore a solution to the problems which have hindered progress in the understanding of what language really is.

Asking such a fundamental question in the twenty-first century may draw criticisms from fellow linguists and semioticians. But, in retrospect, linguists (and semioticians) have come a long way and yet the solution to the question is still not in sight. There are three main reasons:

1. influence of the long tradition;
2. influence from other disciplines;
3. influence of environmental circumstances (especially during World War II and the latter half of the twentieth century).

These reasons are interrelated and overlap to some extent but, for the sake of convenience, they will be itemized for some discussions in Chapter 1.

1 A Brief History of Linguistics: What Went Wrong?

The question 'What is language?' may sound a little superfluous, not only to professional linguists but also to lay people, because 'everybody' is supposed to know what language is. It is a question that may be asked of students taking an introductory course in linguistics. So, why should I ask such a question when the answer seems 'clear' to all? Be that as it may, the truth of the matter is that when the question is pushed hard on anybody, the answer is likely to be quite different from one person to another, depending on who is asked the question.

As a starter, I will cite Brian Stross's quotation of his nine-year-old nephew's definition (1976: 2). When asked, this boy defined language as 'words and ways that we string them together and pronounce them to communicate ideas'. 'Not bad' says Stross, because he thinks like all linguists that the child's definition embodies in simplified terms the technical categories of 'lexicon', 'syntax', 'phonology' and 'semantics'.

But from the perspective of language teaching, a different view can be observed. Here is an example from an American teacher of English in Japan:

> Linguistic theoreticians of the past few decades have proclaimed language to be this or that. They have provided, or at least have in the past, the models of language needed in teaching. The professionals who work in TEFL looked to these models traditionally for guidance in preparing syllabi and developing teaching strategies. All too often the descriptions given have been excessively formal and abstract. Unfortunately, such models are of little heuristic value and some linguists even gloat over the fact that their theories have no pedagogical value. One group of linguists may confidently describe language as oral/aural. Another group may counter with claims that language is rule-governed. Yet another may say that language is interactional. Professional language teachers may say, with some justification, that this situation is simply another case of the blind leading the blind. I think as teachers we can all agree that language is all the above and somehow more. What is needed is not another theory of some part of language but a general framework of language use. That is, a theory which recognizes the 'body' of which phonology, syntax, and semantics are appendages, namely the use of language to accomplish specific rhetorical goals. Pedagogy demands and deserves such a practical, goal-oriented theory. (Wilkerson, 1989: 4)

The aforementioned remarks indicate clearly that language teachers, like Mr Wilkerson, want 'a general framework of language use' badly, but do not care what language really is. However, what they want implicitly suggests that they treat language as 'a thing' or 'a tool', like most people who think that language is simply a 'tool for communication' which can be used, when language is not a thing at all or a tool but behaviour. Their attitude is justifiable, because if they can accomplish the task (using heuristic techniques which to them are 'language') of enabling their students to speak the language they are teaching, their students' brain processes seem of lesser importance. Thus, laying people's views and language teachers' misgivings aside, I will now go back briefly to the history of linguistics, from the Greek period to the twentieth century, in accordance with the three reasons stated earlier, for a short excursion in search of what linguists in the past had thought of language to see what went wrong.

1. The Long Tradition

A cursory look at any textbook on the history of linguistics, such as the one by Robins (1979), will reveal that during the Hellenic period, the Greek scholars thought that language simply consisted of Greek letters; the question of whether knowledge was innate or learned was debated but not a part of the inquiry of language. The evidence was that the term 'grammar' was defined as the correct way of using Greek letters, having nothing to do with meaning or thought.

This is because the first piece of linguistic scholarship in Greece was the development, i.e., the application, of certain consonant signs of the Hebrew system to represent the Greek vowels, and the use of writing (Robins, 1979: 13). The etymon of 'grammar', namely, *grammatikós*, simply referred to 'one who understood the use of letters, *grámmata*, and could read and write during and before Plato's and Aristotle's time'. It was Dionysius Thrax who wrote in *téchnē grammatikē* that 'Grammar is the practical knowledge of the general usages of poets and prose writers' (Robins, 1979: 31) who set the pace for later grammarians as, under such a heading, the debate of nature versus nurture was very much in vogue during the Hellenic period in respect to human knowledge in general. It is interesting to note that Dionysius Thrax's view was echoed many centuries later by the poet Samuel Taylor Coleridge (1772–1834), who said 'prose is words in the best order, poetry is the best words in the best order', a point that was suggested to me by Professor R. Matthews (personal communication).

In addition to, or in the context of, such a debate, the Greek scholars were also engaged in fierce professional argumentation known as rhetoric; that is, they travelled from one place to another to teach others (mostly lay people) how to win an argument or dispute by presenting skilfully worded utterances in court or other public meetings. The professional trade of verbal art became communication in the twentieth century.

The whole Greek tradition continued through the Hellenistic period to the Roman period with little change in thinking except that Latin replaced Greek.

From then on the tradition of language as letters and written words or texts was firmly established, because the study of sounds had not dawned on linguists even during the medieval period and the Renaissance, except that the Arabs had some ideas of the vocal apparatus, which they must have imported from India; the Sanskrit scholars had predated the Greeks to develop a sophisticated grammar based on Sanskrit, as may be evidenced by Pāṇini's famous Sanskrit Grammar, and had had some notions of phonetics and phonology.

The Chinese, on the other hand, were busy preoccupied with three things: (1) exegesis of old texts and deciphering of Chinese characters (e.g., *Shuo Wen Chie Tze* 說文解字); (2) compiling rhyming books by inventing the system of Fan Ch'ie (反切), for instance, *Ch'ie Yün* (切韻) during the T'ang Dynasty (唐朝) because the Chinese scholars wanted to know how to 'transcribe phonetically' the approximate pronunciation of each character for the reader; and (3) compiling dictionaries, e.g., *K'ang Hsi Dictionary* (康熙字典) ordered by the first emperor of the Ch'ing Dynasty (清朝) that bears his name.

Even after the Renaissance in the West, the concept of letters or written texts as language remained. It was on the basis of this concept that Indo-European linguistics was developed. For instance, Sir William Jones' discovery of Sanskrit as being related to Greek and Latin, on the basis of the written texts, marked the onset of philology which became the precursor of modern linguistics.

2. Influences from Other Disciplines

But the concept of letters and written texts as language was intensified, gradually building up to the extent that before Saussure's time the study of language as written words or texts became even more rigorous. This intensification was partly as a result of the influence from philosophy, because of René Descartes (1596–1650), John Locke (1632–1704), Étienne Bonnot de Condillac (1715–80), and physics, because of Isaac Newton (1642–1727) who formulated the binominal theorem, the laws of gravity and motion, and the elements of differential calculus. Newton's laws influenced linguists, as may be evidenced by the vigorous pursuit of Indo-European historical linguistics, such as Grimm's Law, Verner's Law, Grassmann's Law, and other linguistic laws advocated by the Neogrammarians, some with whom Saussure studied.

The influence from philosophy was greater, however, as the issue of the innateness of language was rekindled and hotly debated among philosophers, because the issue was tied to the question of universal grammar during the seventeenth and eighteenth centuries. But the 'Arnauld wing' of Cartesianism had lost its momentum by the beginning of the eighteenth century (see Aarsleff, 1971). The reason was that 'Linguistics', as Bracken suggests, 'ceased to be of major philosophical interest, once it was seen to be merely an empirical science, or at least a science whose *a priori* character could not be as satisfactorily established as geometry's' (see Bracken, 1970b). But Aarsleff counters that 'there is overwhelming evidence that linguistics attracted greater interest among the philosophers in eighteenth-century France than ever before' (Aarsleff, 1971: 5).

In this connection, there are three points which are worthy of mention: (1) the drive towards universal grammar did produce some interesting results; (2) there were studies into the development of various languages; (3) there was great interest in working back to the pre-Babel language, the *real* language – that which God spoke to Adam, just as there was interest arising from study of the kabbalah (Bracken 1970b: 190, quoted in Aarsleff 1971: 5). However, in this vein, according to Aarsleff (1971: 5), 'That statement illustrates the ignorant claims that enthusiasm over universal grammar can be expected to produce.' But the idea of language being a God-given gift was resuscitated by Süssmilch in 1754.

Also of interest is the fact that as the philosophical pursuit of language innateness and univeral grammar waned towards the nineteenth century among the French and English philosophers, the interest in language evolution (or change) and origin in connection with nationalism began to gain ground in Germany, notably among scholars such as Johann Gottfried von Herder (1744–1803), Karl Wilhelm von Humboldt (1767–1835) and August Wilhelm von Schlegel (1767–1845). Some of their ideas were picked up more than a hundred years later by Edward Sapir and Benjamin Whorf, to whom I shall return further below.

One example is Schlegel who in 1818 proposed a typological classification of languages, such as analytic (or isolating) languages (e.g., Chinese), synthetic (or inflectional) languages (e.g., Greek and Latin) and agglutinative (or affixing) languages (e.g., Turkish and Swahili). Many proponents of typological classification went further, because of feverish nationalism or enthnocentricism, by associating excellence and extent of evolution with their classes. For instance, the highest stage of evolution was assigned to inflectional languages as the most perfect form of human language and the lowest (or earliest) stage of evolution was assigned to isolating languages as the most primitive form of human language.

The Marrist aberration of the then USSR went even further to relate linguistic to economic development. N. J. Marr (1864–1934) was a dogmatic, eccentric linguist whose aberrant theory dominated Soviet linguistics 'until 1950 when suddenly Stalin ordained the rejection of the whole Marrist edifice' (Robins, 1979: 225). The idea of classification was then picked up by Fink, who proposed the most complete typology based on grammatical–semantic criteria, and Sapir, who determined the typology from characteristics observed in a wide variety of languages; Greenberg later modified Sapir's approach, a modification that permits classification of languages by selected structural features, rather than by the entire language (cf. Robins, 1979). Nevertheless, Greenberg's notion of language classification, especially the classification of Amerindian languages, was challenged by Americanists.

The important point here, however, is the fact that language as written words and texts was treated just the same by these scholars from the sixteenth to the nineteenth century. This observation may also be evidenced by the vigorous pursuit of Indo-European historical linguistics in the form of linguistic laws.

At the same time, there were also influences from disciplines other than philosophy and physics; namely, from biology and the social sciences because linguists, largely as a result of Sir William Jones' discovery of the relationships of Sanskrit, Greek, and Latin, then began to ponder on *why* a language (whatever it was then, e.g., Latin) could change over time and spread to geographically different locations. This new trend was a 'natural' follow-up, now that the idea of universal grammar and the innateness of language (with a tie to God) was bound to hit a dead end.

These influences were related to some extent. Thus, linguists likened the changes of language to biological factors, and began to talk about 'genetic' relationships among daughter languages from a common ancestral (or parent) language, e.g., PIE and Sino-Tibetan, as if language was an organism. The family trees employed in historical linguistics for various language families were exact imitations from the family trees of various species of animals and plants in biology (zoology and botany, respectively).

August Schleicher's Indo-European family tree was a good example of such imitation. Schleicher was greatly influenced by Darwin and asserted that 'Languages are plant-like, they develop like natural organisms, their relation to each other is identical to the relation of genetically related natural organisms' (Jankowsky, 1972: 106). As a consequence, the term 'genetic relationships' is now used in historical linguistics, a misnomer that has absolutely nothing to do with the term 'genes' in its biological sense, although some believe that language is genetically prewired. At best, it is a misleading metaphor which, if not rectified, will usher in another tribalistic cult.

In so doing, theories of language birth, language growth and language death also began to flourish. And the debate of nature versus nurture was revived, except that it was now shifted to a debate of whether human language was innate or learned. The bibliography of works relating to the origin of language, by one count (Hews, 1974), contains some 10,000 references. Some of them are, from the point of view of neuroanatomy, really hilarious. But some interesting questions were raised. For example:

1. Was the origin of language monogenesis or polygenesis?
2. Were there biological and behavioural prerequisites?
3. Was the origin of language a gradual growth or a sudden jump?
4. Is language species-specific to man?

To this date, however, none of these questions have been answered properly. The intriguing search for the answer to the origin of language peaked in the latter half of the eighteenth century with a prize offered by the Prussian Academy in 1769. The attempt was in part a challenge to Süssmilch's earlier assertion in 1754 that because of the complexity involved the origin of language could only be the direct gift of God. Thus began more than a century of fruitless speculations on language and the mind or language and thinking versus language and culture, which lasted throughout the twentieth century.

Chomsky picked up the philosophical issue of the innateness of language again by invoking Descartes in his *Cartesian Linguistics* (1966) and, as a consequence, voluntarily inherited the notion of language and the mind in his *Language and Mind* (1968) among others. His ideas were rightly refuted by Aarsleff (1970: 46, 570–85; 1971: 1–12, 17) and by Bracken (1970a: 18, 181–92, 1970b: 9, 236–47).

On the other hand, J. G. Herder attended to the questions raised by the Academy and his solution won him the prize, which was published in 1772 as his *Abhandlung über den Ursprung der Sprach.* In essence, Herder advocated that 'language is the tools, the content, and the form of human thinking', an assertion that was to be picked up a century or so later by Sapir and Whorf and known as the Whorf–Sapir Hypothesis.

However, there is a difference. Although the Greeks from Aristotle to the modistae had taken for granted the hierarchical dependence of language on prior thinking and abstraction, Herder assumed the common origin and parallel of language and thought, and asserted their successive stages of growth and maturity together, a novel idea that won him the prize. On the other hand, the Whorf–Sapir Hypothesis tilts language to thought at times and to culture at other times.

In the former, the Whorf–Sapir Hypothesis has two versions: weak and strong. The weak (or broad) version says: the language one speaks shapes the world in which he lives. The strong (or narrow) version says: one cannot think without language. The strong version comes closer to Rémy de Garment's idea of '*on pense au moyen d'images*' (one thinks by means of images), a line suggested by Professor Roger Matthews.

Notwithstanding, there is also a similarity between the Whorf–Sapir Hypothesis and Herder's thesis; that is, both believed that language and thought (or thinking) are two separate faculties (or brain functions in the present context), a common ground that still lingers today in every discipline which has an interest in cognition. I must add, however, that to Herder language was written words or texts but to both Sapir and Whorf language was *not* written words or texts, because both of them had studied extensively Amerindian languages; for example, Hopi, which had not developed any writing system.

This common ground has come down to this date as 'Linguistic Relativity' but will be rejected in this monograph, for language in the brain is memory-governed, meaning-centred, and multifaceted, and thought is none other than an inchoate mass of meanings made up of impulses.

A closer look at Sapir's publications for the latter (i.e., the strong version), moreover, reveals that his thinking at once reflected on two seemingly paradoxical or even contradictory views about language; that is, that language is, on the one hand, a self-contained entity and yet does not, on the other, exist apart from culture. Here are quotations from Sapir (1921 and 1929).

Language is self-contained	**Language is a part of culture**
1. Language is probably the most self-contained, the most massively resistant of all social phenomena. It is easier to kill it off than to disintegrate its individual form. (1921: 206)	1. Language does not exist apart from culture, that is, from the socially inherited assemblage of practices and beliefs that determines the texture of our lives. (1921: 207)
2. It seems that language is that one which develops its fundamental patterns with relatively the most complete detachment from other types of cultural patterning. (1929: 321)	2. Language is becoming increasingly valuable as a guide to the scientific study of a given culture. In a sense, the network of cultural patterns of a civilization is indexed in the language which expresses that civilization. (1929: 322)
3. Linguistics would seem to have a very peculiar value for configurative studies because the patterning of language is to a very appreciable extent self-contained and not significantly at the mercy of inter-crossing patterns of a non-linguistic type. (1929: 321)	3. Language is primarily a cultural or social product and must be understood as such. (1929: 322)

But to explain how the daughter languages became separated from a parental language, other than the family tree model, some linguists proposed the wave theory, headed by Fr. J. Schmidt in 1872, to liken the spread to the waves in a pond when a stone is dropped into it.

As a result, there was growing competition between the theory advocated by the Neogrammarians who claimed that 'language changes according to laws that admit no exception' and the theory advocated by a group of dialect geographers, Wenker for German dialects and Gilliéron and Edmont for French dialects, who claimed that 'every word has its own history'.

The first theory had an interesting variant which developed later in the early part of the twentieth century but, in retrospect, sounds paradoxical today; namely, 'even irregular sound changes are regular', which to them were 'letters'. In either camp, language remained as written words and texts just the same, even though they talked about 'sounds' which to them were the 'pronunciations' of those written words and texts.

The biological influence led linguists in the late nineteenth century to explore the vocal apparatus, thereby forming the beginning of a new discipline now known as phonetics. The Society of International Phonetic Alphabet (IPA) was founded, which asserted initially the notion of 'one sound for one symbol and one symbol for one sound', based primarily on European languages.

No sooner was this notion asserted than members of the Society found through painful experiences that it could not hold water; the reason being that the phoneticians had to contend with the standard of orthographies for European languages. For instance, the word *hat* has its standard of one and only one form in English, British or American, and yet if it was phonetically transcribed as [hæt], [hɛ:t], or even [he:t] for speakers of various regions, deciding which pronunciation should be the standard form became a problem. But it was this new discipline that drew Saussure into his famous dichotomy of *langue* and *parole* as well as his dyadic diagram of the speech circuit, a novel idea that has made him a legendary figure in the history of linguistics.

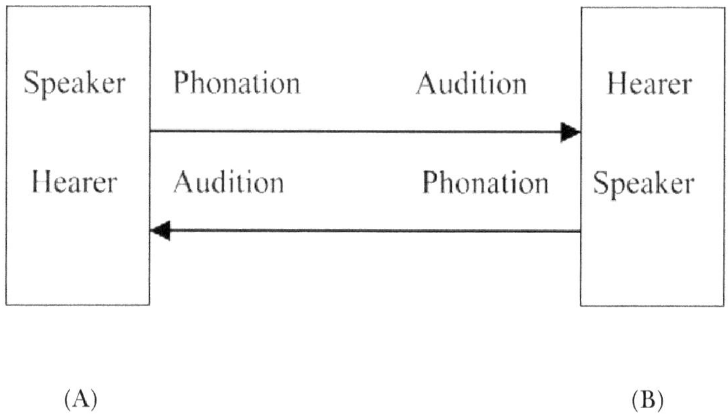

Figure 1.1 *Modified diagram of Saussure's speech circuit between members of a dyad*

Before Saussure's time, however, the innatists as headed by Herder, among others, such as von Humboldt and Harris later, seemed to have the upper hand. The debate, resuscitated from the downturn of the eighteenth century, continued to focus on the origin of language with a tint of nationalism, but the speculation on humans versus non-human primates in respect to language origin remained in vogue for quite some time until it was banned during the conference in 1899 by the Linguistic Society of Paris.

It was 'rekindled' in 1975 in New York at one meeting (22–25 September), sponsored by the New York Academy of Sciences, which I attended; its proceedings were published in one of the Academy's annals (Harnad et al., 1976), promising to revive the zeal for the discussion of language origin. But the zeal of the revival was never followed up; it was short-lived for reasons which will be explained below. However, in 2002, a few geneticists and linguists (cf. *Science*, 2004) revived the issue again, beginning to talk about a language gene for the origin of language, a revival that will not go very far because it is based on a false genetic foundation.

The proponents during the 1975 meeting first hailed the 'new linguistics', which had emerged from the mechanistic techniques in machine translation (MT), as the golden opportunity to revive the issue of language origin. They began to talk about the superior size of the human brain versus those of other primates or animals as the base of the birth of language; some also talked about the limbic system. I objected to both claims during the discussion period, on the ground that it is the complexity of the neuronal circuitry (or networks) that counts, but to no avail. In retrospect, they were barking at the moon or at least barking up the wrong tree, as will be shown later. The evidence is that the conference, though it was also attended by anatomists, biologists and physical anthropologists, besides linguists, was centred on language being an infinite set of sentences governed by rules as the competence of the ideal speaker-hearer, a detrimental premise heralded by the organizers throughout. And that central theme killed the whole zeal because it led to a dead end.

The reasons are manifold:

1. Although some speakers/authors talked about Fossil Record and Neural Organization, and some others talked about Gestural Origin and the Linguistic Competence of Apes, and still others brought in Language and the Human Brain as well as Language Change, there was not a single paper that seriously addressed the question of 'What is language?' Language was taken as a given, based on the then novel notion of an infinite set of sentences. Chomsky's paper 'On the Nature of Language' missed the whole point.
2. The theme was overshadowed by the current of the conference, which was the then prevalent theory in linguistics, a wrong direction that eventually killed the initial zeal.
3. None of the proponents realized the importance of the brain functions of memory in relation to language; the brain functions of memory are *not* species-specific to humans.
4. The prevalent theory at that time was the advocation of the ideal speaker/hearer, a fictional monster that had no brain but, strangely enough, had the knowledge which could enable that monster to produce and understand an infinite set of sentences flawlessly in any language.

It was also well known that Saussure was very much influenced by Durkheim, a sociologist of his time, and his own epistemological view of language (i.e., *langue*). Here, it can be seen for the first time that the long tradition of language as letters and written words was broken. Saussure's theory of *langue* was regarded as a system of pure values and is considered by Thibault in his book as 'a pioneering contribution to the theory of organized complexity in the dynamic, open and evolving relations between a social-semiological system and its environments' (1997: 180). (For a detailed discussion of this view, see my review article (Peng, 2000) which advocates the ontological view of language.)

It is worth mentioning that Saussure's *Cours de linguistique générale* (*CLG*) (1959) has since become a model in the twentieth century for all linguists, at least in the following points:

- the *langue/parole* distinction;
- syntagmatic versus paradigmatic relations, which led to the IC analysis and Halliday's systemics, respectively; IC stands for Immediate Constituents;
- the distinction between synchrony versus diachrony;

- his concept of Thought and Sound;
- his idea of *le signe* consisting of Concept and Acoustic (or Sound) Image.

Both the fourth and the fifth points led to the formulation of A. Martinet's Double Articulation and the formulation of Charles F. Hockett's Duality of Patterning. All these ideas are typical examples of the impact his *Cours* has made.

Note that Double Articulation and Duality of Patterning are the opposite of each other: the former starts from thought (*à la* concept or *signifié*) to grammar as the first articulation and then to sound (*à la* acoustic image or *signifiant*) as the second articulation, whereas the latter starts from sounds to work out sound patterns and then moves on to grammatical patterns via morphophonemics, as in inflection and derivation. For instance, the word *damn* no longer has the sound [n] and yet the sound remains in *damnation*. It is this kind of morphophonemics that draws the attention of historical linguists to sound change and language change for their reconstruction. But, for some peculiar reason, John Lyons in his *Introduction to Theoretical Linguistics* (1971: 54) got them mixed up, by referring Martinet's term of Double Articulation to Hockett's description of Duality of Patterning.

To Saussure, however, thought was an inchoate mass of ideas (or impulses) and sound was just as indeterminate. In this sense, Thibault claims *à la* Saussure that 'the characteristic role of the language system (i.e., *langue*) *vis-à-vis* thought is not to create a material phonic means for the expression of ideas, but to serve as the intermediary between thought and sound ... so that their union necessarily brings about reciprocal delimitations of units' (1997: 167). It is this very characteristic role of the language system purported by Saussure as the intermediary (or, in Hallidayan terminology, social-semiological system) between thought and sound that has influenced and dominated the contemporary theories of linguistics, including, of course, Halliday's theory of systemics.

It was this impact, ironically, that has caused the discipline to have so ably shot itself in both feet and to tilt towards tribalism because of reinvention of the wheel claimed by each tribalistic theory.

To Saussure, moreover, concept and acoustic (or sound) image were intimately linked together, one calling up the other. In his dyadic diagram of the speech circuit, on the other hand, Saussure did mention one direction for speaker and the opposite direction for hearer; namely, psychological phenomenon (concept) to physiological impulses (acoustic image) and then to physical sounds for speaker but the opposite direction for hearer. He depicted the speech circuit as follows: c→s and s→c.

Here, Saussure made two mistakes:

1. He tends to retreat to 'psychology' as a solution for any difficult problem he cannot deal with. What he calls psychological phenomena in the speech circuit are actually neurophysiological in nature, not at all psychological; and he leans to psychology for a solution by saying 'Psychologically ... our thought is no more than an amorphous and

indistinct mass' (Thibault, 1997: 166) when thought in each individual's brain is an inchoate mass of impulses.

2. He uses A (speaker) and B (hearer) to illustrate the speech circuit, and the diagram of phonation and audition seems to balance the two, but unknowingly he favours speaker; that is, hearer is depicted to take what is given by speaker for granted as if the concept in A's brain before the phonation is the same as the concept in B's brain after the audition. The truth is that speaker constructs meaning and hearer reconstructs meaning and the meaning speaker constructs is nine times out of ten *not* the same as the meaning hearer reconstructs.

3. Influences of Environmental Circumstances

Now that Saussure made a significant break from the long tradition about language, linguists in the twentieth century started to push his idea of *langue* and *parole* in every direction. For the sake of easy reference, this section will be divided into several periods.

3.1 The Structuralist Period

The first push was made by the structuralists in the early twentieth century; they defined language as 'a system of arbitrary vocal symbols' largely because of the new environmental circumstances they had to face; namely, the vast number of Amerindian languages which had had no writing systems of their own. So, language as letters or written texts could no longer hold for these languages.

A rather deviant alternative to this structuralist definition of language was stated by Cassirer in *Word* (1945) as follows: 'Language is a "symbolic form". It consists of symbols, and symbols are no part of our physical world. They belong to an entirely different universe of discourse.' If language as defined by Cassirer does not belong to our physical world, it does not belong to any universe of discourse either where individual humans interact with language as behaviour in our physical world.

However, Bloomfield, who also went to Leipzig to study with some of the Neogrammarians, made a significant demonstration of language being oral in his work on Algonquian. (Of course, words and sentences which were uttered by informants had to be transcribed phonetically for analysis.) This drive to study languages which had no writing systems was reinforced by American anthropologists, typically Boas and his student Sapir among others; Sapir also influenced Whorf, the two collaborating to formulate what has been known as the Whorf–Sapir Hypothesis. Its roots, as was alluded to earlier, go back to von Humboldt, Harris and Herder.

Because of the success of analysing unwritten languages, phonemics and morphemics (or morphology) became the centre-piece of linguistics during the first half of the twentieth century. In fact, the classic work of Trager and Smith, *An Outline of English Structure* (1951), set a standard for English phonology in which they proposed four junctures, four stresses and four pitches (called suprasegmental phonemes) vs. segmental phonemes of the overall pattern of nine vowels and twenty-one consonants and three semi-vowels.

In the midst of all this, Bible translators also became involved and were sent to Amerindian territories or overseas as missionaries to study unwritten languages and then translate the Bible (usually the New Testament first) into those languages as part of their mission work. Eugene A. Nida and Kenneth L. Pike were two of the best known Bible translators/linguists and still are. As a matter of fact, Nida's *Morphology* (1949) and Pike's *Phonemics* (1947) were used as standard textbooks in many American and foreign universities as well as missionary-training centres, such as the Summer Institute in Linguistics (SIL), for many years.

Both Nida and Pike studied at the University of Michigan at Ann Arbor. Nida studied English linguistics with C. C. Fries and his doctoral dissertation was later published as *A Synopsis of English Syntax*, using IC analysis which set the standard for later textbooks.

In keeping with this trend of language being oral, Pike's original goal of phonemics for his mission work was to reduce sounds to writing; he studied phonetics at the University of Michigan and his doctoral dissertation was later published as *Phonetics*.

Pike's theory of Tagmemics was originally very much in line with structural linguistics but later became 'contaminated' by the notion of transformation. However, his notion of the emic vs. etic distinction, using baseball for illustration, was patterned after Saussure's notion of *langue* versus *parole*, using chess for illustration.

Meanwhile, in Europe, anthropologists such as Malinowski and linguists such as Firth and D. Jones in the UK, Hjelmslev and Jespersen in Denmark, Jakobson and Trubetzkoy in Prague of then Czechoslovakia, and Martinet in France were developing their own theories of semantics, phonetics and phonology. Malinowski's theory of context of situation, Firth's theory of prosody, Hjelmslev's modification of Saussure's Concept and Acoustic Image as Content and Expression, Jespersen's study of English intonations, Jakobson's early form of distinctive features, Trubetzkoy's principles of phonology and Martinet's functional phonology were also firming up quickly during this period but in different directions.

World War II was another impetus that drove structural linguistics to its height. One driving force was the mobilization of American linguists and anthropologists to the Foreign Service Institute in Washington D.C. to train enlisted men and women as diplomats to 'speak' a foreign language and understand the culture of its people within a short period of time, usually four weeks, before they were sent overseas. Among those linguists mobilized were Charles F. Hockett (for Chinese), Bernard Bloch (for Japanese), Robert Stockwell (for Spanish), George L. Trager, Henry Lee Smith, Jr. (for administration) and Edward Hall (for anthropology), to name just a few. These linguists and anthropologists, after the war, obtained jobs at various universities in the United States, and subsequently trained hundreds of structural linguists by using their experiences and knowledge. I was the first PhD produced by Trager and Smith from SUNY at Buffalo in 1964 and trained by Hockett at Cornell in 1962–63.

The thriving of structural linguistics was carried over into anthropology and influenced anthropologists such as Edward Hall and Birdwhistle. Hall's books, entitled *The Silent Language* (1959) and *The Hidden Dimension* (1966), in which he proposes the concept of proxemics (the study of culturally determined distances that affect human behavioural interactions), were used as standard textbooks in many departments of anthropology throughout the USA. Birdwhistle's work on kinesics (or body language) was in its infancy after the war but has since then become a booming subject in many countries, including Japan where it is now known as 'non-verbal communication'. His work has also influenced many psychologists, such as Paul Ekman, and later child language specialists.

3.2 The Expansion Period

There were three significant post-World War II offshoots (or bonuses) of structural linguistics that are worthy of mention here:

1. Teaching English as a Foreign Language (based on the Michigan Method developed by C. C. Fries);
2. Establishment of the Center for Applied Linguistics in the late 1950s;
3. Inclusion of sign language as language.

Because of the vigorous momentum in studying unwritten languages before the war and the zealous pursuit of Bible translations before and after the war, coupled with the post-war economic boom in the United States, a reverse trend developed; that is, instead of studying 'their' languages, why not teach 'them' our language (i.e., English). Thus, fluxes of foreign teachers and professors of English from Europe, Japan, and other countries were brought to the University of Michigan, at Ann Arbor, under the directorship of C. C. Fries, for training in how to teach English to their students. Through these efforts, courses for training native speakers of English in how to teach English to people in other countries were also developed. The training involved such drills as pattern practices and other techniques, later known as the Michigan Method, which became incorporated in the curricula of many universities for their Freshman English Programs.

The momentum of inviting foreign scholars and professionals to the United States after the war was actually set in motion by what has become known as the Fulbright Act of Scholarships, which was extended to lawyers and other professionals and not limited to language teachers and professors of English; as a result, the Fulbright scholars in Japan, for instance, meet once a year for a reunion sponsored by the American Embassy.

The success of the Michigan Method brought the attention of structural linguists to a new dimension: that of applying structural linguistics to a subdiscipline coined as Applied Linguistics, which was obviously patterned after Applied Mathematics. Structural linguists must have thought that their discipline was rigorous enough, like some kind of mathematics, and therefore could be applied. Here is a quotation from a staunch structural linguist to that effect in 1951:

> The new secretary of the Linguistic Society of America would define linguistics not merely as a branch of anthropology but, more specifically, as a branch of 'cultural anthropology'; another linguist, cited in the same article, speaks of linguistics as a branch of, or rather, a kind of mathematics. (Voegelin, 1951)

The motivation arose in part from the criticism from anthropologists, for example, Linton, who in writing complained that linguistics was of no use to the study of culture and society. In other words, linguistics had been rejected by cultural anthropology as its branch. This negative feeling was nakedly expressed by Linton in the following way:

> Turning to the field of cultural anthropology, and its subsciences, we find that the subscience of linguistics is, at present, the most isolated and self-contained. The study of languages can be and largely has been carried on with little relation to other aspects of human activity ... That linguistics ultimately will be of great value for the understanding of human behavior and specifically of human thought processes can hardly be doubted. However, work along these lines has barely begun and linguistics is still unable to make any great contribution toward the solution of our current problems. For this reason it has been ignored in the present volume. (Linton, 1945)

Thus, in what appeared to be an apparent rebellion against the criticism directed at linguists, under the auspices of the Ford Foundation with a grant, in collaboration with The Modern Language Association, the Center for Applied Linguistics was founded on 16 February 1959 in Washington D.C. with C. Ferguson as its first director. The original aim was to serve as a clearing house for universities, government agencies and other institutions, or individuals concerned with the application of linguistic science to practical language problems (*The Linguistic Reporter*, 1959, vol. 1, no. 1). However, it gradually shifted to promote English teaching or language teaching in general.

In the name of applied linguistics, the International Congress of Applied Linguistics was later formed, which is held every three years. I attended the one held in Greece (1984) and the one held in Australia (1987) under the presidency of Halliday. The point I am seeking to make is that the programmes of both congresses were no longer limited to language teaching; they included among others sociolinguistics, psycholinguistics, computational linguistics, ethnolinguistics and neurolinguistics. In later congresses, however, the agenda became somewhat constricted.

Recall the structuralist definition of language. It was confined to one facet, that is, oral language, by breaking away from the long tradition. Written language was denied, probably as a result of the rebellious attitude to the long tradition, because writing was regarded simply as a surrogate. Sign language was branded. Even Saussure himself denied in his *Cours* the visual facet of language when Whitney suggested it, and dismissed it simply as 'trop absolue' (too extreme or dogmatic) (de Saussure, 1959: 26).

The remark from Saussure is interesting because Saussure's dismissal of the visual facet of languge – for example, sign language – set the pattern for modern linguistics until 1960; before that, sign language had never been considered to be language by linguists. It was in 1960 when William Stokoe, a professor of English at the then Gallaudet College, came to the University of Buffalo to study linguistics with George L. Trager and Henry Lee Smith, Jr. that American Sign Language (ASL) used by students, teachers and staff at Gallaudet was brought up for the first time as a linguistic object of study. Today, no linguist would dare deny that sign language (ASL, JSL, or any other sign language) is language in its true sense.

However, the 'discovery or inclusion' of sign language as language has sparked a new round of debate among linguists over how languages are formed (*Science*, 7 September 2001, pp. 1758–59) when Nicaraguan deaf students were found to have created a new sign language, NSL. Again, its over-enthusiastic adherents miss the whole point, by mystifying and exaggerating NSL as if the origin of language was just discovered, without taking into account the plasticity of brain functions in humans and non-human mammals and the role played by neuroanatomy and gross anatomy in general.

Before the inclusion of sign language, psychologists such as the Hayes had been interested in whether non-human primates could learn an oral language. They trained a female chimpanzee, by the name of Vicki, to talk. After two years of painstaking training, Vicki managed to utter four 'words': *papa, mama, cup* and *up*. I have examined the video tapes recorded by the Hayes in a documentary programme in Japan. From the phonetic point of view, those 'words' were severely 'mutilated', because there was no voicing in the 'vowel' of each 'word' and the nasals were devoiced, not to mention the poor articulation of the 'consonants'. There is a reason for such deficiency. Non-human primates' vocal apparatuses are built differently from the human vocal apparatus, as will be illustrated later.

After the Hayes, because of the 'discovery' of sign language (ASL, in particular) as being language, psychologists such as the Gardners began to train in Nevada another female chimp by the name of Washoe to sign. People around her were forbidden to use English; only ASL was allowed. After one year, Washoe was able to make over 80 signs to interact with humans around her. The training of Washoe was continued later in Oklahoma by Roger Fouts. It was in Oklahoma that I met Washoe for the first time; she did look different from other chimps and signed to Fouts in front of me, begging for food.

In competition with Washoe, Penny Patterson in Palo Alto, California, trained a female gorilla by the name of Koko to sign. Her ASL vocabulary exceeded that of Washoe. Patterson, however, used a different method; she talked to Koko while signing ASL to her. Thus, according to Patterson's report, Koko was not only able to interact with humans by signing but was also able to understand English and yet she would respond in ASL. Koko's ability to understand English, not only from Patterson but also from other humans, makes sense because a non-human primate's auditory system, including the auditory association system in the cortex, is similar to that of a human. There is no reason to believe otherwise – even a lower mammal, such as a dog, can understand its trainer's commands.

Later, Patterson added a male gorilla by the name of Michael to her research, hoping that the two gorillas would interact with ASL and eventually mate to produce offspring to whom the gorilla parents would then teach ASL. But the attempt was not successful, because the two gorillas never 'got married'. I met both gorillas in 1977. Recently, Michael died and Patterson has now acquired another male gorilla from a zoo in the hope to move the two gorillas to Hawaii, the big island, for producing a gorilla colony in a jungle with young gorillas learning ASL.

In addition to chimps and gorillas, a male orang-utan, by the name of Chantek, was trained by Lyn Miles, an anthropological linguist, in Tennessee. Chantek, however, was not as 'smart' as Washoe and Koko. His vocabulary of ASL was much smaller and the pace was slower. (For a detailed report of some of those earlier research results, see Peng, 1978). I also met Chantek in 1979.

Now that all three species of the great apes have been shown to be capable of learning a human language, ASL, there were other attempts to teach chimps: to manipulate coloured chips using a keyboard hooked to a computer in Atlanta, Georgia; and to construct strings of different signs in Kyoto at the Primate Center. All this suggests that cognitive capacity as the other side of the same coin as memory also exists in non-human primates' brains. So long as there are anatomical facets, such as the limbs, the eyes, the ears, the nose, etc., available to non-human primates, there is no reason to exclude cognitive ability from them. In other words, language as behaviour is *not* an exclusive capability of humans; rather, it was the wrong definition of language that caused the confusion among linguists, psychologists, neuroscientists, and, of course, primatologists. More will be said along this line later.

3.3 The Cold War Period

Although structural linguistics was expanding to incorporate other disciplines such as sociology, psychology and computer science as applied linguistics, the scope of the studies within the field itself remained very narrow throughout the first half of the twentieth century; at the annual meetings of the Linguistic Society of America (LSA) the programmes were dominated by papers on phonemics and morphemics and historical linguistics based on them. Then, came a boost of research money from many sources, including the US air forces, navy, army and CIA, among others, because the United States was engaged in a cold war with the then Soviet Union and other communist countries. Recall the boost from World War II to structural linguistics.

The financial supports were prompted by the new technology of computer science and computational programming, because of the rapid advances in computer hardware. Computer scientists and programmers were in great demand for one purpose: machine translation (MT). A journal bearing that name was created by Victor Yngve at MIT; however, it disappeared shortly after its few initial publications, but was resuscitated by a different publisher and a different editorial board. Nonetheless, the fact remains that computers can never replace the human brain for the complex brain functions of language, which are memory-governed, meaning-centred, and multifaceted, as will be shown later.

The research monies were funnelled to various universities and industrial companies, for instance, MIT, University of Texas at Austin, The Rand Corporation, and the Bunka-Ramo Corporation in California, to name just a few. Their works involved developing parsers or software programs for translating Russian and Chinese into English by machine. It was during this cold war period that a drastic change in linguistics took place: Phrase Structure Grammar (PSG) and Transformational-Generative Grammar (TG). MT was primarily based on such notions, even though PSG had its origin in Immediate Constituents (IC) analysis, which was based on Saussure's idea of syntagmatic relation.

In one sense, the drastic change was nurtured by the rebellion or even hostile feelings against the domination of structural linguistics, then the ruling paradigm, for phonology and morphology at the LSA meetings. In another sense, it was the 'yearning' of linguists, then, to be able to align themselves with something 'useful' called computer science as a 'rebuff' of the hitherto isolated status of linguistics labelled against them by attempting something 'mathematical'.

3.4 The Take-Over Period

Because of the drastic change, started in the 1950s, a new brand of linguistics began to emerge within the United States and gradually spread to other countries. Language was redefined as 'an infinite set of sentences'. It was an unfortunate pseudo-mathemetical definition imitating the mathematical notion of Axiom for the initial string #S# which then would algebraically expand into strings of formatives, by Phrase Structural (PS-) rules, until the final strings generate what were thought at first to be kernel sentences, which were said to be finite in number. To these kernel sentences were then applied a set of rules called Transformational (T-) rules, some of which were thought to be recursive, to generate infinitely all and only grammatical sentences of a given language. These PS-rules and T-rules were later claimed to be universal, representing the exclusive human cognitive ability in the brain, thereby reviving the old notion of universal grammar that had been running rampant in the seventeenth and eighteenth centuries in Europe.

Unlike the earlier notion of universal grammar, in which 'infinity' had never been claimed by any of the proponents, during this take-over period the notion of 'infinity' in its version of universal grammar had an interesting ramification which turned out to be quite 'out of touch' from reality, thereby portraying and leaving permanently the impression of mechanistic computer models in all versions of subsequent TG and generative grammar. That is, it was claimed that 'there is no longest sentence in any language, because if someone produces a long sentence, a word can be added to it to make it longer'.

This pseudo-mathematical definition of language has spread to psychology, as may be evidenced by Brown's definition as follows:

> Fewer than one hundred sounds which are individually meaningless are compounded, not in all possible ways, to produce some hundreds of thousands of meaningful morphemes which have meanings that are arbitrarily assigned, and these morphemes are combined by rules to yield an infinite set of sentences, having meanings that can be derived. (1965: 248)

There was no theory of generative phonology at first in this new brand of linguistics, other than the mention of structuralists' morphophonemics, to describe sounds in human language. Halle's *Sound Patterns of Russian,* based on Jakobsonian theory of distinctive features, came out later in 1959a. When generative phonology finally came out, in the late 1960s, possibly because of my critique of the lack of phonology in TG mentioned in my review article (Peng, 1969), it had already made the first major blunder by relying on pseudo-statistics to promote the now defunct notions of accidental and systematic gaps. These notions had been covered in various linguistic conferences and publications (cf. Halle, 1959b, 1961, 1962, 1964; Chomsky, 1965), as if generative phonologists had just made a major discovery in phonotactics. But, quite to the contrary, the notions became a farce in the history of linguistics and will remain so for the following reason.

In generative phonology, /blik/ was said to have an accidental gap and /bnik/ was said to have a systematic gap. The former was defined as 'admissible but non-occurring sequences of sounds in the language' and the latter was defined as 'phonologically inadmissible and therefore cannot occur in the language'. However, when I 'accidently' ran into a lady from New Zealand in the late 1960s, at a meeting of the Association of Foreign Teachers in Japan, who was wearing her name tag showing 'Hazel Blick', I could not help but ask her 'How do you pronounce your name?' She kindly said: /blik/. She added that it is a very old English name. When she was introduced to the Association by its president, an American, as Miss Blick /blik/, which was uttered several times, I was tempted to rise and say: 'Mr President, /blik/ is possible but does not occur in English.'

It was quite ironical that I had to come all the way to Japan to realize that Halle and Chomsky were wrong in the first place. The reason is simple: they were wrong not just because they neglected to check a decent English dictionary but also because they committed the typical error of 'Haste Makes Waste'. Later, I checked my Webster Dictionary (1965), and found out that /blik/ is indeed an admissible and occurring English word, spelled *blick,* which has two entries. The two entries are: *blick,* n, a fish; same as *bleak*; and *blick,* n, same as *fulguration.* Moreover, if /bnik/ is phonologically inadmissible and therefore cannot occur in English, it is *also* phonologically inadmissible and therefore cannot occur in Chinese, Taiwanese, Japanese, and hundreds of other languages. Why should it be so 'systematic' in English? And what was the significance, other than a sheer blunder, of making such a pseudo-statistical statement when Halle and Chomsky had not checked the phonotactics of all these languages in the world? (See Peng (1970: 81–6) for the details of this interesting report and Peng (1974: 81–119) for more details.)

During this take-over period, from the 1960s onward, there was no distinction between linguists trained or even graduate students training at MIT and programmers. IBM was busy hiring linguists who were transformational-generative grammarians to do researches on MT owing primarily to Chomsky's 1957 publication. However, his later book (1965), marked the beginning of fragmentation among members of this new brand of linguistics, known as generativists, nicknamed TG-ers. Transformational rules were replaced by a 'magic wand' called 'Change the category'. (See Peng (1969) for details.)

The fragmentation had to do with or was caused by the notions of deep structure and surface structure within the core group of generativists. That is, the notion split the group into at least (1) the generativist subgroup and (2) the interpretivist subgroup.

The former advocated that semantics was generative in nature, governed by a set of semantic rules which would then generate deep structure as the core from which a set of syntactic rules could be applied to generate surface structure. Surface structure could then be subject to phonological rules to produce the needed pronounceable sentence.

In contrast, the latter advocated that syntax (in the form of a set of rules) was the core of human cognition, which would generate deep structure to interpret meaning, on the one hand, and to generate surface structure to which phonological rules could then apply to produce the needed pronounceable sentence, on the other.

It is worthy of some mention that Chomsky's *Syntactic Structure* (*SS*) was formulated at MIT with a grant for MT headed by Yngve, who later on left MIT and moved to the University of Chicago, abandoning MT altogether. There, he changed his theoretical orientation to what he calls human linguistics, and admitted his mistakes of the past during his presidential address at one of the meetings of LACUS (Linguistic Association of Canada and United States) which I attended. (See his presidential address 'To be a Scientist' (1986) where he proclaims that 'Chomsky's works ... are much more in the realm of philosophy than of science, as has been pointed out more than once in the literature'.)

The interesting point here is that *SS* was a pseudo-mathematics of mechanistic formulation for MT from which Chomsky migrated into philosophy, as in *Cartesian Linguistics* (1966) and *Language and Mind* (1968), both of which, however, have been repudiated as fantasy on philosophical grounds by philosophers of language, as was pointed out above. Yngve states that: 'A competent scientist does not pepper his manuscripts with mathematical notations that serve no good purpose in computation or exposition.' He also adds: 'Mathematical notation is not to be used as window dressing' (Yngve, 1986: 18).

Soon after the take-over, many serious problems emerged largely because of counter-attacks from structuralists and other linguists from Europe. But, in large part, the problems arose from over-zealous attitudes on the part of TG-ers for premature theorizing, such as the notions of accidental and systematic gaps mentioned above. Sociolinguists and some psycholinguists also joined forces for the counter-attacks. The following are the problems.

The first problem was the notion of kernal sentences proposed in *SS*; it was machine-oriented to accommodate the computer, rather than human languages, for no reason other than sheer arbitrary 'convenience' or 'window dressing'. It disappeared from the linguistic scene for a very poor reason: the reason given, informally though it may have been, was that 'It was no longer interesting.' In retrospect, it was erroneously and naively conceived to begin with; its departure was just as unconvincing.

The second problem was the notion of grammaticalness. Because the claim that PS-rules and T-rules could generate all and only grammatical sentences and that there was no longest sentence in such 'grammatical' sentences was found to be untrue, TG-ers at the LSA meetings often had to defend some sentences that were thought to be ungrammatical by others. The solution was a show of hands from the audience; those who said 'Yes' were the minority and usually TG-ers and those who said 'No' were the majority and, of course, not TG-ers.

That the notion of 'grammaticalness' is problematic can be evidenced by the spread of 'Englishes', pidgins and Creoles. These languages were not created by 'rules'; rather, they were created by individual speakers/hearers whose brain functions of memory have enabled them to make proper adjustments to the external and internal environments in their language behaviour.

Let me cite an example from Hawaiian pidgin. In Hawaiian pidgin English, *me no can* for 'I can't do it' can be heard readily. Is this sentence generated by PS-rules and/or T-rules? Or is it generated by the touch of the magic wand 'Change the category'? Mechanistically one can derive it on paper from 'I can't do it' by changing 'I' to 'me' and then delete 'do it' and finally reverse the order of 'can't' to 'no can'. Computers can do that derivation with the right programming. But it would be totally absurd to even contemplate such changes as reflecting the changes (or breakdown) of rules in the brain functions of Hawaiian pidgin speakers. Even if computers could do such changes, is *me no can* a grammatical sentence? If so, by whose standard, American, British, or Hawaiian pidgin speakers?

To justify such a claim, and more importantly to avoid the thorny issues of having to deal with Englishes which are not exactly English, because of pidginization and/or creolization, not to mention the historical changes of modern English, from Old English to Middle English, that has now become a 'creole', a fictional monster called the Ideal Speaker/Hearer was created by Chomsky; the monster became the third problem. It had no human brain but was said to be 'born' with a system of rules of generative grammar the underlying principles of which were purported to be universal and capable of generating perfect sentences, any one of which could be infinitely long, because the monster made no human errors, or was immune from them, in the generation of an infinite set of only grammatical sentences in any language.

It is amazing that linguists, then, TG-ers in particular, could propose and buy such a nonsensical notion as the ideal speaker/hearer that had no brain and was out of touch from reality and yet had the universal ability of generating all and only grammatical sentences that could be infinitely long which were perfect in all varying social contexts of situation. It was and is a hilarious farce and will remain so in the history of linguistics. But this nonsensical notion is now changed to an equally nonsensical substitute called language template by younger innatists on the basis of Nicaraguan sign language, NSL (*The Times*, 9 December 2004).

The fourth problem was the notion of ambiguity; the strength of explaining away certain ambiguity in ambiguous sentences was regarded as a merit of the new mainstream linguistics. But, in MT, post-editing by humans had to be employed to get rid of not only ungrammatical but also ambiguous sentences in the output. Note that ambiguity is a decoding problem and not an encoding one for humans; in human interactions, people usually rely on context of situation to resolve ambiguity for their own purposes, even though such a resolution, nine times out of ten, may not come out right; that is, the result of ambiguity resolution is more often than not incompatible with the encoder's original meaning, as will be explained later on.

The fifth problem was the notion of intuition which was used to defend the second, third and fourth problems, on the one hand, and to guard or strengthen the driving force, called 'mentalism', for the then new brand of linguistics, on the other hand, as may be evidenced by Chomsky's *Cartesian Linguistics* (1966) and *Language and Mind* (1968); he wanted to tie it to his own version of the innateness of language and universal grammar, hoping to justify it by relying on the earlier version of philosophy of language. Other TG-ers followed suit by attacking the structuralists ferociously for 'anti-mentalism'; Bloomfield, in particular, was blamed for being too mechanistically oriented and the methodology employed was 'cursed' as being merely 'discovery procedure'.

The sixth problem was the misnomer of competence and performance which were used to reinforce the notion of intuition. These notions were advocated in the 1960s to replace Saussure's *langue* and *parole*, respectively. Recall that competence was defined as the ideal speaker/hearer's ability (or knowledge) of his/her (or, I should say, its) language, whereas performance was defined as the use of that ability.

These definitions are non-sequitur. For one thing, language is behaviour (not a thing or code that can be used) which must be based only on the brain functions of each individual – which can be active, for production, or passive, for reception, just like all non-language behaviours – not on a fictional monster such as the ideal speaker/hearer.

In either active or passive brain functions what happens in the brain is a transduction of signals (made up of action potentials or impulses) in more than one direction, which must be *all or nothing*. If there are neuronal signals being transduced from one part of the brain to another (which is *all*), the individual's behaviour is being conducted; on the other hand, if there are no neuronal signals being so transduced (which is *nothing*), then the individual's behaviour is not being conducted. There are no such things as 'half-way' action potentials in the brain that can be transduced as signals to be called 'performance'. I shall return to these non-sequitur notions later for more comments when I describe action potentials or impulses which are the only signals the brain recognizes.

That those notions, competence and performance, are a misnomer were pointed out quite early by the structuralists in the 1960s; for example, W. F. Twaddell, one of the leading structuralists at that time. Here is a quotation in full of what he said in 1966 from 'Remarks read at the 1966 Northeast Conference' (1969–70):

[*Abstract*: Comments on the inappropriateness of Chomsky's essay 'Linguistic theory' in the *Reports* of the Northeast Conference. Now printed for the first time, for reasons explained in the added opening paragraphs here.]

For some time I have gotten occasional inquiries about my comments on Noam Chomsky's essay 'Linguistic theory,' pp. 43–9 of the *Reports* of the Working Committee of the Northeast Conference of 1966.

I had not considered it appropriate to publish my comments, since Mr Chomsky's essay and my oral remarks about it seemed best treated as ephemera. However, Mr Chomsky's essay has recently been reprinted (in Mark Lester, *Readings in Applied Transformational Grammar*, New York, Holt, Rinehart, Winston, Inc., 1970, pp. 52–9); this constituted a change in the status of the essay, especially since no indication is given in the reprint of the audience to which the essay was originally addressed. (In the references below to Mr Chomsky's remarks, the page numbers in the forties are those of the Northeast Conference Report; references to page numbers in the fifties are to those in the Lester reprint.)

Quite often, in inquiries and comments, my remarks are described as a disagreement with Mr Chomsky's conception of language.

They were not. Since the late 1950s, I have found Mr Chomsky's publications uninteresting to anyone who is seriously concerned with the real and observable phenomena of human communication via what we usually call language, and I would consider it a waste of my time to pursue the metaphors and speculations of his post-1960 publications.

My remarks were directed at his manners, not his views. To an audience which was overwhelmingly composed of practicing foreign-language teachers, most of them high-school teachers, he presented what I regarded as a supercilious, narcissistic essay. It was bad manners to present, in an off-hand manner, something that was very unfamiliar to most of the readership; it was not quite honest to present it as 'linguistics' when it was only Chomsky's speculations in glotto-psychology.

I thought that it was appropriate for me to apologize for an offensive behavior to my language-teaching colleagues by a *soi-disant* linguist; I also thought it was appropriate to defend the main body of responsible linguists from the misrepresentation of 'linguistics' implicit in Mr Chomsky's essay.

Such was the background. Following are the remarks. 9 March, 1970.

It is not easy to comment on Mr Chomsky's essay to an audience of FL teachers. Mr Chomsky insists that he is not familiar with the teaching of languages, and he doesn't even pretend to be interested in foreign-language teaching. Obviously he hasn't made any effort to communicate intelligibly to this Conference on FL teaching. His special way of looking at 'language' is hard to relate to the real behavior of human beings, and his speculations in this essay are not related at all to the realities of the classroom.

So, naturally, there is little or nothing in the essay which could contribute to more effective FL teaching. Indeed, the essay is more likely to confuse and mislead than to inform.

Few of Mr Chomsky's readers here could know the special focuses and blind spots of his theoretical framework. For example, his dogmatic vehemence (44; 53–54), emphasizing creativeness and denying a habit-structure, reflects Mr Chomsky's current preoccupation with some extremely abstract, unobservable 'linguistic competence' which is somehow very different from any mere 'linguistic performance' that you and I observe in the real world and in the classroom, which does involve habitual behavior. Mr Chomsky several times refers to 'rules that determine the form of sentences' (44, 47; 53, 56–7), whereas in serious scientific investigation the form of sentences would determine the rules. He tells us (47; 57) that the rules of a generative grammar are abstract, but these abstract somethings somehow 'manipulate structures' (47; 57). If we find that metaphor hard to accept, Mr Chomsky scarcely helps us by announcing (46; 56) that 'the native speaker has internalized a generative grammar, a system of rules,' and then tells us (46; 56) that a generative grammar is 'a theory of the speaker's competence.' Putting these two comments together yields the remarkable revelation that the native speaker has internalized a theory of his competence. But although the native speaker has 'internalized this system of rules' (46; 56) he has not learned it (48; 58) and he has no awareness that he has internalized the rules or what their properties are (46; 56).

Whatever all that means, if it means anything, it certainly contributes no guidelines for actual FL teaching.

Similarly, there is no attempt to apply something he calls 'intrinsic organization in cognition' (46, 48; 55, 58) to anything in the classroom.

Mr Chomsky deduces (48; 57) from his theories that 'the underlying principles of generative grammar ... must be universal properties'. Even theoretically, it seems pointless to wonder whether all languages display linguistic characteristics. Anyhow, the guess is worse than useless to teachers who are face-to-face with the real specific similarities and differences of two real specific observable languages.

Mr Chomsky's off-hand remarks about his theories of pronunciation are likely to be misinterpreted, to say the least. To speak, as he does, of 'the intrinsic correlation of sound and meaning in the language in question' (46; 56) is particularly reckless. One of the most astonishing of his unsupported assertions is that 'a decade ago it would have been almost universally assumed that a phonetic representation is simply a record of physical fact' (45; 54). I can think of no meaning for that assertion which would be true.

This audience deserved a more careful and a more relevant statement than a hurriedly assembled collection of authoritarian, unsupported, dogmatic pronouncements, along with supercilious dismissal of the work of Mr Chomsky's

> predecessors and most of his contemporaries. FL teachers will do well to work along with Carroll, Ferguson, and the majority of responsible linguists, and for some time to come not expect any practical help from speculation about 'an internalized but not learned system of rules' which is, or comes from, or leads to, some unobservable abstract 'linguistic competence.' FL teachers need not be awed by a pretentious terminology, or intimidated by a pontifical self-assurance. It is better for us to keep on trying to improve our teaching by cautious and imaginative use of principles that are closer to the mainstream of linguistic theory and research, and formulated by people who have some interest in the realities of the classroom.

The seventh problem was the utterly nonsensical notion of language being 'rule-governed', which has been the basis of generative grammar, as has been succinctly pointed out by Twaddell. It became the crux of the new mainstream of linguistics to justify the now defunct idea of 'generating all and only grammatical sentences' in order to uphold the monster called the Ideal Speaker/Hearer. To the FL teachers in the 1960s, Twaddell quoted Chomsky as using 'the native speaker' but 'the native speaker' was later abandoned, becoming the fictional monster.

The 'rule-governed' notion is meant by the generativists that the finite set of rules as grammar, including PS-rules and T-rules, serves as an interface between semantics and phonology to generate all and only grammatical sentences. This notion still lingers in the literature today of the now mainstream linguistics in at least North America. And, as was mentioned earlier, it was this notion that killed the 'rekindled' zeal of the promise for the pursuit of the origin of language. However, the revival of the issue in the twenty-first century emphasizes the innateness of language by fabricating a non-existing language gene. Language is not rule-governed, nor is it innate; rather, it is behaviour – what the brain does – which is memory-governed, meaning-centred and multifaceted (Peng, 2000, 2001, 2003a, 2003b; Peng et al., 2002).

The 'rule-governed' notion of language (or lexicogrammar) is obviously based on Saussure's social-semiological system of *langue*, serving as the intermediary between thought and sound, thereby giving the impression of the domination of mechanistic and computer models over the past few decades. However, Saussure's notion of 'intermediary' was never intended to be mechanistic. He says, 'Neither are thoughts given material form nor are sounds transformed into mental entities; the somewhat mysterious fact is rather that "thought-sound" implies division, and that language works out its units while taking shape between two shapeless masses' (1959: 112). I should quickly take exception by adding that thought and sound are two different masses of impulses but are *not* at all shapeless, because these impulses are the neurophysiological properties of neurons which are concrete and tangible anatomical structures.

Interestingly enough, Saussure's influence can also be seen in Halliday's systemics. Lamb has picked this up in his stratificational grammar, too; he even goes one step further to claim that his stratificational 'rules' are pathways of the brain. His claim, like those of the TG-ers, is a fiction and will remain so in the history of linguistics.

Ironically, the early TG-ers of the 1960s were attacking the structuralists for 'anti-mentalism' and yet the TG-ers of today have put on themselves an even worse straitjacket of being more mechanistic and 'anti-mentalistic', even though some of them have claimed the representation of rules in the brain by using medical terminology. The use of medical terms does not indicate that the advocates know how the brain functions.

In an attempt to get out of this straitjacket, a group of TG-ers joined the American Academy of Aphasiology, thinking that they could analyse aphasic patients' abnormal utterances to prove that 'language is rule-governed' and that even rules in the brain could be impaired. They tried to 'teach' clinically oriented aphasiologists what language was, that is, 'rule-governed', just like Chomsky was trying to force FL teachers to accept his non-sequitur notions of the ideal speaker/hearer's competence of language, which could generate infinitely all and only grammatical sentences by means of a system of rules that the ideal speaker/hearer had internalized but not learned. Their attitude drove the aphasiologists crazy, in the way in which FL teachers (including teachers of English in Japan mentioned earlier and elsewhere) were driven mad. The TG-ers eventually took over the American Academy of Aphasiology, and the aphasiologists were driven out to form their own separate organization.

3.5 The Neo-Innatist Period

Through such a driving force, the innatism of language was 'triumphantly' brought back to the forefront of the now mainstream of linguistics. As a result, language was said to be born with the child (i.e., 'not learned', as was quoted by Twaddell). This innatism is different from the innateness of language purported in the sixteenth, seventeenth, or even eighteenth centuries. The reason is that practitioners of this brand of language innatism even claimed that the child was born with a copy of Chomsky's *Aspects of the Theory of Syntax* in his brain. There was no learning of language; the child's upbringing served only to trigger or activate the rules that came with birth in the newborn's brain. A typical example of the nonsensical claim of such innatism is the following:

> It is now proposed that, first, children are born with a biologically based, innate capacity for language acquisition; secondly, the best guess as to the nature of the innate capacity is that it takes the form of linguistic universals; thirdly, the best guess as to the nature of linguistic universals is that they consist of what are currently the basic notions of Chomskian transformational grammar.
>
> Metaphorically speaking, a child is now born with a copy of *Aspects of the Theory of Syntax* tucked away somewhere inside. Given the present state of knowledge regarding innate capacity and language universals, the above seem defensible guesses. (Fraser, 1966: 116)

In this view, which is herewith coined as neo-innatism, there was no learning of language, because the child's upbringing served only to trigger or activate the rules that came with birth in the newborn's brain. And yet there was no explanation of how such a brain was supposed to work; nor was there any mention of the interplay of this innate capacity and the environments, which usually would take a lifetime for any individual because of aging and possible brain damage. The reason for the lack of explanation is most likely that such a superchild, with a copy of *Aspects of the Theory of Syntax*, but without any brain, would somehow become the ideal speaker-hearer as a fictional monster.

The fragmentation mentioned above not only split TG-ers into smaller and more and more dogmatic subgroups, each claiming with more minute but trivial 'rules' the 'authenticity' of representing 'human cognition' in the brain, or of 'mentalism', but also drew 'counter-attacks' from other linguists who could not 'stomach' TG. I for one have put forth my repudiations on many occasions (Peng, 1975a, 1975b, 1978). In one sense, such a claim of neo-innatism led to the extreme proclamation of 'universal grammar', going back to Harris, or earlier to Aristotelian doctrine.

Actually, neo-innatism was based on the old idea of 'species-specific' cognitive capacity of language in humans; that is, only humans have language, which is thought to be innate, but other species in the animal kingdom do not. This 'species-specific' cognitive capacity of language in humans has prevailed in anthropology, psychology and some other disciplines, such as genetics and neuroscience, for quite some time; Vicki was presented as evidence for that claim but Washoe, Koko and Chantek were presented as counter-evidence to prove that the great apes do possess sufficient cognitive capacity to learn a human language, that is, ASL, provided that the conception of language is changed or modified, that is, from strictly oral to include sign language.

Put differently, it all depends on what is meant by language. When comparative neuroanatomy and comparative gross anatomy are taken into consideration, each species has its own language. But some geneticists and other neuroscientists, who do not know what language in the brain really is, are still fighting to prove this species-specific cognitive capacity of language for humans.

The fact that we do not know about the intricate nervous system forming behaviour as a language among the chimpanzees and other great apes or even lower forms of animals is not tantamount to the often-heard assumption that they do not have language. Our language is different from theirs, for sure, but that difference is not all versus nil; we just do not know what their languages are like. It is important to emphasize that 'don't know' is *not* the same as 'doesn't exist'. If and when neuroanatomy is taken into account, such an assumption will simply fall apart.

3.6 The Competition Period

On the other hand, the fragmentation stirred up competition from within the United States as well as from Europe. Stratificational theory of language, headed by Sydney Lamb, is one competitor which has its roots in Hjelmslev. Halliday's Systemics is another competitor which has its roots in Saussure's paradigmatic relations and social-semiological system of *langue* for lexicogrammar, but has its roots in Firth's prosody for phonology. (See Peng 1992a for details.) To systemicists, language is now 'a resource for making meaning through choice' (or something to that effect as it is espoused by Thibault throughout his book).

To promote, elaborate, expand and improve the Hallidayan theory of systemics, systemicists annually hold an International Systemic Congress (ISC) which rotates around Australia, Europe, North America and the Far East. It is now called the International Systemic and Functional Congress (ISFC).

I organized the eighteenth (1991) ISC in Japan, with Halliday's support, although I am not a systemicist; rather, I have been sympathetic to their cause and, therefore, felt the need to lend them a helping hand to kick off a new momentum in order to counter TG dominance in Japan. As a consequence, there now exists a systemic organization called Japan Association of Systemic and Functional Linguistics (JASFL), consisting mostly of 'young' linguists and (older) former TG-ers. Even though I am not a member, my daughter who was trained in Australia as a systemicist is on the Executive Board.

As a result of such competitions, a new association was also formed in 1974 called the Linguistic Association of Canada and United States (LACUS – reminiscent of the lakes in Illinois for the logotype). The reason for its formation was that all the other linguistic societies and associations were taken over by TG-ers. Here is a reproduction in full from 'A Mild Proposal . . .' (Peng, 2004) which depicts the strong anti-TG sentiment during that period:

A MILD PROPOSAL . . .

Many linguists of today, whether deeply specializing in some empirical language discipline, or persuaded of the essential unity of language with other human faculties, or both, have found it impossible to accept the so-called Chomskyan, or Transformational-Generative (TG), Paradigm. Indeed, they find hard – precisely because of their particular understanding of the nature of language and because of their individuality – to join the easy chorus that uncritically repeats major tenets of this narrowing and distorting frame of reference.

It has become a common observation that graduate students are indoctrinated with the idea that the TG paradigm alone offers an inclusive, coherent theory of language, an idea that must be rejected on two major counts: first, this paradigm does not by any means cover the full range of language phenomena (despite the brave assertions of its advocates); second, there exist in fact alternative theoretical frameworks though usually unknown to mainstream linguists brought up in the orthodoxy of the reigning paradigm.

Despite the visible break-up from within of the TG movement, the voices dominating current linguistic literature continue to be adherents whether orthodox or apostate, of this particular creed, for one of the major successes of that movement has been to impose its hegemony over organizational linguistics. As a result, dissidents from linguistic establishments, Chomskyite or post-Bloomfieldian, find themselves in the position of dissidents from established religion: hamstrung by their non-conformism, lacking not in scholarly breeding or linguistic training but only in a common voice and group allegiance. The occasional appearance of non-TG ideas in the leading linguistics journals should not be misinterpreted as a sign of significant change within the prevailing establishment; in fact, occurrences of this nature – which make little if any general impact – have the appearance of manoeuvers of deception or attempts to absorb dissident views without much ado.

In view of this present state of affairs in matters linguistic, some of us dissident and dissatisfied students of language, though we may have no particular teacher in common and cherish divergent persuasions, have determined that the era of 'clandestine' manuscripts, dittoed statements, personal correspondence on matters of non-alliance with TG paradigm, and so forth, has been already much too long, and that instead the appearance of a volume of articles by today's yet unorganized dissidents is the order of the day.

The responsibility of bringing out such a volume, edited with scholarly care, and carefully printed, has been assumed by E. F. K. Koerner and J. Peter Maher. It is intended to be in some way re-evocative of the spirit of the Structuralist rebellion against the Neogrammarian domination at the First Congress of Linguists at the Hague in 1928, and earlier still, the 1885 Controversy over the sound-law principle. The proposed title, in fact, of the suggested volume – CONCERNING THE TRANSFORMATIONAL-GENERATIVE PARADIGM: Against the MIT-niks – is inspired by Hugo Schuchardt's insightful polemic in that controversy, *Über die Lautgesetze: Gegen die Junggrammtiker*. Yet above all, the volume is meant to be not merely a collection of negative criticism of particular TG dogmas but a forum for positive theory-construction offering viable alternatives to the one 'theory' which is hardly anything more than a notational apparatus (not without merits) based on false assertions about language in general and used to express many erroneous claims and inept analyses about languages in particular.

We propose to bring the volume out at the earliest possible date, and if the idea catches on another volume is envisaged or more. Our major concern is to attempt nothing less than the RESCUE OF LINGUISTICS AS A HUMAN SCIENCE ...!!!

Since that 'Mild Proposal' was stated, a very fitting critical summary of the TG paradigm over twenty-five years has appeared in *Forum Linguisticum* by J. Peter Maher, entitled 'The Transformational-Generative Paradigm: A silver anniversary polemic' (1980). It contains a detailed analysis of and comments on the contradictions, false claims, among others, of this paradigm as well as comments and critical views from non-TG adherents. Here is a typical contradiction among TG-ers and an interesting self-contradiction in Chomsky's view:

> a grammar may be described as though it were a kind of machine, of whatever sort ... In order that a theory, and therefore also a grammar, be perfectly public and reproducible, but at the same time effective, it is necessary that the predictions afforded by the theory be an automatic consequence of its premises and arguments. If then the appropriate notations be set up, the derivations of its predictions from its premises may be translated into machine terms, and, depending upon how complicated an algebra was employed in the theory, the derivations may be mechanized inside an actual physical machine, such as an electronic computer. (quoted in Maher, 1980: 20)

In *Letters to the Editor of the New York Times*, 5 January 1966, signed by Chomsky, Halle, Fodor, Katz, Kiparsky, Klima and Matthews, the following statements supported the views just quoted:

> We have read the news story in the Times of December 29 referring to a grammar 'is out of The Massachusetts Institute of Technology by a computer' and that purportedly provides the basis for the new English ... As for the work at MIT, we wish to make clear that computers, and modern technology in general, play a very minor role. (ibid.: 16)

But when Chomsky wrote to Ved Mehta in 1971, here is what he said:

> Think of the computer as a model for the human mind. A scientist who didn't know what the program, or input, of the computer was would assume that the only way to find it out would be to analyze the output, language. He would construct an idealization, a model, and develop an explanatory theory in the hope that in time he would be able to deduce the input. (ibid.: 17)

And yet, interestingly enough, in *Aspects of the Theory of Syntax* (1965), Chomsky said something that was quite self-contradictory:

> Linguistic theory is concerned with an ideal speaker-hearer, in a completely homogeneous speech community, who knows its [*sic*] language perfectly and is unaffected by such grammatically irrelevant conditions as memory limitations, distractions, shifts of attention and interest and errors (random or characteristic) in applying his [*sic*] knowledge in actual performance. (ibid.: 23)

> linguistic theory is mentalistic, since it is concerned with a mental reality underlying actual behavior. (ibid.: 23)

By putting all this together, any reader of English can only reach one conclusion: Chomsky's fictional monster was a computer model – it had no brain and, therefore, no memory, but was mentalistic and at the same time possessed a grammar that was mechanistic and universal, which could generate all and only grammatical sentences of any language without making errors; and any one of such sentences can be infinitely long. It was against such nonsensical claims that prompted competitions from non-TG-ers.

However, LACUS was dominated by two groups of non-TG linguists; namely, stratificationalists and tagmemicists, as of 1991; systemicists were a minority, although Halliday served one year as president of LACUS. I was one of its founding members but left the association in 1992 because it was not getting anywhere in terms of the study of how language as behaviour works in varying social contexts of situation.

There were four more organizations, coming from the USA and Europe, during this competition period: Semiotics, Pragmatics, Argumentation, and Child Language Study. The first one started in the USA and attracted many linguists, mostly non-TG-ers. The second one started in Denmark and attracted many former TG-ers who were fed up with the tribalistic and cult-driven trend of current linguistics. It now holds international congresses every two to three years. Each of these two organizations also publishes a journal – *American Journal of Semiotics* and *International Journal of Pragmatics*, respectively.

The third one was started in the Netherlands by communication experts. It has revived the ancient Greek trend of rhetoric and properly calls its activity Argumentation. It has now attracted people from all walks of life, including legal specialists, and formed the International Society for the Study of Argumentation, which holds international conferences every three years.

Incidently, the fifth (2002) conference was organized at Lugano jointly by: the International Society for the Study of Argumentation (Amsterdam), the International Association for the Study of Controversies (Tel-Aviv), and the International Association for Dialogue Analysis (Bologna). It also publishes a newsletter.

The fourth one was started in Italy by a small group of non-TG linguists and psychologists who were interested in child language, although TG-ers were also interested in child language. I organized in 1978 the First International Congress for the Study of Child Language in Japan under the auspices of the International Society for the Study of Child Language. It attracted not only non-TG linguists but also psychologists and language disorder specialists. The proceedings were published in 1979. I would not be surprised, however, that after the first Congress the organization is now contaminated by TG if not dominated or even taken over by TG-ers.

It is of interest to note that these new organizations for the study of language may overshadow the current trend in linguistics. But they are also in need of a strong impetus from the biological as well as the social foundation of language without which they may end up like the current situation in linguistics.

4. The Need for Neuroanatomy in Linguistics

Given the brief sketch of the history of linguistics, from the (ancient) Greek history to the contemporary (recent) history, there should be no denying that linguistics as it has been is in great need of neuroanatomy today. Not only because of the many twists and turns in the long path of linguistics but also because of the fact that linguistics is losing steam everywhere, the need should help linguistics correct its course; hopefully, this time the impetus will move the discipline in the right direction in order to answer the fundamental question 'What is language?' The job will not be easy, because it will take hundreds, if not thousands, of like minds, with multidisciplinary backgrounds, to do a thorough overhaul in the hope that by the end of the twenty-first century, the answer to 'What is language?' can come to fruition. This book is but the first major step in the right direction.

The need for neuroanatomy in linguistics proposed in this book is not tantamount to saying that linguists in the past had not contemplated on acquiring some knowledge of biology or had not thought of the idea of brain functions (or mind capacity) in relation to language. Quite the contrary, linguists in the past had many times tried to link linguistics to brain functions for what they thought was language: for instance, the controversy of nature versus nurture, or rationalism versus empiricism, or single origin versus multiple origins of language, before Saussure, and, when phonetics came into being, the inquiry into the speech circuit by Saussure.

Every attempt failed, because linguists generally do not look deeply into the brain functions for a detailed description of what the brain can do *vis-à-vis* language in the brain as behaviour. For this reason, this book is a first attempt to bring neuroanatomy to the attention of linguists in the hope that the importance of neuroanatomy in linguistics and semiotics can be taken seriously.

2 Historical Perspective from the Semiotic Point of View

If linguistics can claim to have a history of 2,500 years, as was estimated in Robins (1979), semiotics as the study of signs and their uses may also trace its 'roots' back to the Greek period, except that the roots cannot be found in philosophía as in the case of linguistics; rather, the 'roots' are most likely to be found in the Greek form of medicine. As a matter of fact, Hippocrates (*circa* 400 BC), traditionally regarded as the 'father of medicine', wrote about what was then known as 'semiology' in the *Hippocratic Collection*, which comprises a number of his medical works, whereby the term referred to the study of medical diagnosis and prognosis.

In these works, there is of course no reference to any form of study regarding language, except indirectly through the signs observed in diagnosis and prognosis. Something, therefore, must have happened in the history of semiotics as it developed later. That is, the medical term of semiology has changed, and the original medical study of signs ramified, with a bifurcation leading also to a study to include non-medical signs.

1. The Bifurcation of Semiotics

The original medical sense of semiotics may still be found today in medical schools in Europe and Canada; it can also be found in Peirce's usage, expounded by Parret (1984), as one of the two semiotics.

To Peirce (unlike or in contradistinction to Saussure and his follower, Hjelmslev) semiosis itself is an infinite process and semiotics, therefore, does not have a limit; that is, there are no non-semiotic objects, and all sciences and any adequate thought are semiotic. Probably for this reason, Peirce is often regarded as one of the founders of modern semiotics. However, many semioticians are uncomfortable with Peirce because he shifted his stances or theoretical orientations many times, so much so that it is difficult to think which Peirce is meant in semiotics. (See Pula (2001: 141–71) for some interesting discussions).

According to Parret (1984), then, the two semiotics are differentiated in the triadism (in Peirce) versus the dyadism (in Saussure) of the sign-relation which is the philosophy of significance (i.e., sign function). It is the expounding of this paradigm, which is the possibility condition of interpretation of the world and, in particular, of the intersubjective validity of each interpretation, that constitute the differentiation. Be that as it may, every interpretation depends entirely on the individual's brain functions without which nobody can think nor can anybody interpret any sign and, hence, there is no sign function of any kind. For this reason, semiotics is regarded by some as a branch of general semantics.

However, the differentiation is only theoretically distinguishable; in practice, since there is no actual 'school' of semiotics, comparable to the 'Prague School' or the 'Firthian School' in linguistics, it is rather difficult to identify a particular work as being Peircean or Saussurean in orientation, although the Peircean semiotics is supported by Anglo-Saxon semioticians and the Saussurean semiotics has so-called continental followers.

Throughout the history of linguistics and of semiotics briefly sketched above, there are two related common themes that can be detected:

1. Preoccupation with signs or symbols (written or phonetically transcribed texts) which are often collectively called code, so that language is regarded as code.
2. Emphasis on speaker (encoder) at the expense of hearer (decoder).

It is the first common theme that connects linguistics and semiotics (which is regarded by some as equivalent to or includes general semantics), except that linguists are obsessed with signs for the purpose of 'inventing' what they call language structure, on the basis of what they call grammar which they create, and semioticians are not; semioticians are more interested in how to interpret meaning from signs given in varying contexts of situation and how to relate such contexts of situation to the signs to be given by encoder and/or to be interpreted by decoder. Some semioticians would go even further to interpret 'signs' given by animals – for example, chimpanzees or dogs – and call their interpretation 'Zoosemiotics' (Sebeok, 1972). The interpretation, nonetheless, may or may not be right, for humans can 'read' each other's mind better than they can 'read' the mind of a chimpanzee or a dog, although animal trainers, as in a circus, must be equipped with this kind of ability when they train tigers, lions and elephants for the show.

However, I am not sure if semioticians can do any better with the second theme in view of the fact that contexts of situation alone will not help them; moreover, since signs of any kind, such as sounds, have no meanings in and by themselves, unless they take into account neuroanatomy and brain functions when they interpret signs from decoder's point of view and try to predict what the signs to be given by encoder will do to decoder, sooner or later they will run into a dead end just like linguists. The reason is that semioticians, like linguists, are not yet aware that the signs they study have no meanings in and by themselves outside the context of brain functions.

In spite of such a potential danger, many linguists could easily switch or have already switched from linguistics to semiotics, as can be evidenced by the roster of the Semiotic Society of America (patterned after LSA). As a matter of fact, Saussure could easily be regarded as a semiotician, as Parret suggested, if he were around today; this view is reflected in the subtitle of Thibault's book, that is, *The Dynamics of Signs in Social Life* (1997), although Peirce is usually regarded by semioticians as the 'founder' of modern semiotics. Incidently, Peirce is also regarded as a pioneer in Pragmatics, suggesting that semiotics and pragmatics are related, because of his changes of theoretical orientations.

Put differently, unlike linguists, semioticians from Peirce onward are not interested in the structure of language which entails the analysis of texts or signs (written or phonetically transcribed) by way of sentences; rather, semioticians are interested in: how signs are transmitted from encoder to decoder under the circumstances of feedforward, feedback, and the varying social contexts of situation; and what such signs mean or what are intended by such signs under these circumstances. Keep in mind, however, that signs (spoken or written) have no meanings in and by themselves, an important point in neurolinguistics that is totally missing in semiotics for reasons which will become self-evident later.

As a consequence, language is merely a social-semiological system of signs, albeit an important one, among many other systems of signs, verbal or nonverbal. Thus, how language is defined makes no difference to semioticians, except that they are highly interested in how speaker (or encoder) utters signs (sentences or what not) and how hearer (or decoder) interprets or receives such signs irrespective of the phonetic properties, if any, of these signs.

What these interests imply is that semioticians tend to interpret, that is, reconstruct, the meaning of each sign from hearer's or decoder's point of view as if they knew what speaker or encoder had in mind when in fact the sign seen, heard, or touched has no meaning in and by itself. In other words, each sign seen, heard, or touched has no meaning in and by itself unless hearer or decoder has its image already formed in his/her brain for the brain functions of recognition, identification, and coupling. The following is an example which is often encountered by archaeologists:

A foot print found in the wilderness by an archaeologist has to be recognized as a footprint, not a handprint, and then identified as a human footprint or an animal's with the image the archaeologist has in his/her brain. Only when the footprint is so identified can the archaeologist couple the image (as impulses) with the experiences he/she has already had in the brain for interpreting as meaning whether that footprint, if it is a human footprint, was left by a man, a woman, or a child or, if it is an animal's footprint, was left by a chimpanzee, a gorilla, or a monkey. It is in these interests that neuroanatomy will play an important role in semiotics.

Semioticians know very well the importance of how the human brain works in the exchange of signs between the members of a dyad. However, since like most linguists they also lack the knowledge of neuroanatomy, there is a black box in each dyadic member; it pertains none other than to the 'secrets' of brain functions *vis-à-vis* the exchange of signs between the dyadic members.

Usually, because of the importance of these secrets, semioticians would say 'we don't know how encoder's brain works, when he/she utters or gesticulates signs, and how decoder's brain works, when he/she receives or sees signs'. These secrets are exactly the same secrets underlying the brain functions of language which linguists should also know but have no access to other than sporadic uses of medical terms, such as 'pathways of the brain', etc., to cover up their ignorance. It is in this vein that some knowledge of neuroanatomy will be of use in semiotics.

Historically, as was mentioned above, the term semiotics came from semiology which was and is still used by people in the medical corps outside of the United States; for example, Europe and Canada. The term semiology in its original sense is employed by medical people for diagnostic and prognostic purposes as a part of symptomatology. For instance, if a patient is running a high temperature and/or having a sore throat, it is a semiological sign for the physician who has to diagnose what causes it in order to prescribe a drug for treatment; for example, tonsillitis. If the temperature and/or the sore throat persists for months, in spite of the medication, it becomes another semiological sign which tells the physician something else – for example, an early symptom of throat cancer – which requires him/her to do a different examination of the patient – for example, a biopsy. If the specimen is found to be cancerous, then either radiological treatment or chemotherapy will be prescribed, and the prognosis will have to be made for the patient and his/her family members.

2. The Need for Neuroanatomy in Semiotics

When semiotics was taken out of the medical context of semiology, in either sense of the two semiotics, it is no wonder that semioticians are not obsessed with language structure, like linguists. But for some peculiar reason the medical knowledge that physicians have had was not carried over, other than the desire to have it which semioticians still cannot access; it was left behind, as it were. The intent of this monograph is to propose the return of at least some basic neuroanatomical knowledge back to semiotics. In other words, neuroanatomy is needed in semiotics, although it is taken for granted by physicians in the original sense of semiology.

Without some knowledge of neuroanatomy for understanding how the brain works, the functions of which it is to enable the individual to make proper adjustments to the internal and external environments, semioticians will continue to argue in a vacuum about sign-relation in respect to the dyadic members and the social contexts of situation. The need of neuroanatomy in semiotics is even more imperative when semioticians claim that semiosis is an infinite process and semiotics, consequently, does not have a limit, because there are no non-semiotic objects. The reason is that once neuroanatomy is taken into consideration the infinite process of semiosis evaporates.

Be that as it may, I must hasten to add that each object or sign has no meaning, that is, no sign-relation with other objects, unless there is at least a human or a dyad to interpret it in each individual's brain; if there were no humans, as in a ghost town, the objects in the ghost town would most certainly be non-semiotic, and therefore there would be no semiosis to speak of. However, this view was confronted by an Irish philosopher, bishop and writer, George Berkeley (1685–1753), who proposed the theory of the non-existence of external 'reality'.

Even if there are humans, as each individual's human life is finite, never infinite, semiosis *cannot* be an infinite process at all. The notion of an infinite process is reminiscent of 'an infinite set of sentences' proposed by TG-ers. Put differently, semiosis is finite, co-extensive to the availability of humans whose existence depends entirely on their active brain functions, because a comatose or a brain-dead human cannot have any process that can be called semiosis. It is nonsense or a farce to claim infinity of any kind in human interactions. If semioticians claim infinity for their notion of semiosis, as did TG-ers, as if infinity (which is a mathematical notion) were a virtue, in Western cultural value systems, when in reality (i.e., real life) it is not, without taking into account neuroanatomy, semiotics will soon face a dead end, just like linguistics.

3 Historical Perspective from the Medical Point of View

If linguists have been confused about what language really is, it is of interest to know what non-linguists think of language. Three conflicting views can be ascertained in the medical and paramedical fields. The first view is that language and speech are regarded as two separate entities, seemingly unrelated to each other; at least, advocates of this view pretend that they open one eye but close the other. The second view is the opposite, which is to say that language and speech are indistinguishable, because the advocates of this view tend to use the two terms, language and speech, interchangeably. The third view is that the advocates, mostly psychiatrists, tend to think that language is made up of ordinary words; as a result, assignments of abstract notions, names of people, telephone numbers do not belong to it, and balancing a cheque book with complicated numbers has nothing to do with language. I will now go through each of these views, with concrete evidence, to show that medical and paramedical people do not understand what language really is; at least, their views of language are completely different from the two perspectives described above.

1. Language and Speech are Two Separate Entities

This view is held by all aphasiologists and probably by most neurologists. Here is an example of what neurologists think of language:

> It is important to distinguish between language and speech. Language is written marks or sounds by which an understood symbolic meaning is communicated within a cultural group. The human voice is capable of only a limited number of phonemes (the name given to the shortest unit of sound, e.g., 'poo'). It is the culturally determined combination of phonemes that gives language its meaning. Hence a phoneme 'poo' will have a different cultural meaning in Chinese and English. The written symbols also have a different form. A disturbance of oral language is known as aphasia or dysphasia. A disturbance of written language is known as dysgraphia, and a disturbance of the ability to read written language is called an acquired dyslexia. Speech, or articulation, is taken to refer to the motor actions involved in the oral production of sounds that carry the symbolic meaning of language. Disorders of articulation are referred to as dysarthria. The passage of expired air across

the vibrating vocal cords is a necessary part of the production of meaningful sounds. A disturbance of this function is referred to as dysphonia. (Hopkins, 1993: 24–5)

This definition of language has one variant which is probably shared by all aphasiologists or language/speech pathologists. It can be depicted schematically as shown in Figure 3.1

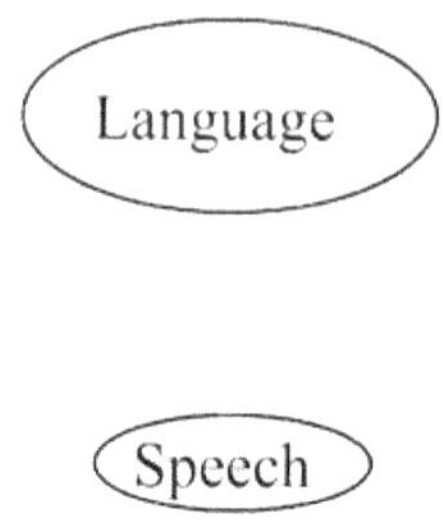

Figure 3.1

However, there is another variant which is held mostly by neurologists. The difference is that in the second variant language is some sort of unknown cognitive process, rather than written marks or sounds (or words).

In April 1995, I gave a series of lectures on the brain functions of memory to a group of neurologists in Seoul, South Korea, at the National Seoul University Hospital. I elaborated on my view that memory and cognition are heads and tails of the same coin and are subserved by the same sets of brain functions. After my lecture entitled 'The Neural Substrates of Memory', one young neurologist raised an interesting point. He said, to him language was some kind of cognitive process in the brain. Since the point raised was in relation to my lecture, I asked: 'What is the distinction to you between memory and cognition?' He could not supply an answer.

In 2000, I gave a lecture entitled 'What is language in the brain like?' at the Medical College in Hualien, Taiwan, to a group of faculty members, medical students, biologists and paediatric neurologists. My main focus was that language consists of two planes, content plane and expression plane (or speech, if you will), and that only by putting the two planes together is there language in the brain. After the lecture, one pediatric neurologist said that speech is the motor functions, saying precisely what Hopkins was quoted as saying above. I then said speech, if you like, is a part of language, and only by putting speech (i.e., expression plane) and content plane together do you have language in the brain. Apparently, he did not catch the punch line of my lecture, and missed the whole point throughout my lecture.

The question is 'Where did these two variants of language and speech being separate come from?' A cursory look at the medical literature will reveal that in 1885, L. Lichtheim published an article entitled 'On aphasia' in *Brain* which proposed a model that has since then become known as the Wernicke–Lichtheim's Model of Aphasias. I believe this model set the pattern for all later neurologists and aphasiologists. More will be said later about this medical tradition in respect to language in the brain. This model is shown in Figure 3.2.

The model has the following components:

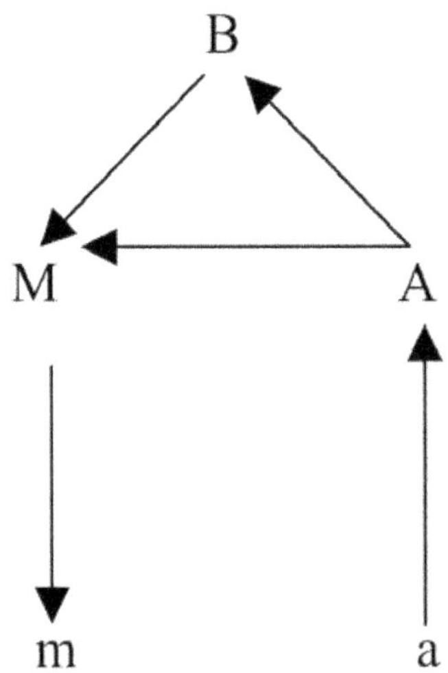

Figure 3.2 *Wernicke–Lichtheim's Model of Aphasias*

1. the auditory centre (centre of auditory images), designated as **A**;
2. the part where concepts are elaborated, designated as **B**;
3. centre of motor images, designated as **M**;
4. an afferent branch of the 'Reflex arc', designated as **a A**, which transmits the acoustic impressions to **A**;
5. an efferent branch of the 'Reflex arc', designated as **M m**, which conducts the impulses from **M** to the organs of speech **m**;
6. the commissure binding the centre of auditory images and the centre of motor images, designated as **A M**.

Note that in this model there was no mention of language other than the part where concepts were elaborated. But before Lichtheim, Wernicke (1874) and Broca (1861) had already published their works: Broca designated the third convolution of the left frontal lobe as the faculty of language for production, which has since then been known as Broca's area which is one of the so-called 'language centres' in the medical literature; to this initial designation Wernicke, some thirteen years later, added the posterior third of the superior gyrus of the left temporal lobe as another faculty of language, this time for reception, which has since then become Wernicke's area. He then speculated that there must have been a connection between Broca's area and Wernicke's area, a speculation that turned out later to be anatomically true; the connection is now known as arcuatus fasciculus, which is the commissure designated as **A M** in Figure 3.2.

However, in 1906, P. Marie re-examined the brain of Broca's patient, Tan-Tan, which had been kept in formalin at a museum in Paris, and declared in *Semaine medicale*, 23 May, that 'la troisième circonvolution frontale gauch ne joue aucun rôle special dans la fonction du langage' (the third, left, frontal convolution plays no special role in the function of language). He thus set in motion a series of debates which, after more than ninety years, is still not yet concluded. I for my part of the debates in the late twentieth century have come to the conclusion that Broca's area is simply the exit of motor impulses and Wernicke's area is simply an entrance of auditory impulses in the brain and not the centres that manipulate language, as had been purported for the past century or so. To me, language in the brain consists of content plane (involving **B**, **B M**, **A B** and **A M** structurally) and expression plane (involving **M**, **M m**, **A**, and **a A** structurally). Functionally, however, these planes are two inchoate masses of impulses which roam around the brain as background noises, each impulse in one plane looking for its corresponding impulse in the other for either production or reception in behaviour, as will be shown later.

Of course, the debates have centred on the issue of 'cerebral dominance', which is often equated with 'cerebral laterality' in neuroscience. To me, the equation is wrong, as will be shown later in Chapter 17. Because the model serves as the precursor, I shall return to it for the critical assessments of such notions. The reason is that the proponents of 'cerebral dominance' assume that there are 'language centres' in the brain and that they tie together the so-called 'language centres' to handedness (hand-predominance), eye-predominance, ear-predominance and leggedness (leg-predominance). But once the concept of 'language centres' is proven erroneous, the issue of 'cerebral dominance' evaporates, although cerebral laterality remains, because animals also have 'handedness', eye-predominance, and ear-predominance. That is, the two hemispheres are functionally asymmetrical (i.e., different), although structurally they are more or less homologous in mirror-image. For this reason, cerebral laterality will be replaced by cerebral asymmetry.

It is of interest to note that William James, a psychologist, reacted sharply and negatively to Broca's and Wernicke's areas as the 'language centres' when he said in *The Principles of Psychology*, 'There is no "centre of speech" in the brain any more than there is a faculty of speech in the mind. The entire brain, more or less, is at work in a man who uses language' (1890: 56). However, James was not alone, for his view did not fall on deaf ears as it was reasserted in 1906 by P. Marie.

2. Language and Speech are Indistinguishable

Because of the purported 'language centres', neuroscientists began to connect the centres with handedness (part of cerebral laterality) and have come to a conclusion that prevails in all medical schools. Medical students are also taught that the two 'language centres' manipulate, in some mysterious ways, language in the brain; later on, in the 1950s, another language centre, championed by the late Dr Penfield of the Montréal Neurological Institute, called supplementary motor area, was added. The conclusion is that most right-handers have the 'language centres' in the left hemisphere and many left-handers have the 'language centres' in the right hemisphere, although some left-handers have the 'language centres' also in the left hemisphere. Ambidextrous people may have their 'language centres' bilaterally represented, even though some of them have the left hemispheric representation.

I have found this conclusion, which has spread to the paramedical domain, such as aphasiology, to be erroneous and will point out the errors in detail in another monograph, *Language Disorders: A Critical Perspectve*, which will be a follow-up to this monograph. The reason is that when language in the brain is regarded as behaviour, like all non-language behaviours, it is memory-governed; as such, it cannot be controlled or manipulated by the so-called 'language centres' as these 'language centres' do not exist in the brain. Before I explicate that reason further (in Chapter 17), let me continue with the second view from the medical perspective.

According to this view, when a right-handed person becomes aphasic, because of a stroke, for instance, the brain damage is in the left hemisphere, which is a regular aphasia. But when a left-handed person becomes aphasic, from whatever cause, and the brain damage is also in the left hemisphere, that person's aphasia is called cross-aphasia; if the brain damage is in the right hemisphere, then that person's aphasia is also a regular aphasia, mirror-imaged to the right-hander's, because of the decussation of fibres in the brainstem.

As a result of the conclusion, the hemisphere that is purported to have the 'language centres' is called the dominant (or major) hemisphere and the other, the silent (or minor) hemisphere. Some prominent neurologists have held the view that the right (or minor) hemisphere was totally 'useless' as far as language was concerned. Because of this prevalent view, the cortex of the 'language centres' is known in brain surgery as the eloquent cortex or simply 'language cortex' or 'speech cortex'.

Thus, neurosurgeons began certain surgical experiments of language/speech arrest, during epilepsy surgery, starting with Penfield at Montréal Neurological Institute in the 1950s; that is, during the operation, the epileptic patient is not put on general anesthesia and, therefore, is able to talk while the operation is going on. There is no pain during brain surgery because the brain itself does not feel pain; the only slight pain felt by the patient is when the dura matter (one of the three membranes under the skull, collectively called the meninges) is pierced. So, the neurosurgeon uses an electrode to stimulate various locations of the area being operated on before an incision is made. If the patient stops talking, then it is claimed that language/speech is arrested at that particular spot. The supplementary motor area of the left hemisphere was found to be sensitive to language/speech arrest; hence, it was added as another 'language centre'.

To these neurosurgeons, there is no distinction of language and speech which are used interchangeably. This procedure of epilepsy surgery is perfectly legitimate and is one of the several surgical procedures for the surgical intervention of intractable epilepsies. I have taken part in pre- and post-operative examination of such epilepsy surgeries in Taiwan. When I reported this participation to the then dean of the College of Liberal Arts at the university I was affiliated with, I was accused of experimenting on humans against the Helsinki Declaration, which allegedly prohibits any such experiments using humans as subjects.

As a result of my participation, however, I have found that all epileptic patients, intractable or not, have serious memory impairment and, therefore, have language disorders of one kind or another (Peng, 1995; 2003a). The memory impairment, in some cases, may progress to the extent that the patient becomes demented, which is too often brushed aside simply as psychosis, a symptom well known in epileptology. I presented a paper, with a clinical case report, at the Fourth Asian and Oceanian Epilepsy Congress, 14 September 2002, Karuizawa, Japan, entitled 'Dementia and Epilepsy: A Case Report' in order to call epileptologists' attention to the relationship of dementia and epilepsy. In fact, the first case of senile dementia having senile plaques at autopsy, reported by Blocq and Marinesco in 1892, was an epileptic patient (Peng, 2003b).

3. Language is made up of Ordinary Words in the Brain

In this third view, speech is not mentioned; perhaps, it is not even important, because this view is taken by psychiatrists in relation to mental retardation or dementia. If speech is not important this view may be a variant of the second view. For the time being, it is treated as a separate third view; it is often associated with patients with Alzheimer's disease (AD) or Huntington's disease (HD), for example, and frequently used to depict the mental state of schizophrenic patients or other psychotic patients for what psychiatrists call thought disorders because of hallucinations (false perceptions) and delusions (false beliefs). For instance, a patient may hear his own thoughts speaking aloud or hear voices discussing him. Likewise, a patient may believe that alien forces are controlling his or her actions or inserting thoughts into his or her mind (Frith, 2004).

Hallucination aside, dementia is actually a neurological disorder but is *not* a disease, although it is customary for many neurologists and all psychiatrists to think that dementia is a (mental) disease. In English, there are four terms that can describe a person's condition: disease, ailment, illness and sickness. In

Chinese or Japanese, there is only one term, that is, *Ping* (病) or *Byoo ki* (病氣), respectively. In Dutch, there is also only one term, *Ziekte.*

Dementia is thus an illness, not a disease. But for some peculiar reason, dementia is often regarded as synonymous with AD, due primarily to the unfortunate twisting of historical facts, as if Alzheimer in 1907 made the discovery of neurofibrillary tangles and senile plaques, when in fact he only made the original discovery of neurofibrillary tangles, in one single case, and not of senile plaques, because they had already been described in 1892 by Blocq and Marinesco, in the brain of an elderly patient affected by epilepsy and confirmed by Redlich in 1898 in two cases. They were also extensively described in 1907 by Fischer in 12 of 16 cases. However, both neurofibrillary tangles and senile plaques are diseases which contribute to or cause neuronal deaths to result in dementia (Peng, 2003b).

I presented a paper, entitled 'Is Dementia a Disease?' in April 2002 in Kyoto, Japan, at the Third World Congress on Vascular Factors in Alzheimer's Disease, in order to bring to the attention of the medical world the historical facts for the correction of the errors made. It is now published in *Gerontology* (Peng, 2003b), after it was turned down by the editor of the Proceedings. I propose that senile plaques (or amyloid plaques, as they are now called) be designated as Fischer's disease (FD).

I also presented a paper in June 2002, during the 83rd Annual Meeting of the Pacific Division of AAAS held in Hawaii, entitled 'Dementia as a Form of Language Disorders', and proposed that, in fairness to Fischer, neurofibrillary tangles and senile plaques should be regarded as two separate diseases, with only the former assigned to AD instead of assigning both diseases to AD as an eponym, a nosological assignment that was politically motivated with no scientific merit whatsoever. My reason is that the wrong nosological classification of two different diseases, that is, neurofibrillary tangles and senile plaques, in AD as one (mental) disease has resulted in a stumbling block with many publications, because of the semantic confusion of dementia being a disease, when it is not, even though both diseases result in dementia. See Peng (2005).

Put differently, Alzheimer never made any original contribution to senile plaques, although he did describe for the first time neurofibrillary tangles. However, the term dementia had already been used in nineteenth-century psychiatric literature as a disease to designate the mental state as a consequence of senile plaques or Pick's disease (known for the presence of Pick bodies).

What then is dementia? It may be redefined as the differential manifestation of deteriorating brain functions over time as a result of cell deaths in the brain caused by any neurodegenerative disease, cortical or subcortical, the prominent symptoms of which are language disorders. If language disorders are considered prominent symptoms in demented patients of any type, it would be better to consider dementia as a form of varying language disorders rather than a disease, because language disorder is *not* a disease. This statement can be affirmatively supported by an interesting article by Snowdon *et al.* (2000) in which the authors report that low linguistic ability in early life correlated strongly with the presence of neurofibrillary tangles and less strongly with that of senile plaques.

Even though dementia is not a disease, nosologically speaking, it is often treated as such by psychiatrists, who would most likely regard it as a mental disease, because of the long history going back to the nineteenth century; mental retardation, on the other hand, is a multifactorial disorder some of which are treated by psychiatrists but others are treated by neurologists. Children with learning disability used to be regarded as mentally retarded, a term that has become a taboo in education. In any event, dementia and mental retardation (or learning disability) are forms of *bona fide* language disorders.

The following quotation about problems with language in AD patients is from the National Alzheimer's Association (quoted in *The Honolulu Advertiser*, 24 July 2001).

> **Memory loss**. It is normal to occasionally forget assignments, colleagues' names, or a business associate's telephone number and remember them later. People with AD might forget things more often and not remember them later.
>
> **Problems with language**. Everyone has trouble finding the right word sometimes, but a person with AD might forget simple words or substitute inappropriate words, making sentences incomprehensible.
>
> **Problems with abstract thinking**. Balancing a checkbook may be disconcerting when the task is more complicated than usual. Someone with AD might forget completely what the numbers are and what needs to be done with them.

Notice that in the third view language is completely separated from memory and abstract thinking when language is actually memory-governed, meaning-centred (of which abstract thinking is only a part) and multifaceted. Without the brain functions of memory there is neither language nor abstract thinking. Without meaning, there is nothing to say, let alone abstract thinking, and without the needed pathways in action for input and output, the individual is either severely handicapped or comatose. Thus, memory impairment and disorders in abstract thinking or in expression are symptoms of language disorders.

It is clear from the historical perspective of the medical and paramedical fields that language is grossly both obfuscated and misunderstood by people in these fields. But, unlike the previous two perspectives, what is needed in the medical and paramedical fields is not knowledge of neuroanatomy; rather, it is knowledge of a new paradigm that is needed. This is not tantamount to saying that linguists and semioticians are well equipped with such a paradigm. Quite the contrary, linguists and semioticians are also in need of such a paradigm which will probably take the rest of this new century to come to fruition. The reason is that the question 'What is language?' can only be answered fruitfully when and only when language is taken seriously as an ontological issue. The following will be an attempt to consider such an ontological issue.

PART II WHAT CAN BE DONE ABOUT THE CURRENT SITUATIONS?

General Remarks

Given the three current perspectives described in Part I, something of course must be done and done quickly, or else the consequences if prolonged are hard to imagine: not only will the future of linguistics as a discipline be doomed, the state of semiotics, albeit booming at the moment, will also become questionable. Moreover, the medical and paramedical sciences, even though a wrong view of language in the brain may not endanger their patients or jeopardize the treatment of such patients, will also have to change their views about language in the brain. In other words, it is imperative to correct the mistakes made in the past, that is, to stay away from the mechanistic and computer models and come to terms with the real issues of language as behaviour, which will also benefit people in the medical fields, medical students and practitioners in particular.

Linguists in the past had thought of enriching their discipline by importing ideas from other disciplines. The motivation was correct but the results were often erroneous because the fundamental issue of 'What is language?' has not been really settled; thus, the consensus of what language is as the core of all concerns, instead of beating around the bush, has not been firmly established, even though tribalistic or cult driven definitions of language can be seen everywhere. Such a fragmentation is very bad for linguistics as a discipline and will affect or spread to semiotics as well if the black boxes mentioned earlier are not faced up to squarely.

What is more disturbing is the fact that when ideas from one discipline, such as linguistics, is transferred to, or taken over by, another discipline, say, neurology, they are completely 'disfigured', such as phoneme being the name given to the shortest unit of sound; for example, 'poo', cited previously.

Linguists, of course, are not entirely innocent. When linguists took over the ideas of family trees from biology to talk about language change, as if language was an organism, such ideas perpetuated even to this date in historical linguistics. One example is the notion promoted by Morris Swadesh in the early 1950s, which is now known as lexicostatistics or glottochronology, attempting to relate it to general linguistics and anthropological theory (Lehmann, 1973: 107); it was patterned after the chemical method of carbon 14 dating of fossils employed in archaeology. It calculates, by way of a mathematical formula designed by Robert Lees, the rate of losses of the so-called basic vocabulary in order to determine how far back in history genetically related languages can be said to have become separated.

When the formula was first published by Robert B. Lees (1953), there were of course many criticisms of this method, mostly from the statistic point of view. More important, however, is the conceptual flaw from the point of view of neuroanatomy. It was totally absurd to treat lexical items as if they were molecules, but this was apparently what Swadesh and Lees thought; and historical linguists have kept using such lexicostatistics to teach beginners in linguistics for dating the fictitious separation of related languages. The reason was and still is inexplicable but their motivation is clear; linguistics has been a discipline that is insensitive to time and they thought they could rectify such a built-in deficit.

Synchronic linguistics is of course totally incapable of assessing, or, rather, unconcerned with the assessment of, time depth. Diachronic linguistics, as in the Comparative Method or the Method of Internal Reconstruction, is interested in the assessment of the time period of the reconstructed proto-forms. But unless written texts are found afterward or as a result of reconstruction, as in Saussure's reconstruction of the PIE laryngeals and the decipherment of the Hittite texts, going back to 1700–2000 BC, there is simply no way in which historical linguistics can assess on its own the time depth of any reconstruction. For instance, Kurylowicz, 12 years after the uncovering of the archives of the Hittite Empire, identified sounds transcribed as *h* and ʔ with reconstructions Saussure made in 1879, when he was only 20 years old, solely on the strength of the Method of Internal Reconstruction, known later as PIE laryngeals. As a result, PIE is now combined with Hittite to become Indo-Hittite going back to 1700–2000 BC.

Swadesh and Lees must have thought that lexicostatistics would give historical linguistics a needed 'tool' which could overcome this built-in time-insensitive deficiency. Their motivation was admirable but the result is erroneous, because language is not an organism and lexical items are not molecules of a fossil. Lexical items are forgotten by people; they do not disappear like molecules of an organism, animal or plant, to be calculated thousands of years later, when it has become a fossil. Language as behaviour changes because individual people change from one generation to another. Put differently, it is people who change, coupled with the environmental changes, that change their brain functions of language as behaviour in various social contexts of situation over time from generation to generation. (See Peng (1976) for this view of sound change and language change.)

If a language has a writing system, the orthography based on it will also reflect the change from one period to another, as in Old English, Middle English, and Modern English, or in Chinese characters from the earliest bone scripts to contemporary non-abbreviated and abbreviated characters used in Taiwan and mainland China, respectively. But there is a contingency involved; the old texts must be found first. Otherwise, there is simply no way of dating the time-depth of any reconstruction. Linguists should stop pretending that they have found such a 'tool' to date the time-depth of language change. The dating of time-depth is, of course, uninteresting to semioticians; they are, nevertheless, interested in meaning change in relation to etymology.

4 A Mild Proposal

In this chapter, I shall propose a remedy to open up a new direction for linguistics, semiotics and neuroscience. Hopefully, the results based on the proposal in this monograph will help pave the way for the correction. The following are some of the ideas I would like to develop in this book as well as in the other monographs of the series mentioned. The ideas are intended for sharing with those colleagues, friends or friends-to-be, in order to jointly build healthy new paradigms in linguistics, semiotics and neuroscience, as the tasks ahead are enormous and may take hundreds, if not thousands, of like-minds to shape up, if we are lucky, during this century:

1. The addition of another core distinction, namely, Individual and Social, to incorporate Saussure's core distinction of *langue* and *parole*.
2. The elaboration of the individual aspect to include neuroanatomy which will benefit not only linguistics but also semiotics and, by extension, neuroscience.
3. The preparation for and establishment of better and more efficient interactions between the social sciences, such as linguistics and semiotics, and the medical and paramedical sciences, such as behavioural neurology and clinical neuroscience, on the one hand, and aphasiology or language/speech pathology, on the other.

1. The New Core Distinction

Recall that linguists after Saussure swung the pendulum of the answer to 'What is language?' three times: for the structuralists, it became 'a system of arbitrary vocal symbols'; for the generativists, it became 'an infinite set of sentences'; and for the systemicists, it became 'a resource for making meaning through choice'. Interestingly enough, only the generativists claim innateness implicit in their definition; neither one of the other two definitions has anything to do with language being innate, for it is learned as it should be, thereby marking a sharp contrast to the generativist definition.

But note that both the structuralist and the generativist views of language do not make specific mention of meaning. The distinction between the two views is clear, however; the former leans towards vocal symbols which are 'arbitrary' in relation to language as a system, whereas the latter is derived directly from computer science, *à la* pseudo-mathematics, such as programming for MT, on the basis of rules (i.e., a finite number of rules to generate an infinite set of all and only grammatical sentences on the strength of recursiveness and transformations).

While the structuralists maintain their stance throughout, the generativists, especially the high priest, changed their stance at least three times, each contradicting the others: at first, it was a pseudo-mathematical stance, based on MT, as expressed in *SS* (1957), with a mechanistic approach; then the stance changed to mentalism, becoming more and more philosophical, as expressed in Chomsky (1965, 1966, 1968). As if the mechanistic and philosophical stances failed to answer the question 'What is language?' because they turned out to be mere fantasy that split the then ruling paradigm, the philosophical stance was then combined with the third stance, a pseudo-biological stance that was at one time heralded blindly and mistakenly by generativists as a revolution (Starosta, 1980). In this third stance, Chomsky claims that language is an organ comparable to the heart, the liver, etc. (Starosta, 1980) and that children do not acquire a language but grow into it; such an extreme assertion is totally false and incompatible with reality, just like the fictional monster, the ideal speaker-hearer.

In contradistinction to the first two definitions, it is the meaning-making feature that characterizes the Hallidayan framework. At one and the same time, it enables Thibault to re-interpet Saussure's thinking in relation to the Hallidayan framework on account of the fact that both the Hallidayan framework and the Saussurean framework emphasize the social aspect of language in terms of the core distinction of *langue* (or social-semiological system) and *parole* (or instantiation), those in the parentheses being the Hallidayan terminology.

In spite of such similarities, moreover, there are problems in both frameworks, which stem from the neglect of the individual aspect of language. The Hallidayan framework does not mention anything beyond instantiations, but 'Saussure also claims that *langue* exists virtually in the brains of an assembly of individuals', that is, '*langue*, for Saussure, also has its material instantiations in embodied social beings' (Thibault, 1997: 25). Thibault quickly adds that 'If *langue* were no more than this, then ... the social-semiological system of *langue* would reduce to the neuroanatomical and neurophysiological capabilities of the individual qua biological organism' (1997: 25).

However, it is precisely these neuroanatomical and neurophysiological capabilities that are missing in both frameworks; the presence of such capabilities, of course, would *not* and should *not* reduce the social-semiological system of *langue* if *langue* really 'exists virtually in the brains of an assembly of individuals', as Saussure once said it does; rather, they should enrich the social-semiological system of *langue*, hence, semiotics as well.

The reason is that such capabilities constitute the 'power plant' of each individual, without which only such a monster like the ideal speaker/hearer lacking the human brain could come out. To substantiate this claim, I have postulated a solution from the neurolinguistic point of view, which will serve as a way out for the current crisis in linguistics and also to help boost the inertia for semiotics in respect to the black boxes mentioned earlier.

The solution so postulated is to incorporate Saussure's core distinction of *langue* and *parole* into another core distinction which has been advocated by me; namely, language has two aspects, social and individual, like the two faces of Janus, one looking outward to society while the other looking inward to the two nervous systems (central and peripheral). (See Peng, 1984 coming out of the Second Internatinal Conference on the Language Sciences, Tokyo, Japan, 22 to 23 August 1982 for an earlier explication of these two aspects of language.)

The two aspects of language, of course, must meet somehow; how they meet will constitute a whole range of new and wide interests that will probably occupy many like minds throughout this century or even longer. This monograph is but the initial first step to open up the door, as it were, toward such a goal. For the time being, the proposed solution may be schematically depicted as shown in Fig 4.1.

SOCIAL	INDIVIDUAL	
I	II	*LANGUE*
III	IV	*PAROLE*

Figure 4.1 *Matrix of the two aspects of language in relation to Saussure's* langue *and* parole: *a solution*

Given the matrix that depicts succinctly the two aspects of language, it not only solves the problems which have been plaguing linguistics for almost a century but may also take care of the 'black boxes' in semiotics so as to enhance the work by semioticians. At one and the same time, the matrix has the capacity of killing 'two birds' with one stone: first, it can be employed to demonstrate what Saussure meant by a plurality of frameworks mentioned by Thibault (1997: 15), which is epistemological; second, it can also be employed to account for the individual's power plant, that is, the brain functions in terms of neuroanatomy and neurophysiology, which is ontological.

In respect to the second point, if neuroscientists are seriously interested in language in the brain, it will change the whole scene in the medical and paramedical sciences. For this second point, the matrix will have to be expanded and greatly elaborated into several books later in order to cater toward the medical and paramedical audiences, the first of these will be the second book of my series *Language Disorders: A Critical Pespective.*

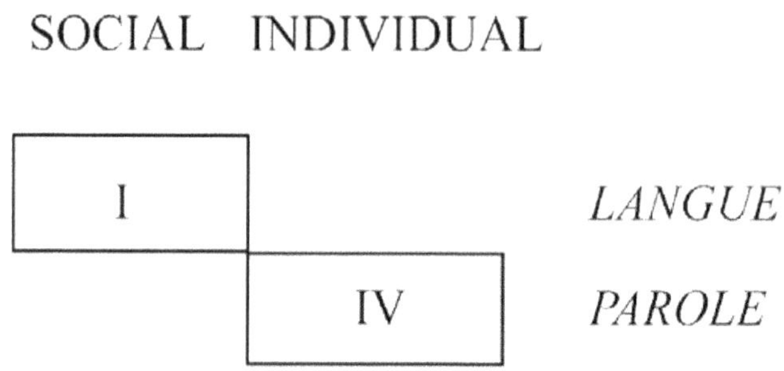

Figure 4.2 *Schematic illustration of the Saussurean perspective*

In terms of this solution, then, several methodological perspectives can be accounted for, starting with the Saussurean perspective shown in Figure 4.2.

In this illustration of Saussure's original conceptions, *langue* is purported to subsume *parole* as the source of raw data whereby the methodology may be said to be concerned with the semiological mediation that is claimed to exist in the individual in order to produce the raw data the speaker wants.

However, when sociolinguistics came into being in the 1960s, the semiological mediation was no longer an important issue or even a concern; rather, it is the social 'topography' (i.e., patterning of when, where, why raw data are or may be produced and who may produce them) that was destined to be foregrounded. In other words, the focus of methodology is on context of situation, even though context of situation has never been claimed to be a part of language in sociolinguistics. Thus, as far as sociolinguistics goes, language becomes something like the following, in Figure 4.3.

On the other hand, in the 1970s, since systemics became known in the UK, making inroads into the then mainstream linguistics in North America to pose a serious competition, language is now completely instituted in the social

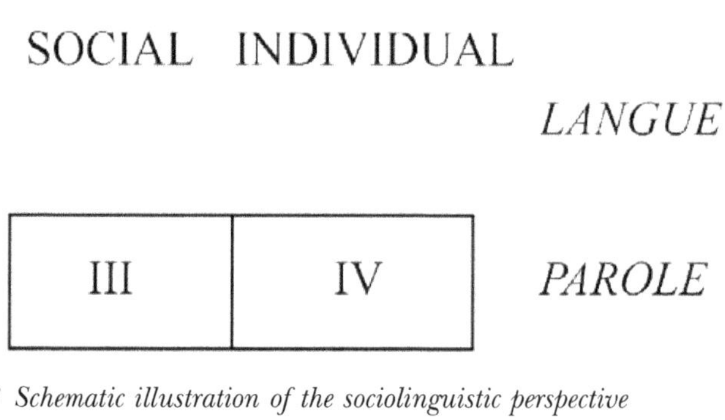

Figure 4.3 *Schematic illustration of the sociolinguistic perspective*

aspect, thereby leaving the individual aspect out of the picture. It is this disconnection of the social aspect of language from the individual aspect that has drawn Halliday into the conceptualization of culture as a network of systems of meaning (or of meaning-making), language being one such system, albeit a prominent one. At one and the same time, it is in this conceptualization that Thibault sees the affinity of the Saussurean framework in the Hallidayan framework. Be that as it may, there exists a difference, as may be seen in Figure 4.4.

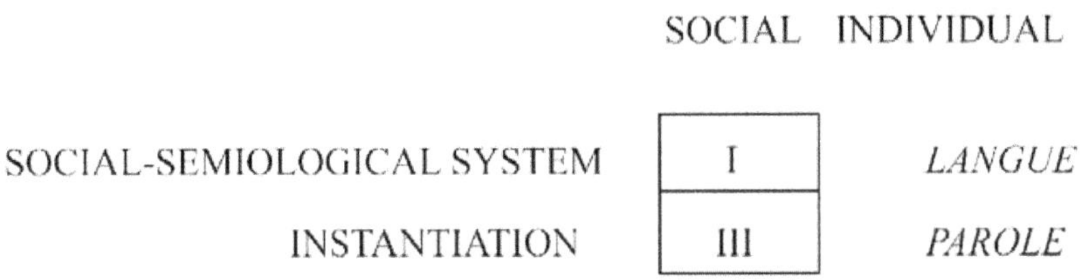

Figure 4.4 *Schematic illustration of the Hallidayan perspective*

The difference is that while Saussure sees *parole* as consisting of individual acts whereby, in Thibault's own words, 'individual language users, in acts of *parole*, use the social-semiological resources of *langue* to express their thoughts, to achieve their purposes and intentions, and so on' (1997: 24), in the Hallidayan framework, instantiations are simply texts which belong to the social domain irrespective of who produced them. Even when the systemic hierarchy (or stratification) goes up to Genre or Ideology (beyond Context of Situation) very little can be detected about the role of the individual aspect of language, although systemicists are very much interested in the development of language in which they talk about functional perspectives on species and individuals (Williams and Lukin, 2004). There is also a sign that Thibault, as a systemicist, may move into or incorporate the individual aspect of language (Thibault, 2004a, 2004b). I would encourage them to go deeper into the individual aspect of *parole* and *langue*.

Incidently, as far as I am concerned, there are no strata beyond the social context of situation which is a significant part of the individual aspect of language as the resource of meaning. It is in the social context of situation as a stratum of the individual aspect of language that semiotics and sociolinguistics can make contact. In Thibault (2004a), however, two new strata are proposed; namely, discourse and context of culture. I have commented on such proposals in Peng (forthcoming), because there is a difference between the stratification in linguistics and the stratification in the brain functioins of language: the former is epistemological while the latter is ontological. The distinction will become clear later. Thibault seems to have mixed the two stratifications together, because this is the tradition most linguists have been following. Nevertheless, in contradistinction to the linguistic tradition, it is important that the distinction is made.

If systemicists continue to pursue Genre and Ideology as the two strata higher than Social Context of Situation, as if they are investigating Saussure's Thought, my misgivings are that in the absence of any concern with the brain functions of language in their framework, they will end up migrating into the realm of philosophy, if they have not already done so, like Chomsky did, thereby forcing systemics to become a pseudo-philosophy. By taking people with language disorders into serious consideration in their theorizing and by concentrating on the patterning of social interactions, verbal or non-verbal (i.e., sign language), among people with or without handicap, they would also have to take the onotological issue of language in the brain seriously in relation to the brain functions of memory, rather than merely philosophizing.

In view of these problems, coupled with the fact that the individual is the 'power plant' without which there is simply no language, I began to develop my own theory of neurolinguistics, the methodological perspective of which may be presented as shown in Figure 4.5.

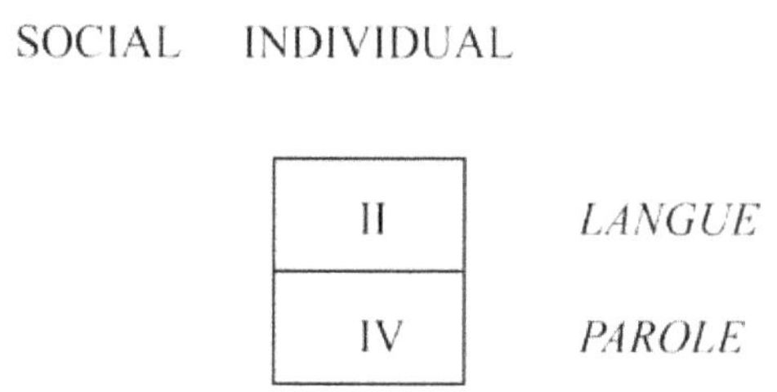

Figure 4.5 *Schematic illustration of the neurolinguistic perspective*

It is on the basis of this perspective that I shall describe the rest of the contents in this monograph.

Mention should be made in passing that there are several kinds of neurolinguistics: some will definitely equate neurolinguistics with language/speech pathology (or aphasiology); some others will treat it as a kind of applied linguistics or an offshoot of 'applied' generative grammar, employing aphasic patients, rather than normal subjects, to elicit their 'abnormal data' to show that rules can be impaired, because to these generativists language is rule-governed. The claim that language is rule-governed is a notion for data-processing in computer science or engineering, because machines have no brain, but is totally false for language in the brain of humans.

There are, of course, other methodological perspectives that can be illustrated by way of the matrix. Examples include anthropological linguistics (or ethnolinguistics), which has the perspective of I and II, and psycholinguistics, which has the perspective of III and II. Since this monograph is concerned mainly with the perspective of neurolinguistics, these extra perspectives will not be mentioned again.

Since none of those other brands of neurolinguistics fits into the neurolinguistic perspective I proposed, because in this perspective language is memory-governed, meaning-centred and multifaceted and not rule-governed, I shall also aim to correct the mistakes made in respect to language by medical and paramedical professionals when the rest of this monograph is explored along the line of the neurolinguistic perspective. It is only when the neurolinguistic perspective, and the Hallidayan perspective are put together can language be properly studied, because it has two faces which may be illustrated as shown in Figure 4.6.

	SOCIAL	INDIVIDUAL	
SOCIAL-SEMIOLOGICAL SYSTEM	I	II	*LANGUE*
INSTANTIATION	III	IV	*PAROLE*
	Systemics	Neurolinguistics	

Figure 4.6 *Schematic illustration of the two faces of language*

2. Elaboration of the Individual Aspect of Language

Since Saussure's distinction of *langue* and *parole* is, for the sake of epistemology, a methodological convenience, there was no need for him to be concerned with the brain functions of language. To him, the object of study in linguistics is not at all the immediately given phenomenon (Thibault, 1997: 14). But the distinction of the Social Aspect of Language and the Individual Aspect of Language I have proposed is no longer an epistemological issue; rather, it is an ontological issue that must be taken seriously. There are pieces of evidence that support this ontological issue.

First, it is individuals who congregate to form a speech community or society, and therefore the individual's nervous system is the 'power plant' (i.e., the source of energy) for human (social) interactions. Without individual humans, who congregate to interact, there is simply no social-semiological system to speak of.

Second, it is the individual who learns the first language from childhood by interacting with other individuals in the same community and then internalizing it in his/her nervous system, the fundamental function of which is to enable the individual to make proper adjustments to the internal and external environments. Making such proper adjustments is innate, because every individual member of a given species of living animals is enabled to do so even before birth (i.e., during the foetal life); language as behaviour during the process of maturation of the individual's nervous system in developmental terms and after it has matured is not innate, however; rather, it is learned, like other non-language behaviour; for example, playing a musical instrument.

Third, innatists making the claim that every individual can learn to speak at an early age without any formal training, and therefore language is genetically wired (or innate), are simply unaware of the fundamental function of the nervous systems, which is not species-specific to humans, and have failed to differentiate such fundamental function and the comparative gross anatomy. Formal education is only a part of the external environments (i.e., experiences) to which the individual may or may not adjust; when the individual adjusts to it, it enriches, not determines, his/her brain functions of language in a way different from the individual who does not need to adjust to it, as in people in a hunting and gathering society.

The enrichment, however, plays a role in later life of an individual if and when all individuals in a given community have equal opportunity to education; if and when some of those individuals drop out, the language behaviour of these drop-outs will be severely affected, making them inferior to the rest of the individuals in the same community. In other words, education in the technical sense of the word is needed in each individual's language behaviour, that is, in the individual aspect of language, for example, to become a lawyer or a physician, if the individual wants to excel within the community.

Fourth, it is the individual who can learn a second language as behaviour of his/her nervous system by interacting with other individuals in another community and then internalizing it while keeping it apart from his/her first language as behaviour.

Fifth, the very production and reception of *parole* (as raw data) must depend on the individual's intact nervous system and other anatomical structures; when the individual's nervous system is damaged, it is that individual's language as behaviour that is impaired while the language of the community, that is, the social aspect of language, remains untainted.

Sixth, when a language is considered dead – for example, Latin, or Hittite – it is because there is no more 'native' speaker left for social interactions involving that language in the community. It can be revived: Hebrew after Israel as a state came into being, or Ainu which has picked up momentum since the 1970s. However, the 'revived' language will not be the same as the 'original' language for obvious reasons because of changes through time and space.

Seventh, on the other hand, an individual may be deprived of his/her first language when he/she immigrates as a child (say, before the age of ten) with the family to another country where a totally different language is spoken, as may be evidenced by children of immigrants coming from Asia as a minority group to the United States or to Canada where the majority of the population speak English.

Eighth, worse still, speakers of a minority language can impose as rulers their language upon the majority of the people whom they rule through political oppression and formal education implemented in the minority language; after half a century or so of such oppression and enforced formal education, the number of individuals who can speak the majority language are likely to dwindle, as may be evidenced by the case in Taiwan where Mandarin as the minority language has forced the people in Taiwan to speak it, thereby depriving the majority of their mother tongues.

It is common throughout the world for the majority to wipe out a minority language – for example, Amerindian languages – but it is very rare for a minority to attempt to wipe out the majority language. Either way, it is known in sociolinguistics as linguistic imperialism or language hegemony in layman's terms.

Given these pieces of evidence, there is no denying that while language has the social aspect, because no individual can live alone – for example, by him-/herself without recourse to social interactions which shape his/her reservoir of experiences in his/her memory – it also has the individual aspect. Thus, other things being equal, I shall now concentrate on the individual aspect of language, from *parole* to *langue*, on the one hand, and point out the remedy for the vacuum left in linguistics and semiotics since Saussure's time, on the other.

3. Intellectual Interactions between Different Disciplines

As can be evidenced by the poor interactions cited above between linguistics and other disciplines, and vice versa, it is imperative that the interactions should improve if the current situations are to change for the better. While this monograph can stimulate certain enthusiasm among the social scientists to pay attention to the medical sciences, I hope that it will also encourage the medical corps to take the social sciences, behavioural sciences in particular, more seriously; at present, people in the medical corps take only passing interest in the behavioural sciences, although some neurologists and psychiatrists have begun to develop a realm of investigation called behavioural neurology.

Such a trend of cross-fertilization is indicative of a healthy development in neuroscience, as may be evidenced by the full-day educational course 'Behavioural Neurology: Issues in Cognitive Neuroscience' at the 55th Annual Meeting of the American Academy of Neurology held in Honolulu, Hawaii (29 March–5 April 2002). It consisted of seven lectures:

1. Functional MRI Studies of Associative Memory
2. Attention to Novel Events (Event-Related Potentials and Patients)
3. Mechanisms of Conscious Awareness
4. Semantic Knowledge (Functional MRI)
5. Language Reorganization After Injury (Functional MRI)
6. Body Schema Representation (Patients and Functional MRI)
7. Cognitive Aging (Functional MRI).

Of course, the practitioners of each discipline have their own pride and attachment to the territoriality which they tend to 'protect'. However, by opening up the invisible boundary that separates one discipline from another, each participating discipline can only benefit from such intellectual interactions. Otherwise, erroneous transfers of ideas from one discipline to another, through imperfect imitation, will result. Such was the case in the past.

It is natural to expect that formal interactions may not be easy, because each discipline prefers to believe that it has all the answers, when in fact it is not the case; very often the intellectual interactions take place through informal, 'private' imitation. If formal training is deemed difficult, informal contact through reading may be of help.

In 1995, I was invited to Timişoara, Romania, by a psychiatrist and a group of neurologists to give a series of three lectures at a hospital. While my lectures were all new to the participants, because the medical people there were more interested in neuropathies (diseases in the peripheral nervous system), rather than in the brain functions of language, I was quite astonished by the chief neurologist during our private conversations in English at dinner time. He could cite examples from Romanian about palatalization, assimilation, or even ablaut and umlaut in Germanic languages, because he could speak perfect German. A psychiatrist with us told me during the conversations that the chief neurologist has read books on historical linguistics.

I was lucky enough to be able to return to my Alma Mater, SUNY at Buffalo, to receive a formal training in the medical sciences, in 1976, when I was already Professor of Linguistics. When the formal training started, the resistance was there, which I could sense first, but I was able to overcome that by submitting myself to the faculty as one of the medical 'students'. Thus, there seem to be two factors involved. First, the factor on the part of the participating individual, from either the social sciences or the medical sciences, is to overcome the overrated 'self-esteem'; it was not easy for a full professor of linguistics to become a medical student in order to learn from the medical faculty members who were assistant or associate professors. Second, the factor on the part of the receiving institution, in either the social sciences or the medical sciences, is to abandon protectionism, so as to enable the participating individual to feel 'comfortable', if not 'at home', in order to benefit from the interactions.

I was not able to interact easily at first at SUNY for my knowledge of the medical sciences was not up to the expected level. However, I was able to raise intelligent questions, either in class or privately with the faculty, which often stunned not only medical students but also their faculty, because such questions could only come from persons with sufficient knowledge in the social sciences.

Moreover, after my initial training, I continued to work in three major hospitals in Taiwan to put my newly acquired knowledge in the medical sciences to clinical practice; as a matter of fact, I was also able to teach linguistic students something about the brain functions of language; I also obtained research grants from Taiwan and Japan to do research, from 1977 to 1989.

It was these experiences that enabled me to further interact with people in the medical corps, now quite intelligibly, by attending professional meetings on not only aphasia but also epilepsy, Parkinson's disease (PD), Spino-Cerebellar Ataxia (SCA), and in clinical neurophysiology, each time either presenting a paper or simply raising constructive questions and comments as a participant in a conference or a workshop and/or symposium. In fact, I presented a paper entitled 'Is Dementia a Disease?' at the Third World Congress on Vascular Factors in Alzheimer's Disease (7–10 April 2002) in Kyoto (see Peng, 2003b). My participation in the general discussions of the congress, in the form of critical comments on historical facts and sharp questions, contributed to the clarification of Alzheimer's disease (AD) as Alzheimer never made any original contribution to the description of senile plaques which have been mistakenly assigned to AD as if he was the first one to make that description.

In any event, it is hoped that this monograph and the other projects which will come out of my research will benefit not only practitioners in the social sciences but also the medical people who are interested in what language in the brain is like. If the book resulting from this research is not up to the level of the medical people, there are other possibilities, which will be graded upward to the level of sophistication for people in the medical corps.

PART III THE INDIVIDUAL ASPECT OF *PAROLE*

General Remarks

There is no denying that the nervous systems (central and peripheral) control behaviour, be it human or non-human. For this reason, scholars in all fields (not just neuroscientists but also philosophers, primatologists, or zoologists, and the like) have for many centuries tried to unravel the 'mysteries' which are wrapped up inside the amazing organ called the brain. But to this date it is not surprising that much of such 'mysteries' remain 'sealed' tight within this organ.

In the past, during the Hellenic period, the Greek philosopher Aristotle did not pay much attention to the brain; in fact, he credited the heart with thinking and sensing and gave the brain the mere servile job of cooling blood. In like manner, the French philosopher and mathematician René Descartes thought that the pineal gland, a small structure about 9mm long, located in the centre of the brain, was the point of contact between mind and body, which he then thought was the seat of the soul. However, modern physiologists are still unable to ascribe a function to this interesting structure of the brain. Although most scholars today will not agree with Aristotle, such expressions as 'kind-hearted', 'broken heart' in English, or '*kokoro no yamai*' (lit. disease of the heart, i.e., mental disease) in Japanese are common metaphors which can still be heard from time to time.

In Part III and Part IV, I shall try to unravel some of the 'mysteries' that have surrounded language in the brain; the unravelling is the main concern of this monograph. Part III and Part IV describe the structure and function of the brain, respectively, with regard to the individual aspect of language.

5 Language Behaviour and Body Movements

Language behaviour, like all other human behaviours, including dancing, playing a musical instrument, or martial arts (e.g., Chinese kung fu, Japanese judo or sumo, and Western fencing), or sexual activity, depends entirely on the individual's brain functions of memory. Such brain functions dictate all movements of any part of the whole body, in production, and process input of someone else's movements, in reception.

Most movements, if initiated, involve not only muscles but also bones to which muscles are attached; some movements, however, do not involve bones, for instance, eye blinking, tongue movements, uvular trills, vibration of the vocal chords and lip movements, or even intestinal movements for the bowels to move and heart beat.

Behaviour is, therefore, the movement the individual intends to accomplish through the body. In linguistic terms, behaviour is emic and movement is etic. Put differently, the individual aspect of *parole* is concerned with human behaviour, language behaviour in particular, in both production and reception, which are made feasible on account of the individual's intact gross anatomy, that is, the whole body which is the locus of various movements.

For production, the purpose of each movement is for the producer to do something with the body to the internal and/or external environment, intentionally or otherwise; on the other hand, for reception, the purpose of processing the input of such movements is to alert the brain through the body, that is, the five senses – the ears, the eyes, the hands, the legs, and the nose, or even the heart and the lungs – to get ready for proper adjustments to the incoming input produced from the internal and/or external environment. In other words, in either production or reception, the purpose of the brain functions of any behaviour is to enable the individual (human or animal) to make proper adjustments to the internal and/or external environments.

In the sense described above, the behaviour in production is called active behaviour and the behaviour in reception is called passive behaviour. Each behaviour involves a great deal of highly complex brain functions, which come from both the central and the peripheral nervous system, as well as body functions. For the time being, body functions will be set aside, until called upon later.

The two nervous systems consist of cells called neurons, along with other supporting cells called glias (or glial cells); the number of neurons are astronomical – that is, billions – only one tenth of which, about 10 billion, are evidently active cells in the brain, although each one of these has actual or potential links with tens of thousands of others; after all, they started from one single conceived cell. The number of glial cells are even larger; one estimation is that there are ten times as many glial cells as neurons in a brain, human or otherwise.

However, the average weight of a human adult brain is only 1.4kg (or 3lb), which is about 2 per cent of the total body weight. But the brain has the priority of blood supply, and therefore a human adult brain consumes 20 per cent of blood pumped out by the heart. This is because these neurons, especially in the brain, are densely packed in the cranium (skull) to form a very complex circuitry with interconnecting pathways, even though they all start from one neural tube which will be described briefly later.

The first aim of this section is to make sure that the concept of behaviour is clearly understood in terms of how these two nervous systems function; that is, they enable the individual to make proper adjustments in his/her behaviour, and since language is behaviour, the functions of these two nervous systems play a vital role in what language is. Misunderstandings of this concept have resulted in various unusual views of language until now. The individual aspect of *parole* hinges entirely on such a concept of behaviour supported by movements of the body.

In the medical field, because of territoriality (technically called specialization) movements are considered to only involve the use of the four limbs, the head and neck, and the torso (or trunk); only when one or more of these body parts are involuntarily impaired, as in Parkinson's disease (PD) and Huntington's disease (HD), because of damage in the basal ganglia, will the resultant symptoms be called movement disorders; such movement disorders are said to be not only permanent but also neurodegenerative. Damage to other parts of the brain, as in cerebral damage as a result of stroke or trauma, may result in hemiplagia, and yet the impairment is not considered a movement disorder on the grounds that it is permanent but *not* neurodegenerative.

However, since many parts of the body, other than the four limbs, the head and neck, and the torso, can also have movements – for example, the vocal apparatus – I have often wondered why medical people have so far ignored the movements, caused by the vocal apparatus in production, as active language behaviour. One reason may be that such movements of the vocal apparatus are for production only but the sounds heard in reception caused by someone else's vocal apparatus are no longer movements to them; as a result, hearing is assigned to audiology for testing, and the reception of sound movements in passive language behaviour is assigned to comprehension in aphasiology, as if only the hearer in reception has comprehension but the speaker in production does not, a strange dichotomy that is the opposite of Saussure's speech circuitry.

As a consequence, behaviour in the medical field also has its specialization, often detached from language behaviour. In other words, language as behaviour is not considered behaviour by most people in the medical and paramedical field. The reason is most likely that language has to do with sounds (production or reception) and some unknown sort of cognitive function – the place where concepts are elaborated in Lichtheim–Wernicke's model – and, therefore, has nothing to do with behaviour which is based on movements involving the use of the limbs, etc. Even so, more importantly, sign language as behaviour has not yet occurred to people in the medical and paramedical field. This is not to say that medical people do not treat patients who are deaf.

Such being the case, language/speech pathology (in aphasia) will have to be changed, because deaf people after a stroke, with hemiplegia as a sequela, do not have speech pathology; they have hand movement pathology instead. In fact, during the Fourth AOEC (Asian/Oceanian Epilepsy Congress) held in Karuizawa, Japan (11–14 September 2002), a paper presented by a Japanese doctor reported three congenitally deaf patients, affected by epilepsy, from a family of five siblings. Their epilepsy was an idiopathic type, so he showed a pedigree of the family's background, indicating the intellectual decline in the patients who developed dementia when they died in their thirties. When asked about the diagnosis of dementia, the doctor simply said they first had sign language but gradually lost it and could no longer sign before their deaths; that is, rather than interacting with them in sign language (JSL) throughout the treatment of their epilepsies, the doctor simply watched or observed that the patients could still sign each time they were treated but they gradually lost the ability to sign before death.

In *Journal of Speech, Language, and Hearing Research*, an official organ of the ASHA (American Speech, Language, and Hearing Association), an article by Ronnie B. Wilbur and Les Petersen (1998) showed how the authors used two groups of normal (i.e., hearing) subjects: ASL-English bilinguals and signed English users who know no ASL.

This article proves that language/speech pathologists would have no way of handling deaf persons who became hemiplegic, as these patients could not talk before the illness and could no longer sign properly after the illness. That is, would they treat hemiplegic deaf persons with 'sign therapy' comparable to 'speech therapy' for language rehabilitation? Language/speech pathologists avoid the issue by referring it to communication disorders, a 'waste basket', to shelve the problems of having to deal with the individual aspect of language as behaviour. Communication disorders include autism, dementia, mental retardation (now called learning disability), among others, which are actually none other than various forms of language disorder. Incidently, both Wilbur and Petersen are linguists who have specialized in sign language research.

Fortunately, some neurologists calling their specialization 'behavioural neurology' have begun to take interest in language as behaviour. However, unless they have come to grips with what language as behaviour is, especially what the individual aspect of language is, the goal is still far away for them. I have already cited a few examples in which language is detached from memory and abstract thinking, both of which are important brain functions pertinent to language as behaviour. Below are some more examples from *The Honolulu Advertiser* ('Warning signs of Alzheimer's disease', 24 July 2001) to support my point.

> **Difficulty performing familiar tasks**. Busy people can be so distracted from time to time that they may leave the carrots on the stove and remember to serve them only at the end of the meal. People with AD could prepare a meal and not only forget to serve a dish but also forget that they made it.
>
> **Disorientation of time and space**. It's normal to forget the day of the week or your destination for a moment. But people with AD can become lost on their own street, not knowing where they are, how they got there or how to get back home.
>
> **Poor or decreased judgment**. People can get so immersed in an activity that they temporarily forget a child they're watching. People with AD could forget the child under their care entirely.
>
> **Misplacing things**. Anyone can temporarily misplace a wallet or keys. A person with AD may put things in inappropriate places; an iron in the freezer or a wristwatch in the sugar bowl.
>
> **Changes in mood or behavior**. Everyone becomes sad or moody from time to time. Someone with AD may have rapid and mood swings for no apparent reason.
>
> **Changes in personality**. Personalities ordinarily change somewhat with age. But a person with AD can change dramatically, becoming extremely confused, suspicious, or fearful.
>
> **Loss of initiative**. It's normal to tire of housework, business activities, or social obligations, but most people regain their initiative. People with AD may become very passive and require cues and prompting to become involved.

It is of significance to point out that all the items quoted pertain to behaviour as defined above, because they are the functional results of the two nervous systems as manifested in active and/or passive behaviour which may be normal or abnormal. However, as can be seen in the separation of 'Changes in mood and behaviour' from the other items, neurologists and/or psychiatrists tend to treat the other items as something else, totally unrelated to behaviour, when they are behaviour *par excellence.* More importantly, it should be added that all items have something to do with passive behaviour, or else the clinician or family members are unable to detect the symptoms of AD, except that 'Misplacing things' can also be observed in active behaviour of the patient. Why do AD patients behave differently? The answer is that their brain functions of memory are severely impaired and the impairment is neurodegenerative, because the brain functions of memory control all behaviours, language behaviour in particular.

Recall that, in the same vein, neurologists/psychiatrists separate language, which is behaviour *par excellence,* from abstract thinking, which is also behaviour *par excellence.* It should be clear now that the brain functions of memory govern not only language as behaviour but also all behaviours which may in some way pertain actively or passively to language behaviour, or else the observer (clinician or otherwise) has no way of knowing or detecting any changes in behaviour, normal or abnormal, in daily social interactions. Such being the case, I shall leave the abnormal behaviour until the publication of *Language Disorders: A Critical Perspective* and concentrate only on the normal behaviour. For this reason, I shall now delve briefly into neuroanatomy (histology first) and later into gross anatomy.

6 The Physical Basis of Life

In order to demonstrate that language in the brain is behaviour, I will begin with the cell which has structure and function essential to life itself. Many self-proclaimed geneticists have overlooked this important fact and claimed that they have found a language gene that separates humans from non-humans. Many linguists, who are innatists and have little knowledge about the cell's structure and functions, have asserted on many occasions that language is innate or an organ, like the heart, or a set of rules, and therefore genetically transmitted. In this monograph, especially Chapter 16, I intend to refute such claims once and for all.

Why do I mention cells, neurons in particular, when my task is to describe briefly language in the brain (or the individual aspect of language)? The reason is that I want to tie neuroanatomy with behaviour, because language in the brain is the most complex human behaviour, the total revelation of which could take the cooperative efforts of hundreds, if not thousands, of like minds throughout the twenty-first century to accomplish; I simply take the first step here towards that eventual goal. That is, I take the following approach:

Cells → Tissues → Organs → Organisms → Behaviours

In so doing, questions about cells will reveal answers to questions about tissues (which are masses of similar cells connected together); questions about groups of tissues of similar functions, likewise, will reveal answers to questions about organs; and questions about complex groups of organs and tissues (their differences in particular) will reveal answers to questions about organisms (their similarities and differences in particular); and finally questions about and concerns with such similarities and differences among various organisms, hopefully, will lead to the answers to questions concerning their behavioural similarities and differences of which language as behaviour is the main focus. A clear understanding of such behavioural similarities and differences, it is hoped, will shed some light on the origin of language which will have to be differentiated semantically from one species to another, each having its own ontological criteria for the existence of its language.

Because this monograph, which has been expanded from my various research reports, is for linguists and semioticians, only the essential physical basis of life, a phrase first used by the eminent British biologist Thomas Henry

Huxley is briefly described here from the point of view of linguistics and semiotics; namely, first, life begins with one conceived cell, second, cell structure, and third, cell divisions. This monograph, therefore, is not intended for medical students and/or professional neuroscientists, although they may benefit from it as well. For this reason, this chapter is organized differently from an ordinary textbook of cytology.

1. Life Begins with One Conceived Cell

When I returned to the Medical School of SUNY, Buffalo, for medical training in 1976, I attended the class of physiology for the first time. The professor was an elderly lady who opened up her lecture with this statement: 'Life begins with one cell.' She was talking about cells in general. I then raised a question about the differences between cells in general and germ cells (i.e., egg and sperm) in particular. She thus corrected herself and said 'Life begins with one conceived cell.'

After the conception, cells can be divided into three types:

1. stem cells (which are undifferentiated cells);
2. germ cells (which are specialized for reproduction);
3. differentiated cells (which are specialized for specific body parts).

At these cellular levels, physiological (i.e., functional) and morphological (i.e., structural) phenomena are much the same.

1.1 Stem Cells

Stem cells are partially developed cells which exist in early embryos, foetal tissues and several adult tissues, for example, bone marrow. They can change course and become different types of cells, for instance, a proto-brain cell developing into a muscle cell, or a bone marrow cell, usually expected to become a blood cell, developing into a liver cell. Exciting researches are currently testing the potential abilities of stem cells for clinical applications in order to cure diseases such as diabetes, heart disease, Alzheimer's disease, Fischer's disease, and Huntington's disease. Expectations are such that worn-out, defective cells could then be replaced, or even new organs inserted, and impossible illnesses cured. For this reason, President Bush signed in July 2001 the authorization to allow research using stem cells. These expectations run parallel with expectation in gene therapy.

1.2 Germ Cells

Germ cells are already specialized for reproduction only. But they still undergo maturation to be fertile; that is, during childhood, germ cells are immature. It is during the maturation that each germ cell, egg or sperm, can go through the process of cell division in the course of reproduction.

1.3 Specialized Cells

A cell once fully developed (or specialized) is destined to fulfil its role until it dies or is damaged; in other words, a fully developed cell cannot undergo the process of cell division again to replace an organ, with some exceptions, such as the liver cells which can still go through cell divisions to multiply after a surgery or transplantation, or the blood cells, the hair cells and the nail cells. In some lower forms of animal, however, cell division is still possible after a part of the body is severed to grow the same part of the body.

Neurons are fully developed brain cells or nerve cells, the number of which are determined at birth; that is, after birth, neurons have reached their peak in number but their functions continue to grow through arborization (i.e., connections of fibres among themselves to constitute a highly complex circuitry or network of connections) and myelination (i.e., connections with supporting cells, called glial cells) until the age of 18, which is the peak of neural functions; after the age of 18, neural functions start the process of aging because of neuronal losses. (See Peng (1981, 1995) for a detailed analysis and clear evidence of this view.)

2. Cell Structure

Since this monograph is for linguists and semioticians, I shall limit my description of cell structure to that of the fully developed animal cell, even though there are certain features common to all cells, plant or animal. In so doing, the description will be confined to only a few components relevant to this monograph for linguists and semioticians (see Figure 6.1).

2.1 Protoplasm

The protoplasm comprises the total substance of the cell and is wrapped up in a flexible membrane. Protoplasm was aptly called by the eminent British biologist Thomas Henry Huxley 'the physical basis of life'. And the flexible membrane accounts, in part, for the various forms and shapes of animal cells.

2.2 Cell Membrane

The cell membrane is an important part of the cell; it protects the cell's substances and permits certain chemical substances, typically ions, to move in and out of the cell. It is this function of the cell membrane, especially the neurons (i.e., nerve cells), that enables cells to communicate with one another, thereby allowing each cell to transduce signals to its neighbours for active and/or passive behaviour.

The mechanism of the transduction of signals depends on the differences between the concentration of such substances in the cell and the concentration of the same substances in the area surrounding the cell. In this case, the

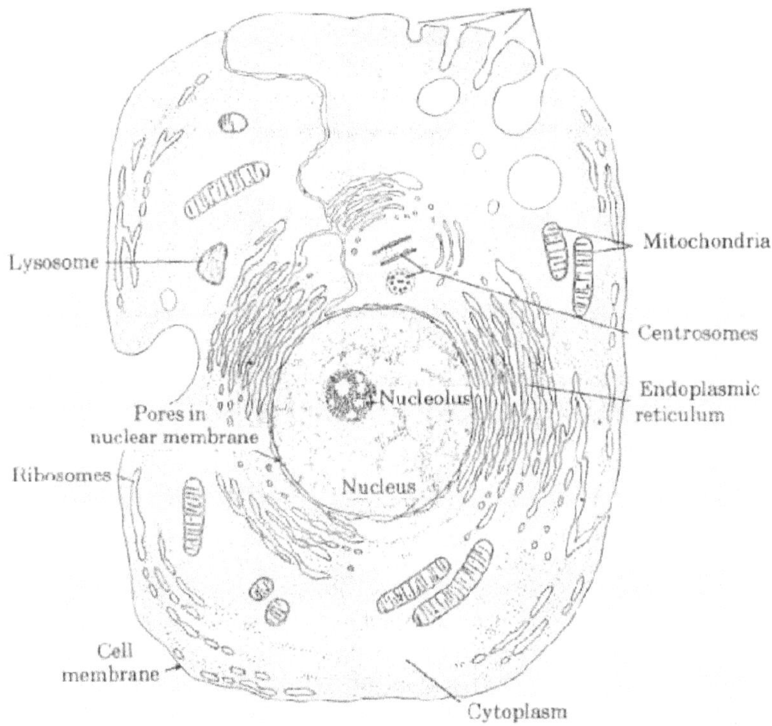

Figure 6.1 *A schematic representation of some of the components of a typical animal cell* (Reprinted from *Dorland's Illustrated Medical Dictionary*, 25th Edition, edited by W. A. Newman Dorland, copyright© 1974 with permission from Elsevier)

flow of ions is from the area of their higher concentration to the area of their lower concentration.

Thus, in the resting stage, sodium is in higher concentration outside the cell, while potassium is in higher concentration inside the cell. So, the cell interior is negatively charged in respect to the outside of the cell. Under these circumstances, the cell membrane inhibits the passage of sodium and potassium ions. However, when stimulated, the sodium ions and potassium ions exchange through the cell membrane; that is, sodium ions flow in and potassium ions flow out of the cell. This exchange, once it reaches the threshold, alters the electrical potential across the cell membrane, in an all-or-nothing manner, a physiological phenomenon that is called depolarization, which results in action potentials or electrical impulses that are the only signals the nerve cells recognize. Moreover, once the cell membrane is depolarized, the action potentials maintain the same strength until they reach the targeted neighbouring cell, although they can be inhibited.

These electrical impulses are divided into three types in terms of functions: excitation, inhibition and disinhibition. These functions are the neural properties of specialized neurons because of the kinds of neurotransmitters these neurons emit in their neuron-to-neuron communication and of the particular interconnections of certain neurons in the circuitry. More will be said about these functions later.

2.3 Cytoplasm

The cytoplasm is all the protoplasm of the cell minus the nucleus. Under a light microscope, the cytoplasm appears as a transducent, granular and fairly homogenous substance. However, under an electron microscope, it can be shown to contain various cytoplasmic components, each one of which plays an important role to synthesize chemical compounds needed for the life and activity of the cell. But only a few of such cytoplasmic components will be described here: mitochondria, lysosomes, Golgi bodies, endoplasmic reticulum and ribosomes, and centrosome.

2.3.1 Mitochondria

Mitochondria are the principal sites for the generation of energy, resulting from the oxidation of foodstuffs; hence, the mitochondrion is the 'power house' of the cell. It is an organelle with a spherical structure containing mitochondrial chromosomes, and is a site of energy production for each cell. If and when it is disordered, the consequence is called mitochondrial disorders (formerly called mitochondrial encephalopathy, a rare disease), which occur mostly in children and occasionally in young adults and affects all the mitochondria in the body. The patient becomes mute and immobile.

The disorders have a molecular basis, the exact cause of which is not yet clear; but the discovery of an impressive and ever expanding number of mutations of mitochondrial DNA coupled with clinical and molecular observations have recently indicated that many syndromes are caused by abnormalities in nuclear genes related to oxidative phosphorylation. (For the details, see Zeviani and Klopstock (2001)). I have encountered one case which is reported briefly below.

The case was an 11-year-old girl whom I examined on 28 February 1992 in Taipei. The initial symptoms observed by me and reported by her parents and relatives accompanying her were: epileptiform seizure, rigid muscle tone in all four limbs and torso, mutism, loss of memory, inability to walk or stand still on her own because of motor impairment arising from rigidity, inability to eat (i.e., to masticate) on her own and possibly dysphagia (i.e., difficulty in swallowing), and in need of assistance for urination and bowel movement. The first symptom was reported to me by her parents and could be as a result of secondarily generalized seizure.

Since mitochondria are the 'power plants' of life, it is to be expected that any failure in them will lead to serious behavioural and mental problems which are degenerative. What is of significance is the speed at which her conditions deteriorated.

According to her parents her conditions had begun to deteriorate only six months prior to the examination when she was compelled to leave school. The reason was that she could no longer follow any instructions in class. At that time, she was still able to 'speak' (albeit with limited capacity, according to her parents). Obviously, the illness had been going on for quite some time, the onset being around the age of seven. The important point is that during the six-month period she completely lost her ability to speak (i.e., total mutism), to walk and to masticate, mainly because of two factors: serious impairments of her brain functions related to language behaviour; and loss of all muscular movements because of rigidity, so much so that she could not even sit up while being examined and had to be carried about (horizontally) from one place to another. In fact, she was carried in that way by three or four adults. She also lost her reflexes because her parents tried several times to sit her up, but as soon as her upper body was put upright she would slowly fall backward or sideways (left or right) down on the sofa.

2.3.2 Lysosomes

The lysosomes are spherical bodies which contain digestive enzymes for the process of localized intracellular digestion and, therefore, are seen in many types of cells. They break down fats, proteins, and other large molecules into smaller compounds upon which other enzymes of the cell can act. The supplemental dietary pills, called Lysines, which many Americans take when they have fever blisters on the lips, contain just this kind of digestive enzymes.

2.3.3 Golgi Bodies

A Golgi body is also called a Golgi complex or a Golgi apparatus. It was first described by the Italian histologist Camillo Golgi (1843–1926), co-winner, with Santiago Ramón y Cajal, of the Nobel Prize for medicine and physiology in 1906. The Nobel Prize was in recognition of their work on the structure of the nervous system.

The Golgi bodies are stacks of membrane-bound sacs which are the main sites responsible for packaging substances for transport outside the cell. They synthesize certain carbohydrates. Deficiency of carbohydrates causes bad breath. It is, however, of interest to note that their views on the brain were diametrically opposite; while Cajal advocated the view that the brain was made up of millions of brain cells, called neurons, which were divided by clefts, later on known as synaptic clefts, Golgi insisted on the traditional view that the brain was an integrated whole. Cajal eventually won the argument and his view became known as the Neuron Theory, which also led to two more Nobel Prizes: for Charles Scott Sherrington (1857–1952) on synaptic changes, physiology of the nervous system, co-winner in 1932 with Edward Douglas Adrian, and for Sherrington's student John Carew Eccles for discoveries concerning the ionic mechanisms involved in excitation and inhibition in the peripheral and central portions of the postsynaptic nerve cell membrane, co-winner in 1963 with Alan Lloyd Hodgkin and Andrew Fielding Huxley.

2.3.4 Endoplasmic Reticulum and Ribosomes

This is an extensive network of tiny interconnected 'canals' which extend throughout the cytoplasm. Two forms have been differentiated: *granular reticulum* and *agranular reticulum.* The former is lined with tiny particles called ribosomes which are the main sites for synthesizing enzymes and other proteins. It exists in nearly all cells of higher plants and animals. The latter contains no ribosomes.

2.3.5 Centrosome

This is a small, round structure which is located near the cell nucleus. Its function is very important to cell division, for either meiosis or mitosis; during cell division, the centrioles, which are two small dots in the centrosome, become clearly visible within the centrosome and act as part of the apparatus that divide the nuclear components, as will be shown further below.

2.4 The Nucleus

The nucleus is the largest structure within the cell; it is generally located somewhere near the cell's centre surrounded by the cytoplasm. It has a nuclear membrane of its own and is the first structure to undergo division.

The nucleus controls the metabolic activities of the cell and carries all the genetic information about the cell in the important (ultimate) nuclear component called DNA (deoxyribonucleic acid), which is a special type of nucleic acid of which genes are composed. A DNA is a long, twisted, double coil molecule consisting of many nucleotides which form two parallel chains. A nucleotide consists of a special kind of complex sugar (deoxyribose), a phosphate, and one of four nitrogen-containing bases, that is, A (adenine), T (thymine), G (guanine) and C (cytosine). Each one of these is a molecule. The repeated sugar-phosphate linkages constitute the chains which wind around each other and twist in a spiral fashion to form a double helix. Thus, it is each sugar-phosphate linkage that is tied to a base.

When the linkages repeat, the various combinations of the bases also repeat. But since the altering sugar and phosphate molecules are the same all the time, the representation in DNA of the molecules is usually written as follows:

```
Sugar-Phosphate-Sugar-Phosphate-Sugar-Phosphate
   |                  |                |
  Base               Base             Base
```

As there are two molecular chains, their representation, by skipping the sugar-phosphate linkage, can be written in an abbreviated fashion. The dotted lines between the bases are the hydrogen bonds; they indicate weak chemical bonds that hold the two chains of DNA together.

T-A-A-T-T-G-C-G ......

. . . .

. . . .

. . . .

A-T-T-A-A-C-G-C.......

The ordering of the bases in a single chain of DNA is not restricted; however, the ordering must obey two restrictions if and when the chains are paired:

1. Every T base in one chain must correspond to an A base in the other chain;
2. Likewise, every G base in one chain must be paired with a C base in the other chain.

It is according to these principles that the precise order, which is the genetic message or information, varies from gene to gene. The DNA replicates in the process of cell division (cf. mitosis), by separating the two chains to build a complementary chain along side each of the originals.

Each segment of the combinations contains a different genetic (i.e., functional) instruction to direct the destination and determine the structure and function of the cell when the cell multiplies to form tissues and eventually to become organs, such as the brain, the tongue, the lips and so on. Thus, a gene is a functional concept, not a structural one, such as a molecule or even a nucleotide. Put differently, a molecule like A or T or C or G is not a gene; it is the strict pairing and a different combination each time of these molecules in a segment of a double helix that are collectively called 'a gene'.

When there is an alteration in the combinations, it is called a mutation; it is a stable but heritable change of the nucleotide sequence in a DNA, a change that typically results in a new allele or even a new phenotype. Any of one or more of the alternative forms of a given gene is called an allele; the phenotype is defined in medical terms as 'the observable characteristics of an organism, either in total or with respect to one or more particular named characteristics'.

If and when the alteration expresses itself to cause a defect in an organ affecting the organ's function in an organism, as in cleft palate, or affecting the organism's behaviour, it is called gene expression. Thus, the phenotype of an organism may also be regarded as the manifestation of gene expression in that organism, for instance, Spino-Cerebellar-Ataxia (SCA) now with 25 types, each one of which may cause or result in dementia affecting the patient's language behaviour. However, many people may have poor genes (i.e., defective combinations), such as in diabetes, or are gene carriers, but will not have gene expressions if they eat properly and do sufficient exercise. In the case of SCA, it is the repeats of trinucleotides – for example, CAG – beyond the normal range (32–57) that cause the gene expression to result in SCA.

It is, therefore, totally wrong for linguists, who are innatists, to think and believe that language is genetically transmitted, because language is *not* a structure, like an organ (as Chomsky claimed) or an organism which is formed by genetic instructions during cell divisions and multiplications. It is equally wrong for naïve geneticists to think that they have found a language gene in a family of English speakers, just because some of these speakers make grammatical mistakes in the tense markers, and therefore assert erroneously that the 'language gene' they have found determines or evolved to result in the development of language or grammar in humans.

Language in the brain is behaviour, not at all an organ or an organism, and therefore absolutely cannot be genetically transmitted, because there is no language gene in humans any more than there is grammar in the human brain. Only structures, such as cells, tissues, and organs or defects in them, such as cleft palate and SCA, not behaviours caused by movements of them, are formed by instructions to show the phenotype, that is, characteristics of the organism. How many trinucleotide repeats are expanded that can be found in the individuals who were purported to make grammatical errors? If there is a language gene in them, which has formed their language but is now claimed to be impaired, the number of trinucleotide repeats must be calculated first. It took geneticists ten years to work out the exact trinucleotide repeats in many pedigrees in many countries in order to determine the gene that causes Huntington's disease.

On the other hand, a genetic defect can cause language disorders, such as nasality in a person with cleft palate, or mutism in a person with mitochondrial disorders, or dementia in a person with AD, HD, SCA, FD, or Pick's disease (each one of which may be genetically induced). (For those interested in the genetic factor of cleft palate, see Mehmet *et al.*, 2001.)

In this vein, it is of considerable significance to mention that dementia is a form of language disorders *par excellence*, that is, abnormal language behaviour and not a disease as is so believed by many a practitioner in the medical corps. (See Peng, 2003b, 2005.) I have also found that patients with all forms of epilepsy have language disorders of varying degrees, because each form of epilepsy causes memory impairment in the patient and language in the brain is, by definition, memory-governed. However, temporal lobe epilepsy may be caused by stroke, trauma, or encephalitis during childhood, in which case, it is not genetically induced. Some forms of epilepsy are genetic (i.e., idiopathic), as in cerebral dysplasia (resulting in double cortex, megaloencephaly, schizoencephaly, hemiatrophy, or similar) that causes epilepsy.

Some geneticists have also erroneously believed and asserted, by identifying a gene in chromosome 7, that language disorders are genetic, because they equate dysfunction with loss of the origin of function; hence, on account of language disorders (i.e., abnormal language behaviour) they have come to assert that language in the brain is innate, which is species-specific to humans. They are wrong, as will be shown in Chapter 16, for two reasons:

1. Causing language disorders, because of defects in the tissues or organs, neural or otherwise, resulting in a peculiar phenotype, has nothing to do with language being innate.
2. A defect, genetic or acquired, in the tissue of an organ may result in behavioural alteration which has nothing to do with language being innate; the behavioural alteration of an organism is not tantamount to the defective tissue or organ alone being responsible for the original intact behaviour.

Behaviour is the totality of many body movements, which is intentionally enacted or 'secretly' and 'unilaterally' perceived. Unaware of this, the erroneous equation just pointed out has been committed by neuroscientists in the past, thereby causing unnecessary confusion, as was mentioned earlier.

As have been shown above, all cells produce energy for a host of activities; they also manufacture proteins for survival. Animal cells, in particular, produce energy from food and apply this energy to special purposes for the body in accordance with the specialization of each type of cells: gland cells for chemical substances; muscle cells for mechanical movement; nerve cells for impulses (or action potentials) to produce motor actions or sensory perception; and kidney cells for excretion, and so on.

3. Cell Divisions

In this section, I shall now describe why all cells produce energy, since they all come from one conceived cell. Cells are microscopic units that support all forms of life with the exception of viruses; viruses are an exception because they stand between the living and the non-living. In such cases, all life functions, such as reproduction, metabolism and response to stimuli are performed by and within a single cell. However, a high degree of specialization develops, if and when a single cell can multiply in number, because a single cell may constitute the entire body of a plant or of an animal. It is the multiplication of cells leading to various functional specializations that distinguish one species from another; as such, functional specializations become more and more complex in both phylogenic and ontogenic terms, because of interconnections, through two important processes: Meiosis and Mitosis.

Perhaps, Darwin's theory of evolution (in his *The Origin of Species*), in relation to language origin, can be accounted for on the basis of the cell's ability to multiply and specialize in each species of animals. I shall, therefore, briefly explain what these important processes are.

3.1 Meiosis

Meiosis is a process that occurs during the maturation of germ cells and germ cells only. Thus, before puberty and after menopause (for women) meiosis does not take place, that is, germ cells are not fertile, although they exist in those individuals; in men, however, sperms continue to be fertile.

During the process, the chromosomes, each of which contains the DNA in the nucleus of each developing egg or sperm, are reduced from the number characteristic for the species. In humans, the characteristic number is 46 (or 23 pairs). In chimpanzees, it is 48. When a person has one extra chromosome, that is, 47, as in children with Downs' Syndrome, that person becomes mentally severely retarded and his/her language behaviour is disordered. Put differently, having more chromosomes than the characteristic number the species is entitled to will do more harm than good to the individual having that extra chromosome. In addition to the nucleus, chromosomes also exist in each mitochondrion.

For that reason, the DNA is an important structure that must obey the strict species-specific order of the characteristic number of chromosomes and/or their genetic code; it is wrapped by a sheath of proteins to constitute a chromosome. That is, if a chromosome is stripped of its proteins, the DNA in the form of a double helix can be seen under the electron microscope. Any violation of this strict species-specific order of the characteristic number of chromosomes will result in abnormal behaviour, developmentally, if the individual is born; even cloning, as in the late 'Dolly', the famous sheep first cloned in the UK, cannot guarantee that the cloned animal or human will remain the same as the original or even normal in behaviour.

The characteristic number of chromosomes in a species is called the diploid number; it is reduced to one-half which is called the haploid number. In humans, the diploid is 46 and the haploid is 23. These chromosomes are conventionally numbered according to the sizes and the position of the centromere on each chromosome; the centromere is the point where a chromosome is attached to a spindle fibre during cell division. The convention was established at a meeting of human cytogeneticists in Denver in 1960, and is thus known as the Denver classification (Nora and Fraser, 1974).

According to the Denver classification, in the case of Down's syndrome, it is the twenty-first pair that become aberrant during the process of meiosis. That is, the twenty-first pair of one parent's chromosomes fail to separate, a failure which is called non-disjunction, thereby resulting in the occurrence of that particular chromosome in triplicate, rather than duplicate, in the offspring.

Although the aberration does not imply that Down's syndrome is a hereditary condition, it can be said that it is not the transmission of a defective gene that causes the condition; rather, it is a disturbance in the reproductive process of meiosis of the parent that results in the condition which can be abolished during the early foetal life. The method is called amniocentesis, which is to take a sample of amniotic fluid from the mother's uterus for analysis in order to find out whether or not there are possible chromosomal aberrations, a test that allows termination of a pregnancy to avoid the birth of a child with the conditon. Or else, the child, if born, will have difficulty learning a language; even if some rudimentary vocabulary items may be acquired, the child, with an IQ between 20 and 49, physically marred by abnormal characteristics in the facial features, will certainly develop serious language disorders, typically in ideational discourse with short sentences. Children with Down's syndrome look more alike with one another, because of the abnormal characteristics in the facial features, than with their siblings.

In human males, one pair of the chromosomes, the twenty-third pair, are different, while the remaining 22 pairs have both members of each pair alike. The twenty-third pair have two different chromosomes, one of which is called the sex-chromosome, also called the Y chromosome, while the other chromosome in the pair is the X chromosome; the rest are called the autosomes which are the 22 pairs. In human females, however, the twenty-third pair have only the X chromosomes, to differentiate from the male, while the rest are all autosomes.

Chromosomal aberrations are not limited to autosomes; the X and Y chromosomes may also result in aberrations. For instance, a 47,XXY sex chromosomal constitution in a baby will result in Klinefelter syndrome, the extra X chromosome being considered inactive; or males with the 47,XYY chromosomal constitution will appear taller and more aggressive than males with normal XY. Although it is not clear how consistent this feature is, the aggressive and antisocial behaviour of XYY males leading to imprisonment may be one of the more important discoveries in human behavioural genetics (Nora and Fraser, 1974). In either case, autosomal or sex-chromosomal aberration, it is called trisomy. So, Down's sydrome is a trisomic disorder.

In spite of the potential risk just described, the reproductive process of meiosis is a must because when an egg is fertilized by a sperm, the two haploids will join together to result in a new diploid in the fertilized cell, called the zygote, with a correct number of chromosomes; hence, life begins with one conceived cell. From that point onward, a constrastive kind of cell division begins, called mitosis by means of which the cell multiplies leading to eventual specializations.

3.2 Mitosis

Mitosis is an important process of cell division for all forms of life, in which the nuclear material, including the chromosomes, is divided evenly between the two new cells, called the daughter cells, each of which has the same number of chromosomes as the parent cell. The process has five stages: Interphase, Prophase, Metaphase, Anaphase and Telophase.

3.2.1 Interphase

When an egg is fertilized by a sperm to become a zygote, the zygote has all the structural components described above of a cell which is said to be 'resting'. This is the stage of interphase (Figure 6.2). The chromosomes as the genetic materials form a mass of chromatin wrapped inside the nuclear membrane. The nucleolus, which manufactures substances needed for synthesis of cell proteins, is put near the middle of the chromatin. The two centrioles needed for nuclear division during mitosis are contained in the centrosome.

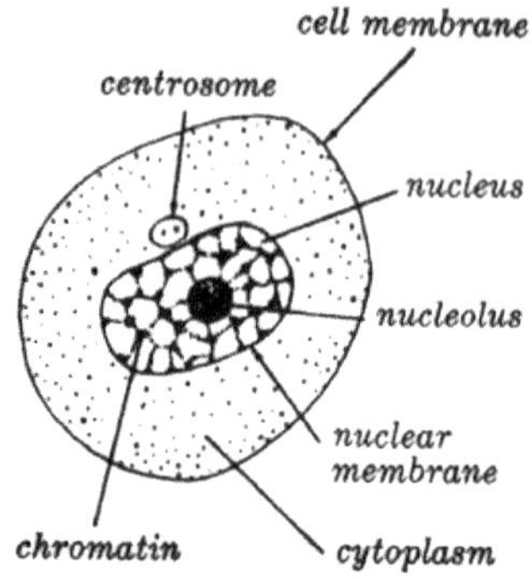

Figure 6.2 *Interphase of the cell before cell division* (From *The Encyclopedia of Health and the Human Body*, edited by Gerald Newman, copyright 1977 by Franklin Watts. All rights reserved. Reprinted by permission of Franklin Watts, an imprint of Scholastic Library Publishing, Inc.)

3.2.2 Prophase

When the fertilized cell begins the process of mitosis, structural components mentioned above start to change. The two centrioles inside the centrosome appear, each moving to opposite sides of the nucleus, but they are connected by filaments called spindle fibres, with short fibres called asters radiating from each centriole. At the same time, the diffuse chromatin begins to condense, taking shape to become distinctive forms as chromosomes. At this time, each chromosome has already duplicated itself and consists of two chromatids which lie parallel to each other and are connected at one point by the centromere; near the end of prophase (Figure 6.3), the nuclear membrane disappears and the chromosomes become associated with, or anchored by, the spindle fibres.

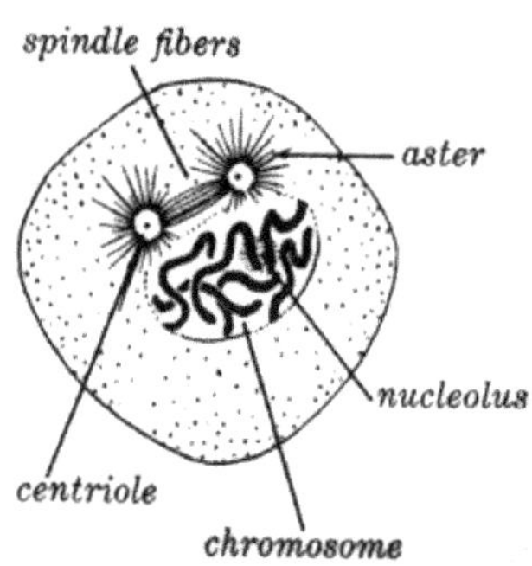

Figure 6.3 *Prophase of cell division as the cell enters mitosis* (From *The Encyclopedia of Health and the Human Body*, edited by Gerald Newman, copyright 1977 by Franklin Watts. All rights reserved. Reprinted by permission of Franklin Watts, an imprint of Scholastic Library Publishing, Inc.)

3.2.3 Metaphase

The chromosomes now line up and separate into two sets of chromatids through the centre of the cell midway between the two asters during metaphase in an equatorial plate; each chromatid is attached to a spindle fibre which will then pull it towards the centriole on its respective side (Figure 6.4).

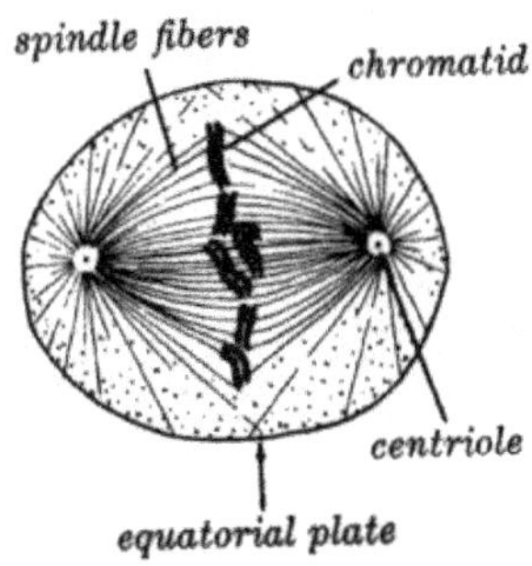

Figure 6.4 *Metaphase of mitosis* (From *The Encyclopedia of Health and the Human Body,* edited by Gerald Newman, copyright 1977 by Franklin Watts. All rights reserved. Reprinted by permission of Franklin Watts, an imprint of Scholastic Library Publishing, Inc.)

3.2.4 Anaphase

The spindle fibres to which the chromatids are connected pull the two halves of each chromosome in order to separate them, each half moving to the centriole closest to it to become one complete set of 'daughter' chromosomes. Near the end of this stage of mitosis, a constriction appears at the upper and lower edges of the cell along the equatorial plate (Figure 6.5).

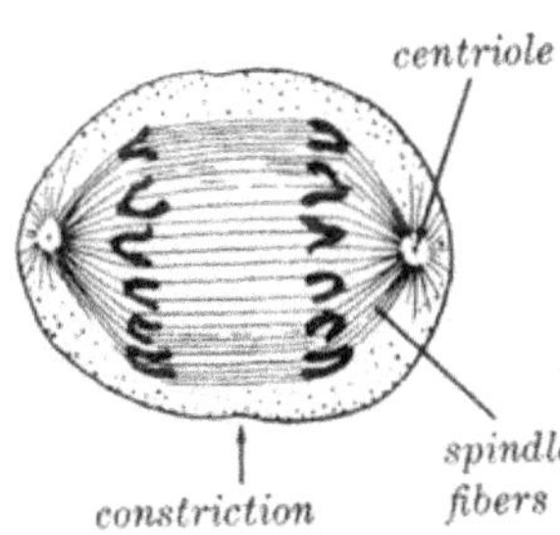

Figure 6.5 *Anaphase of mitosis* (From *The Encyclopedia of Health and the Human Body,* edited by Gerald Newman, copyright 1977 by Franklin Watts. All rights reserved. Reprinted by permission of Franklin Watts, an imprint of Scholastic Library Publishing, Inc.)

3.2.5 Telophase

When the chromosomes on each side complete their movement, they become less distinct and form chromatin again. At this time, a nuclear membrane develops around the two new groups of chromosomes, surrounding each group as chromatin, and the spindle fibres disappear while each centriole also divides into two to become a new centrosome for each group of chromosomes. At the end, a cell (i.e., cytoplasmic) membrane forms to surround the protoplasm of each daughter cell along the equatorial plate, thereby completing mitosis, and the two new cells enter the interphase for the next cell division (Figure 6.6).

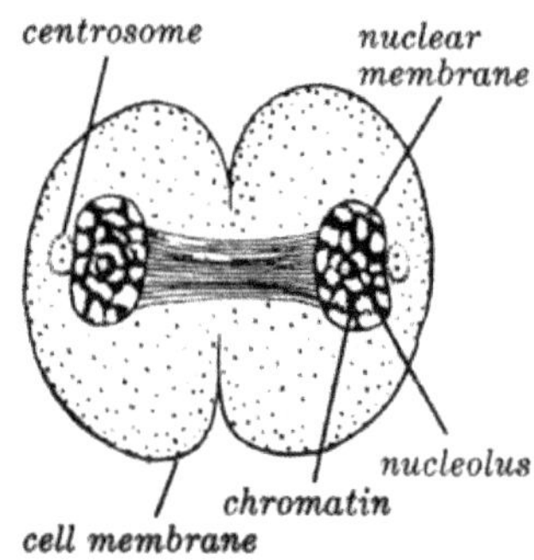

Figure 6.6 *Telophase of mitosis* (From *The Encyclopedia of Health and the Human Body*, edited by Gerald Newman, copyright 1977 by Franklin Watts. All rights reserved. Reprinted by permission of Franklin Watts, an imprint of Scholastic Library Publishing, Inc.)

7 Embryonic Development of the Nervous System

As the zygote (conceived cell) multiplies through the process of mitosis, it takes place first in the fallopian tube in five stages within a short period of time (usually about four days). Every woman has two fallopian tubes that connect the ovary to the uterus. The five stages are:

1. fertilization of an ovum to become a zygote for 12 to 24 hours;
2. two-cell stage, approximately 30 hours after conception;
3. four-cell stage, approximately 40 hours after conception;
4. early morula (a solid ball of eight cells resulting from division of the zygote), approximately 80 hours after conception;
5. advanced morula, approximately four days after conception.

At that point, the advanced morula must enter the uterus to become the blastocyte, approximately five days after conception. After that, the blastocyte becomes the embryoblast in the uterus, thereby starting the embryonic development. If, for some reason, the advanced morula does not enter the uterus in time and develops into the blastocyte in the fallopian tube, the consequences can become detrimental for the mother, because the blastocyte being prevented from entering the uterus becomes embryoblast in the fallopian tube, an abnormal condition that is called tubal pregnancy. It can cause the fallopian tube to burst, resulting in heavy bleeding which requires immediate major surgery to evacuate the accumulating blood in the abdomen, or else the mother will die.

The blastocyte, in a matter of less than a week, is a structure which is a mass of non-specialized aggregated cells and develops into the embryoblast that is the early form of an embryo, although the mother is still not aware that she is pregnant. In this chapter, I shall describe briefly the fascinating development of the embryonic nervous system. As language learning does not begin post-natally but starts from the embryonic life for reception and becomes sophisticated during the foetal life, this is a useful stage with which the child language expert should become more aware.

1. The Initial Development

After conception, as the conceived cell begins the process of mitosis to multiply into two, four, eight cells, and so on for its embryonic growth to become an embryoblast, it is now a six-day-old embryo which is an egg-shaped 'lump' from a back (dorsal) view (Figure 7.1). In neurophysiological terms (EEG), however, the gestational age (GA) refers to the time from the first day of the mother's last menstrual period to birth (Hughes, 1982: 69). For this reason, the mother is still not conscious of the existence of an embryoblast. Not until her menstrual period stops will she become aware of the pregnancy. By that time, the embryoblast has become a fully fledged embryo that is several weeks old in GA. For the sake of continuity, I shall resume the description from the stage of a six-day-old embryoblast.

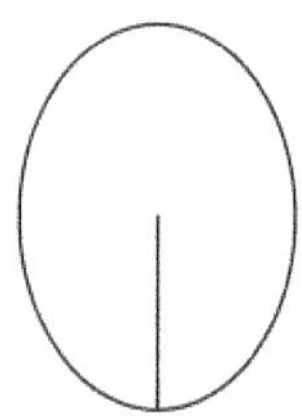

Figure 7.1 *A six-day-old embryoblast*

At this stage, with the exception of a 'cleft' in the centre, it shows few signs of brain or cord. But note that the rostral (top) end is bulging and the caudal (tail) end is elongating and that the neural plate develops first before any part of the body appears.

By 20 days after conception, the neural plate shows a groove in the middle by folding the outer layer of cells into parallel waves to form the first sign of a tube on the neural plate (Figure 7.2).

The parallel waves gradually close to form the neural tube, which is the beginning of the central nervous system (Figure 7.3). Notice that the tube will

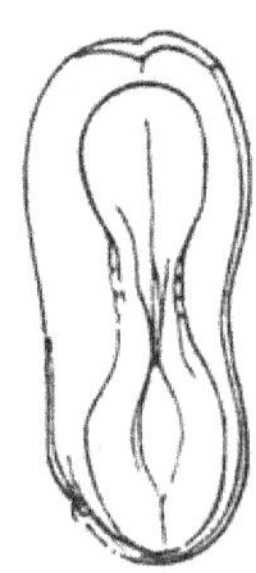

Figure 7.2 *A 20-day-old embryo* (From *The Brain: A User's Manual*, copyright © The Diagram Visual Information Group Ltd. Used by permission.)

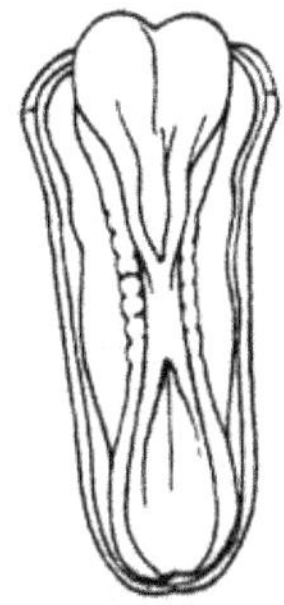

Figure 7.3 *A 22-day-old embryo* (From *The Brain: A User's Manual*, copyright © The Diagram Visual Information Group Ltd. Used by permission.)

also form the central canal in the spinal cord and the ventricles in the brain for the flowing of CSF (cerebrospinal fluid), which is essential for the survival and activity of neurons. After birth, the brain and the spinal cord literally float in CSF, which serves not only to 'lubricate' the surface of the nervous system but also protect it as a 'cushion'. However, if CSF is blocked or obstructed in the brain, after birth, the consequence becomes serious. A disorder called obstructive hydrocephalus will then arise, which requires brain surgery, a procedure called Ventrico-Peritoneal (VP) shunt to drain from the ventricles the accumulated CSF, with a pump buried inside the scalp and an artificial tube buried inside the skin of the chest, into the peritoneal cavity. Without this procedure the brain becomes enlarged and pressured inside the skull and all brain functions will be jeopardized, if not stop completely.

Only one day after that, the embryo develops paired structures; three weeks or so after conception, the embryo is just about 3mm long, with the top part bulging from the neural tube, while closing the parallel waves (cf. Figure 7.3), because the brain begins to take shape. If for some genetic reason(s) the parallel waves fail to close to form the paired structures (Figure 7.4) at the top

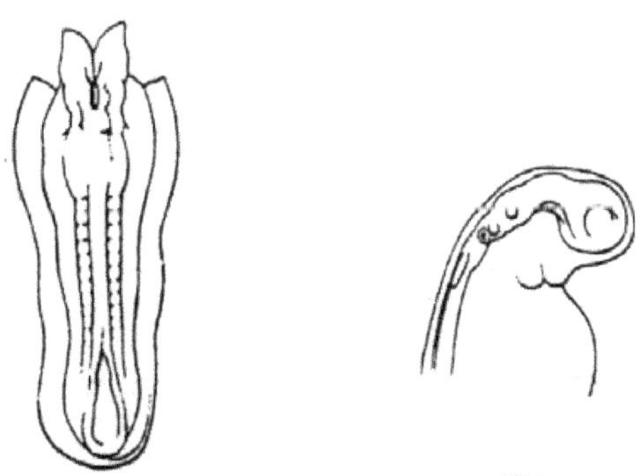

(A) **(B)**

Figure 7.4 *A 23-day-old embryo: (a) dorsal view; (b) lateral view* (From *The Brain: A User's Manual*, copyright © The Diagram Visual Information Group Ltd. Used by permission.)

end of the neural tube, the consequence is called anencephaly (i.e., an undeveloped brain) and the embryo either dies or will develop into a deformed foetus; if born, the infant will develop pediatric epilepsy and be short-lived.

It should be noted that the 'top end' will become the 'front end' because the neural tube will bend, for mammals, so as to increase the complexity of the circuitry of neuronal interconnections. The embryo of a lower vertebrate – for example, chicken – will not bend the 'top end' of the neural tube. The bending increases its angularity as the embryo grows; however, the angularity varies from one species to another, with the human brain being most pronounced or extensive.

2. Further Development of the Nervous System

The paired structures, that is, the enlarged sections, will now change into an embryonic brain showing stages of developmental divisions some of which, even after birth, are still used by neurologists; such developmental divisions are often mixed with structural divisions, causing some terminological confusion unless care is taken to discern them.

The embryonic brain, only after 25 days of gestation, has now three main vesicles which are the precursors of the forebrain (prosencephalon), the midbrain (mesencephalon), and the hindbrain (rhombencephalon) (Figure 7.5). The forebrain begins to bend down more.

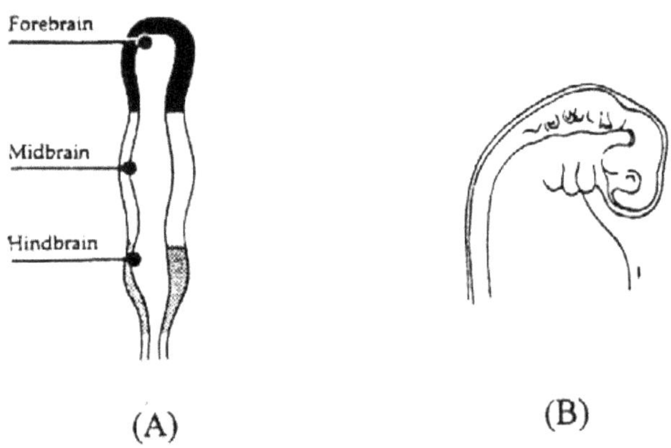

Figure 7.5 *Three vesicles of the embryonic brain: (a) dorsal view; (b) lateral view* (From *The Brain: A User's Manual,* copyright © The Diagram Visual Information Group Ltd. Used by permission.)

Later, the three vesicles will become five as prosencephalon (forebrain) further divides into telencephalon (end brain) and diencephalon (between brain), and rhombencephalon (hindbrain) divides into metencephalon and

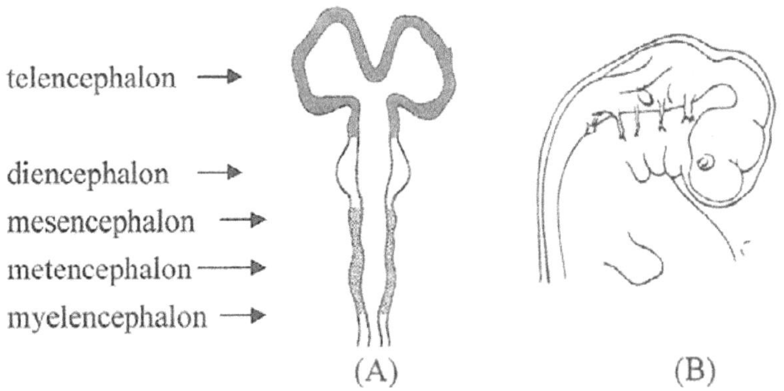

Figure 7.6 *Five vesicles of the embryonic brain at five weeks: (a) dorsal view; (b) lateral view* (From *The Brain: A User's Manual*, copyright © The Diagram Visual Information Group Ltd. Used by permission.)

myelencephalon (Figure 7.6a). During this stage, in the lateral view (Figure 7.6b), notice that a deep crease has developed, which is the demarcation of telencephalon, where the two cerebral hemispheres grow, and diencephalon, where the hypothalamus (an important structure for the limbic system) and thalamus (an important structure in the limbic system for relay and integration of brain functions) are formed. It can also be seen that an eye bud is growing from the end brain; the retina in a fully formed eye is a part of the brain. Several cranial nerves are sprouting. The upper limbs begin to show, too.

Telencephalon is then divided into two halves which will become the two cerebral hemispheres with inner structures: each half contains a cavity which is designated as the lateral ventricle, the two cavities making up the first and second ventricles each of which is an enlargement of the original central canal for the flowing of CSF (Figure 7.7a).

The bulge below mesencephalon is the beginning of the cerebellum (dor-

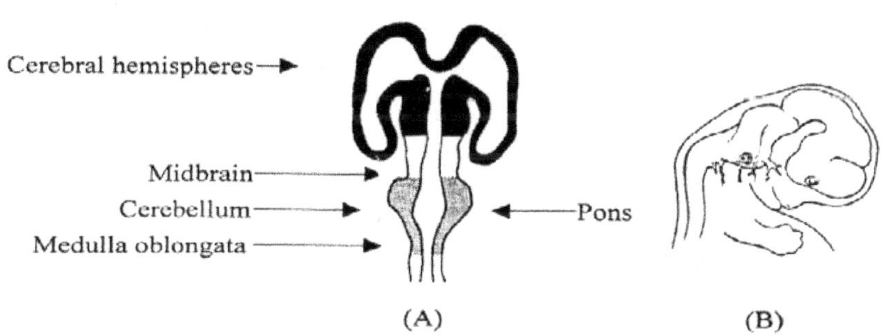

Figure 7.7 *Further development of the embryonic brain at seven weeks: (a) dorsal view; (b) lateral view* (From *The Brain: A User's Manual*, copyright © The Diagram Visual Information Group Ltd. Used by permission.)

sally) and the pons (ventrally); that is, metencephalon differentiates into the dorsal enlargement which will become the cerebellum and the ventral enlargement which will become the pons (Figure 7.7b).

The myelencephalon then develops into the medulla oblongata, which is continuous with the spinal cord below the hindbrain in the original neural tube. In the developing embryonic brain, the demarcation of the medulla oblongata and the spinal cord is vague; however, when cervical, thoracic and lumbar nerves develop from the embryonic spinal cord, the demarcation is marked by the decussation of the nerve fibres, that is, neuronal axons which will be introduced later.

8 Foetal Development of the Nervous System

At 11 weeks, the embryo is now a foetus on the following grounds: first, telencephalon has overlapped diencephalon and the cerebellum begins to take shape, because the two hemispheres have outgrown other regions by multiplying more cells more rapidly; second, the facial features, such as the eyes, the nose, the mouth, and the ears, as well as the tongue (not shown), are clearly formed, because the twelve pairs of crainial nerves are also in their appropriate positions; and, third, most of the viscera, especially the heart, the bladder, and the like, are formed and begin to function. The lungs, however, are formed but flattened, because there is no need for them until after birth; the foetus literally lives in 'water' (amniotic fluid) but does not drown. And the stomach and the intestine (the gastro-intestinal tract) are formed but not used, because the foetus gets its nourishment from the mother and the oxygen through the umbilical cord (see Figure 8.1).

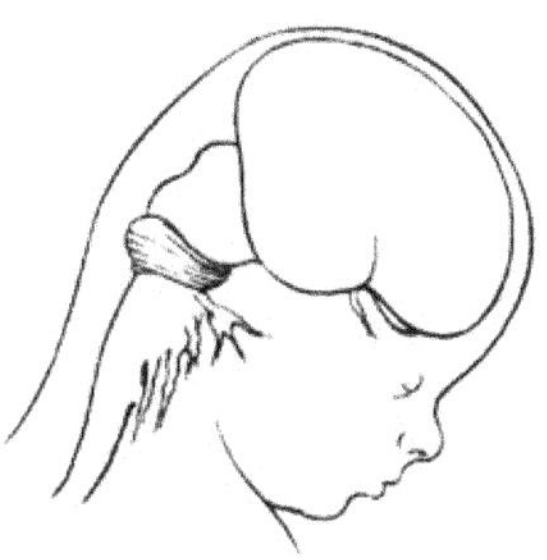

Figure 8.1 *11-week-old foetal brain* (From *The Brain: A User's Manual*, copyright © The Diagram Visual Information Group Ltd. Used by permission.)

It is important to note that major regions of the human brain develop from embryo to birth in a sequence reminiscent of its phylogenic development; that is, it treads the path of evolution. At four months, telencephalon and the cerebellum have already met and one of the cranial nerves, the optic nerve is well developed, even though it is completely dark in the uterus. However, the acoustic nerve, a part of the eighth nerve (vestibulo-cochlear nerve), not only is well developed but also functions quite well, so much so that the foetus can literally hear the conversation between the mother and the father; the acoustic effect is not 'ideal' through the mother's skin and the amniotic fluid, for it is constantly overshadowed by the rhythmic noises from the mother's blood flow and heart beat. Moreover, the lateral (i.e., Sylvian) fissure, one in each hemisphere of the cerebrum (from telencephalon), has formed a groove, thereby beginning the second step in the increase of the complexity of networks in human neuronal interconnections in evolutionary terms, that is, in comparison with vertebrates and other mammals (see Figure 8.2).

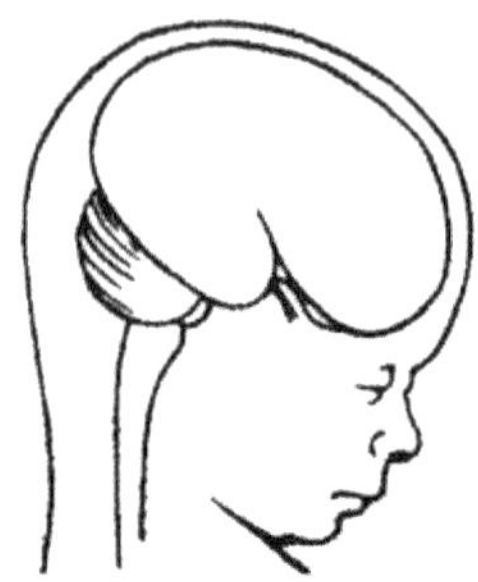

Figure 8.2 *Four-month-old foetal brain* (From *The Brain: A User's Manual*, copyright © The Diagram Visual Information Group Ltd. Used by permission.)

Because of these developments, some neuroscientists believe that pre-natal (i.e., foetal) education through the mother will benefit the baby's post-natal accomplishment in cognitive capacity. For instance, during pregnancy, if the mother listens to music more often or reads and writes more frequently, her behaviour will influence the brain functions of the foetus; if the mother likes to play the piano, she can play the piano more diligently during her pregnancy, thereby increasing the child's potential of becoming a good musician, if not a great pianist.

Likewise, because the foetus literally lives in 'water', there is a method of delivery which is quite popular in Japan, whereby the mother delivers the baby in water (usually in a bath). The baby, after the umbilical cord is cut, can be placed in a pool and can swim without drowning. It is for this ability that the Russians, according to a report, train their Olympic swimmers quite early, usually from infancy at the age of four months; the theory behind this training method is that infants are so accustomed to water that they are not afraid of it if the training starts early enough before they forget the 'joy of living in water'.

In Japan, there were also experiments to test infants' prenatal memory. One such experiment was to play a tape-recorder that had recorded the prenatal 'noises' of the mother's blood flow and heart beat to a two-day-old infant who was crying; in a matter of seconds, the infant stopped crying, as if it just heard a 'lullaby' which put it to sleep in comfort.

9 Phylogenic and Ontogenic Origins of the Complexity of Neuronal Circuitry

In order to pave the way for a solution to the tangled up intrigue of language origin and to refute the neo-innatism and the recent claim that 'A GENE that controls the development of speech and language has been identified for the first time in a break-through that will transform understanding of an uniquely human ability' (*The Times*, London, 10 April 2001), I shall now move to a new section by incorporating the remaining foetal development and post-natal development of the nervous system. This chapter is also intended to refute the nonsensical claim that 'a language gene emerged 200,000 years ago' (*The Daily Yomiuri*, 20 August 2002).

In so doing, I shall summarize several neuroanatomical steps in the increase of the complexity of neuronal interconnections; the increase of the complexity in my view has in both phylogenic and ontogenic terms led eventually to the elevation of brain functions in humans compared to other species in the animal kingdom. Every species in the animal kingdom has its own language, which is behaviour, suitable for members of the species to make proper adjustments to the internal and the external environments (i.e., context of situation). It is the insistence on human language as the standard (or yardstick) for judging other species that has led, in the past and even today, to so many futile and nonsensical semantic confusions in the literature concerning language origin.

1. Bending of the Telencephalon

I have mentioned above that mammals (which are also vertebrates) differ from the lower forms of the vertebrate during the embryonic stage in one important aspect – the bending of telencephalon – in both phylogenic and ontogenic terms when the three vesicles have become five. A vertebrate is distinguished from an invertebrate by the possession of a spinal column (i.e., backbone). The subphylum Vertebrata includes mammals, birds, reptiles, amphibians and fish.

This development is particularly important for 'packing an astronomical number of neurons in the cranium, which have evolved over millions of years'. To understand the dimension of this important development, imagine a 30cm cylinder, 5cm in diameter, in which a wire of one metre must be packed. If the wire is inserted straight, it will *not* go in. The solution is to coil the wire, like a shock absorber for a car, so that it will fit in neatly.

But this development alone will not account for the enormous human brain functions. There are four other factors which are equally important. All of them are not unique to humans but vary in degree from species to species among mammals; one of them is particularly significant in terms of language as behaviour; all of them, however, overlap to some extent. I shall now describe them below.

2. The Formation of Gyri

The formation of gyri (neuronal folds, or 'wrinkled up' neural tissues) also separates mammals from vertebrates; a lower vertebrate's brain has no gyri. More importantly, the neuronal folds increase in mammals from one species to another on the evolutionary scale, with the human brain being most 'wrinkled up'. An adult human brain, if 'stretched out' flat, can cover an entire sheet of an opened up newspaper.

The formation of gyri starts from the 'groove' which first appears in a human foetal brain when it is only four months old. After that, it increases quickly as a result of the rapid multiplication of neurons. In 1970 two British researchers, John Dobbing and Jean Sands (The Diagram Group, 1982: 48), discovered two main phases of such multiplication:

1. The first phase of proliferation starts when the foetus is 15–20 weeks old. Notice that this phase falls between the appearance of the cerebellum (11 weeks) and the appearance of the first 'groove' (the lateral fissure) at four months.
2. After the first phase, at 25 weeks (see Figures 9.1 and 9.2), another spurt begins; this time, it persists less intensively to birth (see Figure 9.3) and continues after birth for a year and beyond. Dobbing and Sands surmised that this spurt coincided with the growth of the supporting cells (glias which means 'glue') and not so much of yet more neurons. However, they were only partially right, because the number of glial cells continue to grow until birth and beyond, and the growth of glial cells is accompanied by the next factor, myelination, which goes through the development when the baby learns to crawl, babble, walk, talk and run. Keep in mind that the human baby during the first two years of childhood is less advanced cognitively compared to a chimpanzee at two years of age, even though the human baby may have more gyri in the brain than the chimpanzee baby.

The formation of gyri, however, is not limited to the cerebrum. The cerebellum is even more 'wrinkled up' than the cerebrum, although it is smaller in size. Even so, if the outer layer, that is, the cortices, of the two human cerebral hemispheres is flattened, its total surface area will cover an entire sheet of an

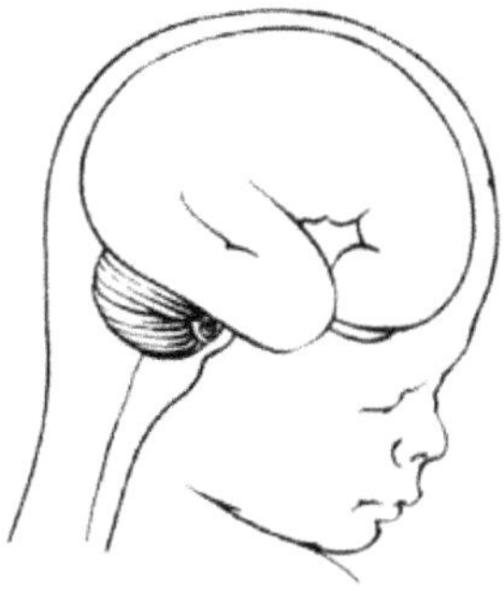

Figure 9.1 *Six-month-old foetal brain* (From *The Brain: A User's Manual*, copyright © The Diagram Visual Information Group Ltd. Used by permission.)

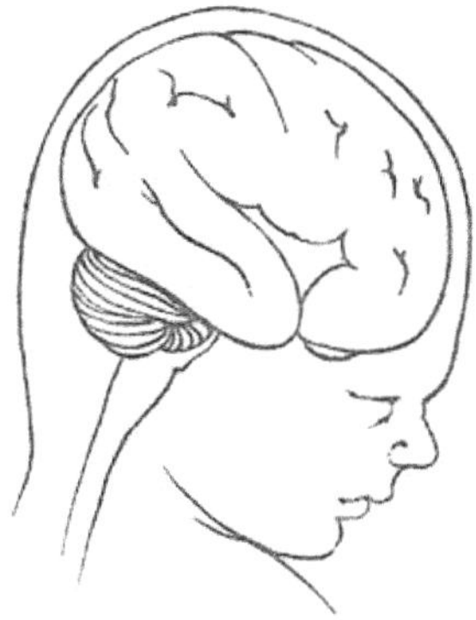

Figure 9.2 *Eight-month-old foetal brain* (From *The Brain: A User's Manual*, copyright © The Diagram Visual Information Group Ltd. Used by permission.)

opened up newspaper; one of them will yield roughly the same surface area as the cerebellum when it is flattened. More exactly, 'Flattening out the human cerebellum yields a sheet with an average area of 1,128 square centimeters – slightly larger than a record album cover. That is more than half the 1,900 square centimeters of the surface area of the two cerebral cortices added together' (Bower and Parsons, 2003: 42).

But the important point here is that when the cerebellum is folded, that is, 'wrinkled up' with folds called 'folia', it takes up much less space than a single cerebral hemisphere, suggesting that the cerebellum is much more neatly packed, that is, with more 'wrinkled up' folia, as a brain structure. Indeed, the cerebellum's most remarkable feature is that it contains more individual neurons than the rest of the brain combined (ibid.: 42), probably because the cerebellar granule cells are packed together at a density of six million per square millimetre (ibid.: 43).

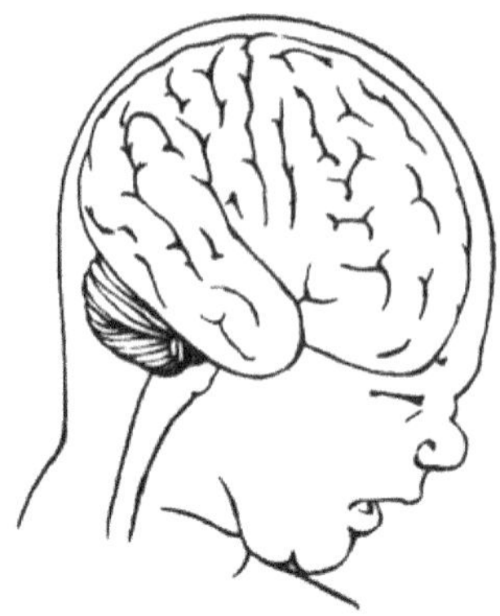

Figure 9.3 *Newborn infant's brain* (From *The Brain: A User's Manual*, copyright © The Diagram Visual Information Group Ltd. Used by permission.)

The corollary of this intricate and highly complex packaging indicates that the cerebellum should have crucial functions for the brain, which have been overlooked but are beginning to be revealed, albeit gradually, as will be shown further below. For instance, the Purkinje cell is one of the largest neurons in the nervous system, which receives about 200,000 inputs; these inputs come primarily from granule cells which also communicate with the stellate, basket and Golgi cells, the three other types of neurons in the cerebellum that help modulate the signals (i.e., impulses) emitted by both the granule and the Purkinje cells.

3. Myelination: To Strengthen All Axons and Speed Up Signal Transduction

Myelination is a process that together with the growth of neurons and glial cells in number increases not only the size of the brain before and after birth but also its weight before and after birth. The growth of neurons in number stops at birth in all mammals but myelination begins after birth in humans; it varies from species to species among mammals. Human myelination, I have speculated, continues until the peak of the brain functions at the age of 18 (Peng, 1995). The reason is that myelin (consisting of oligodendrocytes in the central nervous system but of Shwann cells in the peripheral nervous system) is very important in the transduction of impulses (or action potentials) to electrical signals. Impulses can be excitatory, inhibitory or disinhibitory in motor or sensory neurons. When a neuron is excited, if its excitation is stopped by the impulse of another neuron, the second neuron has the inhibitory function. However, if the inhibition is removed by a third neuron, the first neuron's excitatory function will resume and the third neuron is said to have the disinhibitory function.

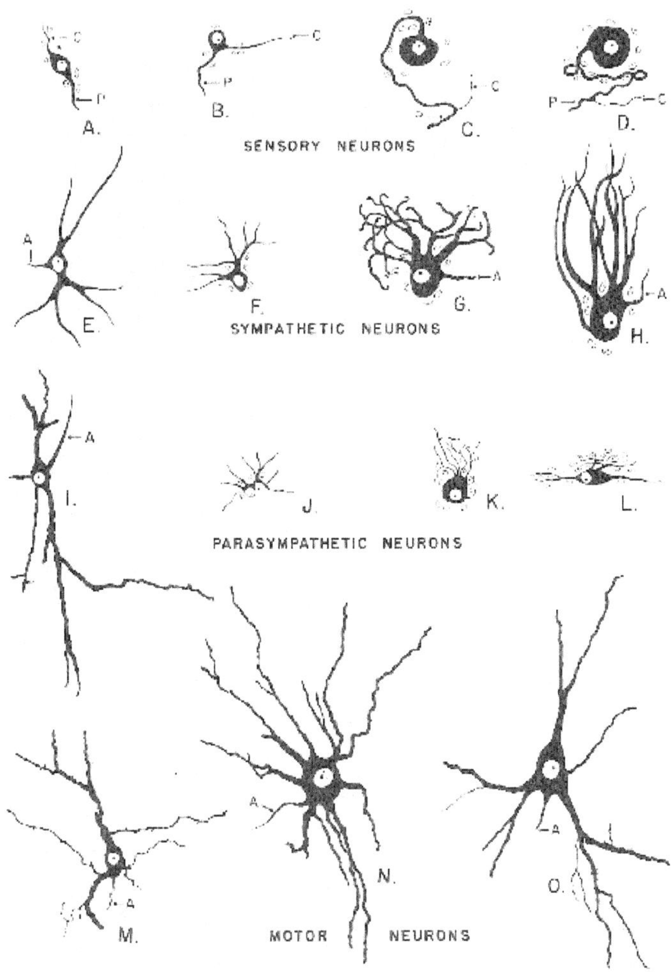

Figure 9.4 *A few varieties of neurons: (A) Bipolar neuron; (B) Pseudounipolar neuron; (C) Unipolar neuron; (D) Unipolar neuron; (E, F, G, H, I, J, K, L, M, N, O) Multipolar neurons* (From Malcolm C. Carpenter, *Human Neuroanatomy*, 7th Edition, copyright © Lippincott Williams and Wilkins, 1976. Used by permission of Lippincott Williams and Wilkins.)

Disinhibition, however, may be accomplished inadvertently by a surgical means. I encountered an intractable temporal lobe epileptic patient who was tested preoperatively by me. My job was to supplement the findings from EEG and other tests in order to help ascertain whether the epileptofocus was in the left or the right hemisphere. My conclusion was that the patient had bilateral epileptofoci while the other findings all indicated the left temporal lobe to be the only epileptofocus. A left anterior temporal lobectomy was performed. The patient seemed temporarily seizure-free post-operatively.

One week later, I tested the patient post-operatively. In the midst of the testing, she had a seizure attack, attesting that indeed she had had the bilateral epileptofoci. The reason why pre-operatively the other (i.e., the right) hemisphere had not seemed to be affected was because it had been inhibited by the epileptiform discharges from the affected (i.e., left) side. Epilepsy by definition is an abnormal discharge of electricity in the brain. So, when the left epileptofocus was surgically removed, the inhibition upon the right hemisphere was disinhibited, thereby leading to the resumption of the abnormal discharge of electricity in the right hemisphere, which was the manifestation of a new seizure attack.

I have in pages 76–83 described in some detail the various functions of the cytoplasmic components. In neurons, however, there are important ramifications of the cell function; unlike other fully developed cells, nerve cells (brain cells in particular) have more varieties in shape, size and function than other cells (Figure 9.4).

There are four types of tissues: epithelium (e.g., muscles); smooth tissues (e.g., viscera); connective tissues (e.g., bones and blood); and neural tissues (e.g., brain and nerve). Only neural tissues in the central nervous system have the supporting cells (glial cells or neuroglial cells). The neuroglial cells are of three types: macroglias (also called astroglias or astrocytes); oligodendrocytes (also called oligodentroglias); and microglias.

All these supporting cells are supportive (i.e., neuroprotective), when and if they function normally, but can become troublesome when their functions go wrong. Glial cells can become tumours which are collectively called gliomas. A glioma is a tumour composed of neuroglial cells and fibres, most commonly found in the brain. They are either astrocytomas or oligodendrogliomas. Microglia, if reactivated, can revert to phagocytes (cells that eat neurons) following injury to the nervous system, thereby leading to cell deaths (i.e., neuronal losses), technically called apoptosis (for any cell death, not just neuronal death). Reactivation of microglia also causes inflammation in the brain, especially in the midbrain (from mesencephalon), because there are more microglias in the midbrain than in the cortex, thereby resulting in Parkinson's disease.

Neurons also vary in size and shape. The main differences between neurons and other cells are that:

1. a neuron has one or more processes and other cells do not;
2. neurons can initiate and receive impulses because of the presence of neurotransmitters (which are chemical substances) and other cells cannot initiate impulses but may (as in muscle tissues for contraction) or may not (as in connective tissues) receive impulses;
3. a neuron has more mitochondria than other cells (because of the processes and myelination of its axon);
4. intracellularly all neurons have neurofibrills (which are concerned with metabolism and the transport of materials).

Neurofibrills can become tangled up, resulting in neurofibrillary tangles which are the cause of Fischer's disease (FD), purported by Alzheimer in 1907 in a female patient in 1907 in a female patient whom he had observed for several years (from ages 51–55). After her death, Perusini autopsied her brain and stained the nerve cell bodies by employing the newly available Bielschowsky's silver staining method to show extensive neurofibrillary tangles. In the same year, Fischer also described such neurofibrillary tangles, but his description was brushed aside by Kraepelin.

However, Alzheimer called her symptoms senile psychosis in contrast to senile dementia, a term that had been used in the nineteenth-century psychiatric literature for patients with senile plaques. See de la Torre (2002) who inadvertently calls AD including both neurofibrillary tangles and senile plaques, 'a vascular disorder with neurodegenerative consequence', rather than a neurodegenerative disorder with vascular consequence. What he should have said was that senile plaques, which I have proposed to call Fischer's Disease (FD), are a vascular disorder with neurodegenerative consequence, without grouping both neurofribrillary tangles and senile plaques together under the 'umbrella' of AD, because neurofibrillary tangles are not vascular in nature; they are intracellular, while senile plaques are extracellular.

Incidently, AD has been mistakenly regarded by medical people to include both neurofibrillary tangles and senile plaques (which are now changed to amyloid plaques probably because they are located extracellularly, outside the neurons, involving glial cells). For instance, 'In 1907, German physician Alois Alzheimer first described two features that have come to be the diagnostic hallmarks of AD: amyloid plaques and neurofibrillary tangles' (Margolis and Rabins, 1998); and also see McKhann *et al.* (1984, 34: 939–44). Worse, some neuropathologists have gone even further to regard senile plaques alone as AD (see Mandybur and Chuirazzi (1990)).

This unfortunate twisting of the actual historical facts is a mistake that is taught as such at medical schools, from one generation to the next, throughout the world, and even presented at major conferences of neurology. Examples are: 'Dementia Update' during the Education Program at the 55th Annual Meeting of the American Academy of Neurology held in Honolulu (29 March–5 April 2003) which I attended (see Juan C. Troncoso in the program); and The Alzheimer's Association International Conference on 'Prevention of Dementia: Early Diagnosis and Intervention' (18–21 June 2005), which I also attended. Such teaching makes Alzheimer look like he discovered both neurofibrillary tangles and senile plaques, when in fact he *never* made any original contribution to the description of senile plaques.

Neurofibrillary tangles and senile plaques were debated by neurologists and psychiatrists in 1907–11 as to whether they constituted the same 'mental disease' called senile dementia or were different diseases, each resulting in dementia. It was Alzheimer's powerful boss, Kraepelin, who arbitrarily designated neurofibrillary tangles as presenile dementia and later on changed his mind to call neurofibrillary tangles Alzheimer's disease, an eponym, to differentiate neurofibrillary tangles from senile plaques, that ended the nosological dispute. Senile plaques were first described more than a decade before, by Blocq and Marinesco in 1892, and confirmed by Redlich in 1898 (cf. Amaducci et al., 1986; Peng, 2003).

However, this historical fact of the eponym, for some peculiar reason, has been twisted. This twisting of historical facts, if continued, would literally do Alzheimer a disservice, rather than honouring him, as if he committed plagiarism by default when he and the proponents of the eponym had no intention of taking over senile plaques as his own discovery.

In fairness to Fischer and to give him proper credit, which is long overdue, for his contributions to the extensive description of senile plaques in 1907, I have proposed on several occasions at meetings and in writings to call senile plaques Fischer's disease (FD) so as to separate it from AD (see Peng, 2003b). It is time that people in the medical world face the historical facts and come to terms with the scientific truth and fairness in medical science and ethics. After all, in science people want to know the scientific facts and not fabrication or politics. Facing the scientific truth may even solve or, better still, remove the stumbling block that has been hindering progress in researches on AD, despite thousands of publications on that subject, because it contains two different diseases in one nosological classification from two different sources one of which is actually FD and not AD which should designate, as was intended originally, only neurofibrillary tangles.

4. Neuronal Shapes, Myelination and Demyelination

Neurons also vary in the number of processes they possess, one of which in a neuron is called axon and the rest, dendrites. Thus, there are: unipolar neurons, bipolar neurons, and multipolar neurons (cf. Figure 9.4). Unipolar neurons are found in sensory ganglia (clusters of nerve cells). Bipolar neurons, which have two processes, are located in the retina (a part of the brain), olfactory membrane, and ganglion of the auditory nerve (a branch of the eighth cranial nerve); one of the two processes is the axon and the other, a dendrite. And multipolar neurons, which have three or more processes, are located in the central nervous system (the cerebral cortex, the cerebellum, and the spinal cord) and autonomic ganglia; one of the processes is the axon, and the rest are dendrites.

Myelination takes place as a result of neuronal growth (which reaches its peak at birth) but has an important function for both pre-natal foetuses (for non-human mammals, in particular) and post-natal human individuals (infants, children and adults). It occurs in both the central and peripheral nervous systems.

Myelination also differs among non-human mammals. Many mammals, after birth – for example, gnus, giraffes – must be able to stand up and walk immediately or even run, shortly afterward, for reasons of survival; in the case of kangaroos, the newborn infant must be able to crawl with its forelimbs by itself from the mother's genitalia all the way to her pouch in order to suckle from the mother's nipple to survive until its hindlimbs grow. It is interesting to note that the hindlimbs will start to grow post-natally but will become bigger and stronger than the forelimbs, which started to grow pre-natally.

Human infants, however, can neither stand up nor crawl after birth, although they are able to move their limbs, toes and fingers. This is because the brain and other parts of the nervous system in both humans and non-human mammals grow faster before birth and in the early years of life than muscles, genitalia or other body parts. In the case of humans, their infants will take several months to a year or more after birth to be able to sit up, crawl, babble, talk, walk and run. The differences seem to reflect the phylogenic order.

Myelination is, therefore, the wrapping of the axon with two coverings: myelin (fatty substance) and a sheath of Schwann cell (in the peripheral nervous system) which forms part of the myelin as it circumnavigates the axis cylinder of the axon; in the central nervous system, Schwann cells are replaced by oligodendrocytes for similar functions.

When the sheath of Schwann cell circumnavigates the axonal axis cylinder to form the myelin, there are spots where the axonal fibres are *not* myelinated; these spots are called Nodes of Ranvier. Nodes of Ranvier are very important for the transduction of impulses: they facilitate (i.e., speed up) the impulses in milliseconds; the fastest nerve can transduce impulses at the speed of 130 metres per second or 13cm per millisecond.

Such a speed is important for many behaviours: 100-yard dash for athletes, fingering and bowing for violinists, and of course speaking in language behaviour, for production; it is also very important for reception, as in fencing or kung fu and, most of all, listening (in debates, for instance). Imagine what will happen if a person takes minutes to complete a 100-yard dash or ten seconds, if not one minute, to utter a word. Or, if a person in fencing takes five seconds to see or even realize that the opponent's sword is coming, can he/she survive without being killed? But if an athlete has Parkinson's disease, like Mohammed Ali, the former heavyweight champion in boxing, he can no longer box. Or, if a debater takes several seconds to realize what the opponent is saying, can he/she win the debate?

Be that as it may, high speed is not needed in cortico-cortical connections, especially for the short fibres (i.e., between gyri), where the axons are not heavily myelinated. I am inclined to speculate that there are two interdependent behavioural reasons: function enhancement for meaning, and abstract thinking for meaning. Both are pertinent to the brain functions of memory and cognition because neuronal axons are myelinated, subserved by CREB (cAMP-responsive element-binding) proteins at the same time. The former has to do with the functions of the six layers of cerebral cortex while the latter has to do with the extra-pyramidal looping, the cerebello-cerebral circuit, and the Papez circuit.

There are numerous publications regarding cognitive functions of the cerebellum which had been assigned to a mere function of voluntary motor control in the past. For instance, in 1958, Ray S. Snider wrote an article in

Scientific American, introducing the cerebellum to its readers, by saying 'In contrast to the cerebrum, where men have sought and found the centers of so many vital mental activities, the cerebellum remains a region of subtle and tantalizing mystery, its function hidden from investigators.' The mystery has continued to be hidden beneath the notion of movement, never going beyond the assertion, 17 years later, by Rodolfo R. Llinás who confidently stated in the second *Scientific American* article on the cerebellum that 'There is no longer any doubt that the cerebellum is a central control point for the organization of movement.'

In 2003, however, there is a third article, by Bower and Parsons (2003: 41–7), in which they report that 'the cerebellum's function has again become a subject of debate'. On the basis of numerous sophisticated cognitive studies by cognitive neuroscientists, they also report that damage to specific areas of the cerebellum can cause unanticipated impairments in non-motor processes, especially in how quickly and accurately people perceive sensory information.

The point in focus here, which is not mentioned by Bower and Parsons, is that the cerebellum is also heavily myelinated, although it has been known for decades that a single Purkinje cell in the cerebellum receives 150,000 to 200,000 inputs from the cerebrum, the pons, and the spinal cord through its peduncles, while the Purkinje cell provides the sole output of the cerebellar cortex. These inputs and outputs form enormously complex aborizations (interconnections of cerebellar neurons) which enable the cerebellum to play important roles for the proper adjustments to the internal and external environments beyond the mere motor control. These adjustments include memory and cognition, attention, emotion; other findings indicate the adjustments for the ability to schedule and plan tasks in dealing with the sensory inputs just mentioned and in processing information from such inputs. (See also the References in Schmahmann (2003)).

Meanwhile, it is worthy of mention that in neuroscience, neuropsychology, or cognitive psychology, cognition is traditionally thought to include thinking, learning, and memory; that is, memory is a part of cognition. In this view, then, the complication lies in the clinical practice which presupposes that while a patient with memory impairment may have intact cognitive function, conversely, another patient with cognitive impairment may preserve intact memory. At the same time, it is also often claimed that 'while strokes in the medial temporal lobes causes memory impairment, it usually takes bilateral lesions for serious and permanent memory problems' (Hachinski and Munso, 2000).

The interesting point here, in neurolinguistic terms, is that it is then asserted that certain cognitive impairment has nothing to do with memory impairment, a peculiar belief that leads to a strange predicament that is inexplicable in any scientific way. Medical people and psychologists do not seem to realize such a predicament. But here lies a stumbling block in the relationships of memory and cognition, because memory impairment is the cornerstone of dementia. That is, what is the consequence of cognitive impairment that is not memory impairment? Presumably such a cognitive impairment refers to impairment in thinking and/or learning. Is this condition possible without memory being impaired as well?

The answer, however, raises more questions:

1. Is thinking possible as an important brain function without the brain functions of memory involved?
2. Must learning always precede memory which is regarded by some as the recollection of that which was once experienced or learned?
3. Is there a time factor involved in the relationships of memory and cognition such that memory deals with the past and the past in the present (never with the future, which can only be talked about on the basis of the past and the present) while cognition handles the goings-on of the here-and-now? That is, how much will the time factor involved in the relationships of memory and cognition affect the brain functions of memory (or language in the brain)?

Current theories of memory, such as working memory and the like, have all failed to address these important questions.

While the answers to these questions were briefly offered in my keynote lecture 'Memory and cognition: what are they?' on 16 June 2003, during the 84th Annual Meeting of the AAAS, Pacific Division, in San Francisco, and more details of the answers will be presented in a later book in this series *Language and the Brain Functions of Memory*, cursory answers will be presented further below as well as in Part IV. Before these, I will briefly touch on demyelination and its consequence.

By now, the importance of myelination is clear. But what if myelin is damaged or destroyed? It is a condition of the nervous system known as demyelination. When a nerve is demyelinated, the consequence is a neurological disorder because the nerve becomes hardened, leading to a disease called multiple sclerosis (often abbreviated as MS). It may present many symptoms including: cognitive impairment (or difficulties), depression, impaired body movements, sexual dysfunction, slurred speech (because of impaired body movements), fatigue, dizziness or vertigo, bladder and bowel dysfunction. The individual can no longer walk, or use his/her arms (or hands), or talk, depending on where in the brain the demyelination takes place.

When demyelination takes place in one of the temporal lobes (or in both lobes), causing sclerosis of the mesial part of the lobe, involving the hippocampus, the result is called mesial temporal sclerosis (or hippocampal sclerosis), which invariably triggers temporal lobe epilepsy (often abbreviated as TLE). The seizure attacks may vary from once a day or once a week to several seizure attacks per day. If the seizure attacks cannot be managed by medication, the epilepsy becomes intractable and requires surgical intervention, which may range from anterior hippocampectomy, or amygdalohippocampectomy, to temporal lobectomy, in order to make the patient seizure-free. Either pre- or post-operatively, the patient (intractable or non-intractable) has serious memory impairment; hence, he/she has language disorders ictally (i.e., during a seizure) or interictally (i.e., between seizures).

Even though myelination and demyelination can change the brain functions of memory, it should be cautioned that myelin is not the source or origin of the brain functions of memory. It would be absurd to correlate or associate, as many neuroscientists would do, a particular lesion or lesioned site in the brain (e.g., a hardened neural tissue in the case of MS) with a behavioural deficit or a group of such deficits (as indicated above), as if the lesioned site (i.e., demyelination) was originally responsible for the lost functions when it was intact. Apparently, this is what some geneticists have done when they attempted to associate the mutation of FOXp2, claimed to be the language gene they discovered on chromosome 7 in a small pedigree of English speakers, with the grammatical errors of the tense markers some of the speakers made and erroneously jumped to the conclusion that they discovered the language gene.

What I am proposing is the idea that myelination facilitates the brain functions of memory and demyelination hampers the brain functions of memory, because the brain functions of memory are the responsibility of the entire brain, involving the functions of many parts of the brain, and therefore govern all behaviours, including language behaviour. I will now delve into this realm of investigation briefly by returning to the relationships of memory and cognition before continuing with aborization.

It is now known as a result of researches on PD that there are two loops in the functions of the cortical and subcortical connections. Coupled with these connections are the increasing awareness and knowledge of the many significant roles played by the cerebellum in the brain functions of memory and cognition.

The two loops are part of the cortico-bulbar pathways and the cortico-spinal pathways. In these pathways, the loops, one in each hemisphere, are called cortico-striato-pallido-thalamo-cortical loops (or basal ganglionic loops). It is in the looping, as I have proposed in the literature (Peng, 2000, 2001; Peng *et al.*, 2002), where thinking takes place; in other words, thinking in the looping is modulated or assisted to a great extent by the cerebello-cerebral circuit and by the Papez circuit, both of which also go through the thalamus, involving the limbic system for the memory of emotions and affect; these two circuits will be introduced later.

In my view, without the proper brain functions of memory, there is no appropriate thinking; insanity is the result of inappropriate thinking. One good example of inappropriate thinking is schizophrenia, although psychiatrists may prefer to call the cause of schizophrenia thought disorders. This issue will be discussed in great detail in a later book *Language Disorders: A Critical Perspective.* However, it should be emphasized that as long as a person can move around, even when he/she may go berserk, there are some brain functions of memory remaining in his/her brain, which are nonetheless disordered, thereby leading to inappropriate thinking; hence, impaired cognitive behaviour in the here-and-now. When a person has lost his/her brain functions of memory *in toto*, that person is either comatose or brain-dead.

Most psychologists prefer to think that memory is the result of learning, as if memory is 'a thing' or 'an event' which can be put away on a shelf, like a book in a library, for safe keeping. However, I take exception to this static view, because I regard the brain functions of memory as a dynamic tripartite system in the brain, consisting of brain functions of memory as content, brain functions of memory as capacity, and brain functions of memory as mechanism.

My theoretical construct, therefore, takes exception to any traditional view available in the literature, which asserts that memory and cognition are subserved by different brain structures; for example, memory by the two hippocampi and cognition by the neocortex as a whole, especially the frontobasal systems. My theoretical construct takes the stand that memory and cognition are actually two sides (heads and tails) of the same coin, when the time factor is taken into consideration, for they are subserved by the same sets of brain functions. Put differently, in my view, memory is a dynamic tripartite system of brain functions and, therefore, it cannot be confined to the two hippocampi, nor is it a part of cognition; rather, it is widespread throughout the entire brain.

For this reason, I have advocated that language in the brain is memory-governed. And as heads and tails of the same coin, the brain functions of memory are often called upon to become the brain functions of cognition in the here-and-now in order to handle problem-solving, decision-making (regarding, e.g., what to say and what not to say), judgement, our ability to orient ourselves in space and time, and most of all our ability to think in order to utter and understand sentences and words for proper adjustments to the external and internal environments in human interactions.

5. Aborization: Formation of Neural Networks for Function Enhancement

When neurons increase in number before birth, they are not well connected, although in lower animals the interconnections (axonal and dendritic) are pretty well complete at birth. In humans, it takes many years to complete; I suspect that its completion coincides with the peak of brain function at the age of 18 (Peng, 1995).

One important aspect of aborization is that all neurons must be in their proper places before birth in order to be ready for the total aborization after birth. During foetal life before birth, neurons become specialized; those which have similar functions 'stick together' to form a cluster or a layer (especially in the cerebral cortex and the cerebellum) or a ganglion (in the basal ganglia or the peripheral nervous system).

I have already mentioned gyri, each one of which is a strip of neurons sticking together to form a fold. As there are many such folds, they are divided by ditches, so that the folds look like 'wrinkles' (Figures 9.5 and 9.6). The more wrinkled up the brain surface is the more advanced the brain functions

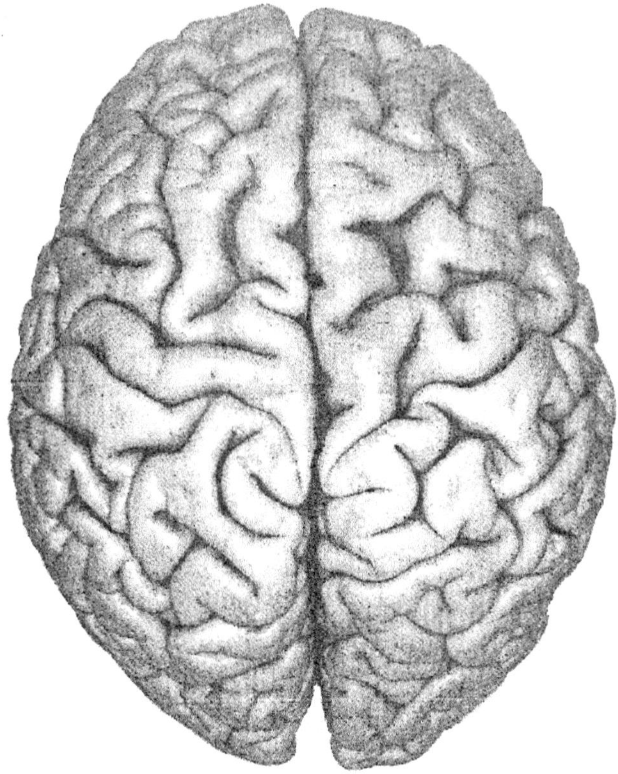

Figure 9.5 *Dorsal view of the human brain* (From *Structure of the Human Brain: A Photographic Atlas,* 3rd edition, by S. J. DeArmond and M. M. Fusco and M. M. Dewey, copyright © 1974, 1976, 1989 by Oxford University Press, Inc. Used by permission of Oxford University Press, Inc.)

are. Thus, the brain of a lower form of vertebrates, such as a chicken, does not have gyri and an adult chimpanzee's brain has far fewer gyri (cf. Figure 11.2) than does an adult human brain.

Within each gyrus the neurons have come into their respective positions lined up in the cerebral cortex or stratified in six layers during foetal life. Mechanically, it may be thought that neurons of the first (top) layer will take their position first and neurons of the last (bottom) layer will take their position last. However, it has been found recently by researchers from Stanford that the actual ordering of layers in foetal life is the reverse of the 'common sense' mechanical ordering. It was shown at one of the annual conferences of the American Epilepsy Society with a video taken from a lab that neurons of the bottom layer take their position first and neurons of the fifth (i.e., second to the bottom) layer take their position next, and so on, and finally neurons of the first layer take their position last. After that, all neurons

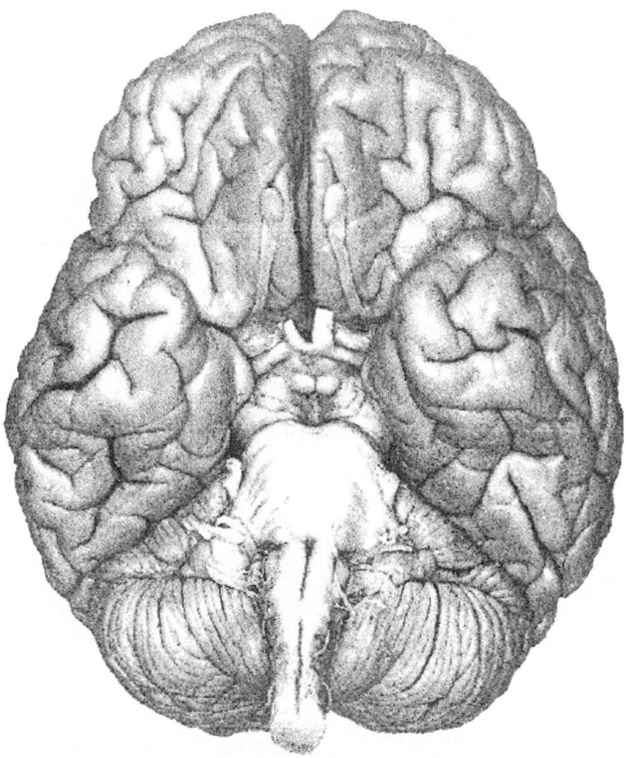

Figure 9.6 *Ventral view of the human brain* (From *Structure of the Human Brain: A Photographic Atlas*, 3rd edition, by S. J. DeArmond and M. M. Fusco and M. M. Dewey, copyright © 1974, 1976, 1989 by Oxford University Press, Inc. Used by permission of Oxford University Press, Inc.)

begin to aborize, that is, extend their processes vertically and horizontally, to interconnect with one another. (See Figures 9.7, 9.8 and 9.9.)

Now, what will happen to the foetus if neurons during the developing stages, collectively called neurogenesis, are misplaced, or do not get to their appropriate positions in time, or are overproduced? It is known that the growth in all animals takes place in two processes: the cells within the organism increase either in number (through mitosis), called hyperplasia, or in size, called hypertrophy. The brain is no exception. But the neurons in the brain, in addition, must migrate to their appropriate positions in time. If not, the consequences are very serious. Examples are cortical displasia, as in double cortex, megaloencephaly (enlarged cortex), or schizoencephaly (one oversized hemisphere), or progeria (premature aging syndrome, which is caused by a mutation in DNA arising from unknown factors).

In the case of cortical displasia, the newborn will develop pediatric epilepsy and may not live very long. Progeria, however, is a very rare disease, one in

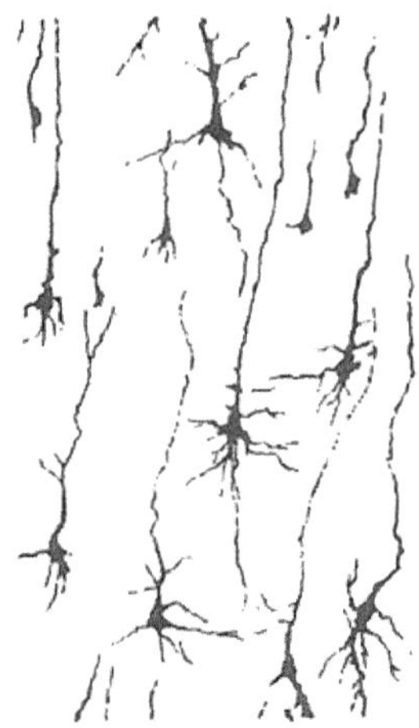

Figure 9.7 *Well-spaced neurons in the cortex at birth* (From *The Brain: A User's Manual,* copyright © The Diagram Visual Information Group Ltd. Used by permission.)

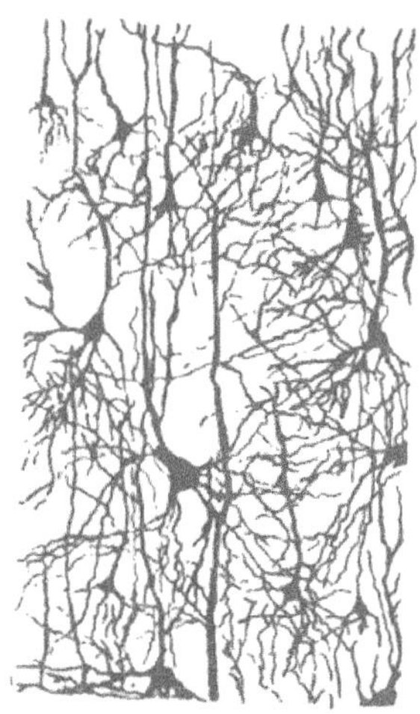

Figure 9.8 *Interconnections of the well-spaced neurons in the cortex by six years of age* (From *The Brain: A User's Manual,* copyright © The Diagram Visual Information Group Ltd. Used by permission.)

every eight million infants, and there are only about 40 such reported cases. The newborn at first looks 'normal' but ages very fast, at the pace of one year equivalent to 8–10 years in normal aging. Thus, a child with progeria at the physical age of 10, if he/she lives that long, would look like an old person of 80, although that individual would have no problem learning the rudimentary form of a language so long as there is no other neurological complication in

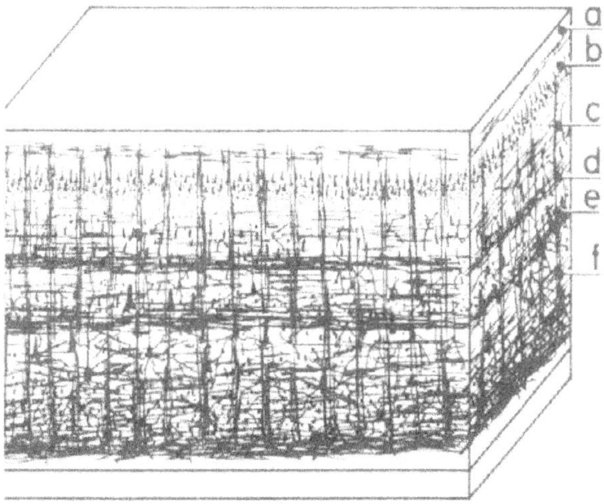

Figure 9.9 *The six layers of neurons in the contex of an adult brain N.B. (a) (Outer) molecular layer. (b) External granular layer. (c) Outer pyramidal layer. (d) Internal granular layer. (e) Ganglionic layer. (f) Multiform layer.* (From *The Brain: A User's Manual*, copyright © The Diagram Visual Information Group Ltd. Used by permission.)

his/her brain, for instance, a stroke, just as an old person has learned his/her language but may have a stroke; the difference is that the child with progeria has reached the age of 80 ten times faster than a normal person.

10 Species-Specific Formation of the Human Vocal Apparatus

I have mentioned that the sequencing of the various stages in the growing brain is reminiscent of its evolution; that is, the brainstem develops first, because it supports life, to a certain extent, and is common to all mammals; the brainstem of an adult cat is very much like the brainstem of an adult human being. Thus, a human infant without the cerebrum, with just the brainstem, can survive for just a short period after birth but not the other way around; no vertebrate or mammal can survive with just the cerebrum, because the neural plate does not develop that way.

In the 1980s, a newspaper from Florida published a picture of an infant with just the brainstem, that is, just the diencephalon, the mesencephalon and the rhombencephalon (without the cerebrum, i.e., without the telencephalon and hence without the cerebral hemispheres). The newspaper also published a plea from its mother to the district court, requesting permission to put the 'infant' to sleep, so that the mother could donate the infant's other organs to those in need of them for transplantation. The court did not grant euthanasia, so the mother filed for a court injunction. During the legal process, ten days after birth, the 'infant' died.

The point here is that the brainstem, coupled with the appearances of the 12 pairs of cranial nerves, is very important to the formation of the vocal apparatus in all vertebrates and mammals but that the importance is associated closely with the above-mentioned factors; namely, the bending of telencephalon, the formation of gyri, myelination and aborization. All cranial nerves belong to the peripheral nervous system. I will now explain these cranial nerves below.

1. Appearances of the Cranial Nerves

The 12 pairs of cranial nerves do not appear together during the embryonic development of the brain. The appearances are ordered as follows.

The first cranial nerve (olfactory) appears when telencephalon gives rise to the cerebral cortex and basal ganglia; the nuclei of the two olfactory nerves are attached to the two olfactory bulbs, which are also part of the brain belonging

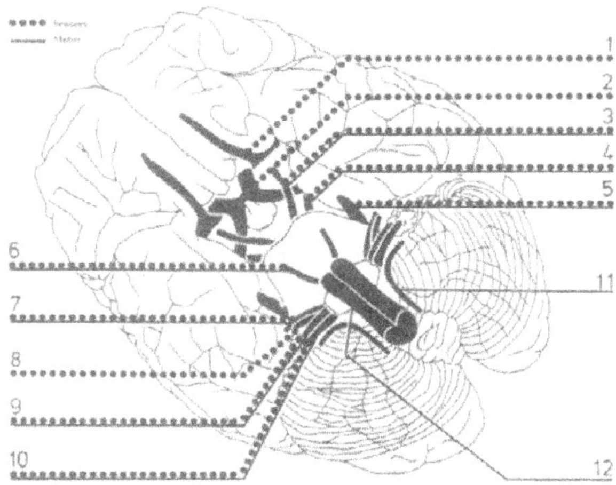

Figure 10.1 Ventral view of the brain showing all the cranial nerves (From *The Brain: A User's Manual,* copyright © The Diagram Visual Information Group Ltd. Used by permission.)

to the limbic system, and buried inside the ventral portion of the cerebral cortex.

The second cranial nerve (optic) enters diencephalon, from the retina which is a part of telencephalon, when diencephalon splits into two halves with a mid-line third ventricle, which is a slit that communicates with the lateral ventricles (i.e., first and second ventricles) by way of the interventricular foramen. Diencephalon is further divided into (a) the epithalamus, (b) the dorsal thalamus (i.e., the thalamus proper), (c) the subthalamic nucleus, and (d) the hypothalamus.

The nuclei of the third cranial nerve (oculomotor) and the fourth cranial nerve (trochlear) are formed dorsally within mesencephalon which, centrally, contains a rather constricted part of the ventricular system, namely, the cerebral aqueduct that communicates with the third ventricle; however, the two cranial nerves are associated with the midbrain ventrally in a different way; that is, the oculomotor 'pierces' through mesencephalon to come out ventrally but the trochlear comes out dorsally first and then 'swings' around, coursing the surface of mesencephalon, to come out ventrally.

The nuclei of the fifth cranial nerve (trigeminal), the sixth cranial nerve (abducens), the seventh cranial nerve (facial), and the eighth cranial nerve (vestibulo-cochlear) are also formed dorsally but within metencephalon when it differentiates into the cerebellum dorsally and the pons ventrally. However, all of these four cranial nerves attach to the pons.

The nuclei of the ninth cranial nerve (glossopharyngeal), the tenth cranial nerve (vagus), the eleventh cranial nerve (accessory), and the twelfth cranial nerve (hypoglossal) are somewhat complicated, even though they are all associated with the medulla oblongata which comes from myelencephalon.

The complication lies in two factors: (i) intermingling with the autonomic system (sympathetic and parasympathetic) and (ii) innervation of the tongue which receives the facial nerve for taste buds on anterior two-thirds of the tongue, the glossopharyngeal nerve for taste buds on posterior third of the tongue, the vagus for muscles of the pharynx, larynx, and esophagus and taste buds on epiglottis, and the hypoglossal nerve for muscles of the tongue. For these reasons, the tongue is the most movable body part. (See Barr (1974: 119–41)).

2. Formation of the Vocal Apparatus

The vocal apparatus exists in all reptiles, vertebrates and mammals. However, because of the differences in the genetically determined ontogenic appearances of the cranial nerves, coupled with the differences in the also genetically determined phylogenic development of the central nervous system for differentiation and encephalization, its formation also varies from species to species. There are two aspects in the variation: shape and timing.

2.1 Shape

In linguistics (or, rather, phonetics) vocal tract shape is concerned with the function of the vocal apparatus; that is, how various linguistic sounds (not at all other sounds like yawning or sneezing or laughing) are produced and heard is the main concern. Thus, the shape of the vocal apparatus is too often taken for granted by many people (linguists or otherwise, like psychologists, e.g., the Hayes); any failure to make proper linguistic sounds is, therefore, blamed on the individual's cognitive inability; for example, Vicki's ability to learn only four 'words'.

However, because of the differences in the complexity of the neuronal circuitry, the formation of the vocal apparatus in humans is closely (i.e., genetically) tied to the phylogenic and ontogenic development of the nervous system. In non-human animals, the formation is completed before birth; after birth, the vocal apparatus may grow larger because of mitosis, but its shape is definitive at birth. In humans, however, the vocal apparatus not only grows in size but also changes its shape from foetal life through the first two years of post-natal life (Figures 10.2 and 10.3).

2.2 Timing

What are the reason and the course of such differences? The reason is genetic and greatly determined by the bending of telencephalon, the formation of gyri, myelination and aborization in both the cerebrum and the cerebellum; in other words, it is closely related to the increase in complexity of the neuronal interconnections in the brain. Thus, there are phylogenic timing and ontogenic timing.

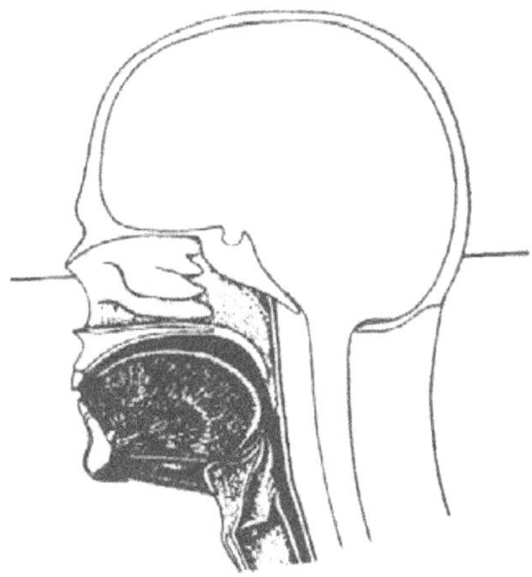

Figure 10.2 *Lateral view of the adult human vocal apparatus* (From E. Lloyd du Brul, *Evolution of the Speech Apparatus,* 1958. Courtesy of Charles C. Thomas, Publisher, Ltd, Springfield, Illinois.)

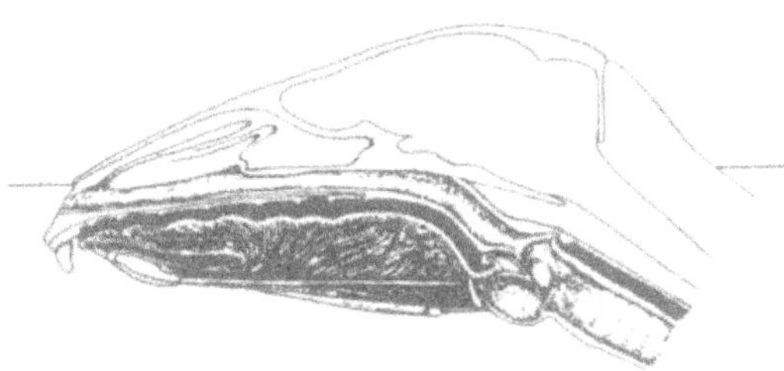

Figure 10.3 *Lateral view of the adult monkey's vocal apparatus* (From E. Lloyd du Brul, *Evolution of the Speech Apparatus,* 1958. Courtesy of Charles C. Thomas, Publisher, Ltd, Springfield, Illinois.)

2.2.1 Phylogenic Timing

This timing refers to the length of gestation in humans, that is, nine months, during which time the human brain develops in a sequence reminiscent of its phylogenesis. The length of gestation in dogs is two months; the length increases in non-human primates, that is, monkeys and apes. Because of the longer gestation in humans, the cranial nerves also take longer to complete their development.

Because of these differences, in reptiles the vocal apparatus (from the mouth to the trachea) forms a straight tube; the epiglottis is underneath the velum inside the tube, like a valve, so that it can open and connect the larynx to form a direct path to the nasal cavity, as there is no pharynx, but close the larynx completely when swallowing food, if necessary; and the tongue is highly prehensile as in a snake or a frog. For this reason, reptiles such as crocodiles and snakes have teeth and yet they can swallow food, such as a fish whole, but cannot chew it; a snake can swallow another snake larger than itself whole but cannot chew that snake.

In lower mammals, however, the vocal apparatus forms a downward angle at the junction of the pharynx, which is very small, and the larynx, but the epiglottis can still connect the nasal cavity with the larynx to form a bypass for nasal ventilation, when necessary, by contacting the velum, and the tongue remains very prehensile. The prehensile function of the tongue is important for survival in the case of four-legged mammals when they eat grass – for example, cows and sheep – or lap (not drink) water – for example, dogs and tigers – against the gravity.

In the case of non-human primates, the vocal apparatus forms even a greater downward angle at the same junction (see Figure 10.3). Notice that the epiglottis can still contact the velum and bifurcate the pharyngeal cavity, which is still small, into a direct bypass from the larynx to the nasal cavity for ventilation, when needed, and the direct path also from the larynx to the oral cavity. When the epiglottis closes the trachea, the closure allows a direct passage of food from the oral cavity into the esophagus.

Notice also the texture of the tongue; from the point of view of gross anatomy, the tissues are thin and the tongue tip is long, suggesting the retention of its prehensile function. Notice moreover that the oral cavity is very narrow and the pharyngeal cavity is very small, if it exists at all, with little room for the tongue to move around inside the mouth. For these gross anatomical reasons, a non-human primate, not to mention other mammals, does not choke when swallowing food, because it masticates food while closing the velum with its epiglottis, thereby preventing the food from going down the 'wrong pipe'.

In humans, however, the downward angle of the vocal tract is now even greater (see Figure 10.2); the oral cavity is at right angles with the wind pipe, so much so that the epiglottis is lowered to a position that it can no longer touch even the uvula, let alone the velum; there has now grown a distance of 3cm between the tip of the epiglottis and the velum in the pharyngeal cavity, which has become larger and wider, creating a room that is big enough now for the various tongue movements for proper articulations. This change of developmental course has a price to pay: the danger of choking. Only humans can choke to death.

When masticating food, especially soft and sticky food, such as rice cake (*mochi* in Japanese), a human must raise the back of the tongue to block the food until the food particles become small enough for swallowing, as the epiglottis can no longer touch the velum to form a temporary blockage of the oral passage to the esophagus. But when an elderly person's epiglottis becomes weak, and there are few teeth left, as he/she attempts to swallow the mochi; which is not well chewed, the food can easily get stuck in the air pathway, between the epiglottis and the trachea, thereby suffocating the person to death. Such deaths during the New Year's celebration, which is the time for eating *mochi* and *ozooni* (*mochi* cooked with other ingredients such as pork and vegetables in soup), are occasionally reported in Japan.

It should be reminded that the human vocal apparatus in a newborn is different; it developed differently before birth during its foetal life. The vocal apparatus at birth is just like that of a chimpanzee; it has all the characteristics of a non-human primate's vocal apparatus mentioned above. Recall the reminiscence of evolution in the embryonic and foetal development. The human vocal apparatus takes up its own ontogeny after birth, or else the ontogenic development after birth is phylogenetically determined; hence, there is this ontogenic timing.

2.2.2 Ontogenic Timing

This timing refers to the schedule of changes and growth in the shape and function of the human vocal apparatus after birth. While a chimpanzee's vocal apparatus may grow bigger in size during its foetal life, its shape, as was described above, and function remain unchanged after birth. However, the human vocal apparatus has a rigid timetable to follow after birth, which is genetically pre-determined.

First, a newborn infant's brain has reached one quarter of its adult weight, even though the infant is only one-twentieth as heavy as the adult it will become, as a result of the completion of neuronal growth during its foetal life, because muscles, genitals and other body parts are lagging behind in ontogenic development. However, the tongue is an exception, for at birth it is almost as big as an adult's full-size tongue; hence, there is no room for manoeuvre in the mouth. It has also lost its prehensile function during the foetal life; that is, the human tongue can lick and suck after birth but can no longer wrap around an object and pull, nor can it lap.

With little space for manoeuvre inside the mouth, the tongue height (i.e., position) is at the level of the ears if the infant is held with the head up. That is why newborn babies are likely to catch cold more often; when the immune system strengthens, as the infant grows, it becomes stronger.

On the other hand, an adult's brain is only 2 per cent of his/her total body weight, and yet the brain consumes 20 per cent of the total blood supply, partly because the vocal apparatus which utilizes the cortico-bulbar pathways in production occupies a good portion of the five million fibres in the pathways compared to the fifty thousand fibres in the cortico-spinal pathways for the other body parts in production (Nauta and Feirtag, 1979). However, neuroanatomists such as Carpenter (1976) have a different estimate of around one million fibres, which are still far fewer than the fibres in the cortico-bulbar pathways.

Second, as the gyri increase, myelination and aborization progress, and glial cells grow in number for the cerebrum and the cerebellum, the baby's brain weight doubles within the first six months of life. This doubling of brain weight is accompanied by or coincides with the changes in the formation of the baby's vocal apparatus for its shape and function. The baby begins to babble at the age of six months, the babbling being the baby's way of learning to articulate, or reassuring itself of what it had 'learned' during its foetal life, 'testing the waters' as it were, in order to now really form 'words' to its liking, which is still far from meeting the standard of adults. This learning (or, practising) of articulation actually started during the baby's foetal life inside the uterus, as will be mentioned below.

Third, at the age of six months, the baby's vocal apparatus begins to change in four directions:

1. the vocal tract bends more;
2. as a result, the larynx starts to descend in order to pull the epiglottis away from the velum;
3. the pharyngeal cavity as a consequence is gradually enlarged;
4. the tongue becomes thicker and more movable, especially its posterior movements because of the enlarged pharyngeal cavity, even though it has phylogenetically lost all of its prehensile functions.

From the age of six months onward, the baby learns to utter words more frequently, through imitating the sounds heard around it. Even during its foetal life the foetus had already heard sounds from the outside world; it has already learned some abilities for articulation by using its now fast developing facilities, from one-word to two-word utterances, and so on, which are not quite up to the adult's liking and are subject to correction from time to time; such corrections are consciously or unconsciously engrained in the baby's central nervous system (through its peripheral nervous system) by its developing brain functions of memory.

Formal training, as in education, later in different stages, from nursery to college or higher, for societies which have such educational systems, will expand and/or regulate the child's brain functions of memory and cognition in ways different from those of other individuals in hunting and gathering societies. Having or lacking formal training (or education) have nothing whatsoever to do with language in the brain being innate, for the individual's brain functions develop and mature as a direct result of the brain's interactions with the environments; the deterioration of the individual's brain functions, however, is an ontological issue, arising from normal aging, other genetic factors (as in hereditary diseases), or environmental factors (as in injuries caused by traumas), which must also be taken into account for language in the brain.

Fourth, the changes of the vocal apparatus continue until the age of two, at which time the child's vocal apparatus has reached a stage comparable to that of an adult (see Figure 10.4). The child, facilitated by the newly developed vocal tract, can now utter longer sequences of words which may not be quite accurate by adult standard, in terms of wording of the varying meanings in the social contexts of situation. I have used the term 'wording', in lieu of 'grammar' which, contrary to the traditional view, does not exist in the brain, a controversial view that will be explicated in detail later. The reason is that

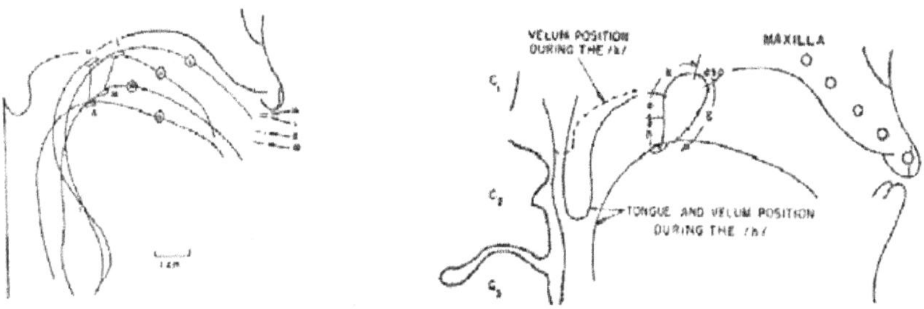

Figure 10.4 *Some instances of human vocal behaviour: vowels and consonants* (From Joseph S. Perkell, *Physiology of Speech Production: Results and Implications of A Quantitative Cineradiographic Study*, Cambridge, MA: MIT Press, 1969. Copyright © 1969 by MIT Press. Used by permission.)

grammar is a creation of linguists, as an epistemological issue, not an ontological given in the brain.

But recall that during the first two years of life, the changes are accompanied by the development of the baby's many behaviours as a human individual. The baby has begun:

1. to first strengthen its head, so that the head is not wobbly, that is, the neck is strong enough to hold the head up,
2. to turn its body,
3. to crawl,
4. to stand (with help),
5. to stand up on its own,
6. to walk, and
7. to run.

Such behaviours are possible all because of myelination and aborization. That is, all the neurons in the developing post-natal brain must already have migrated to their appropriate positions for interconnections by way of the various steps in neurogenesis and synaptogenesis (through sprouting dendrites and their contacts with the axons of other neurons). In other words, according to recent studies, dendritic spines can change their shapes in a matter of minutes, thereby playing an important role in the increasing brain functions of memory.

As a consequence, the child's language behaviour increases by leaps and bounds, so much so that the mother can hardly keep it quiet. If the child is not full of curiosity from within and cannot be intrigued by new things from without, the child has autism, a multifactorial disorder of the nervous system that will prevent him/her from learning the first language.

The changes and the accompaniment are important for language being multifaceted. But it should be pointed out that because of these changes, which are preceded by the foetal development, language in the brain is behaviour. Innatists have often asserted that language is not learned, because a child can speak without formal training or education. But I should hasten to counter that formal training or education is required for writing and reading, because writing and reading belong to a different facet from that of speaking and hearing; however, speaking, hearing, writing, and reading are the brain functions for the internal and external environments to which the individual (throughout its infancy, childhood, and later adulthood) is enabled to make proper adjustments.

In fact, hearing in early childhood is a brain function that began in early foetal life. Speaking, although the foetus cannot make sounds in the amniotic fluid, is also forming as a brain function during foetal life; in Japan, I have a video tape of ultrasonic recordings of a foetus practising articulation by moving the lips and sticking out the tongue, urinating in the womb, and even sucking one of its thumbs. The recordings were shown to a mother, holding her baby who was also sucking his thumb. The mother was asked why her baby was sucking the thumb. She said perhaps the baby just wanted to play with something readily available nearby. When she was told that her baby was the foetus on the video tape, she was astonished that the baby had picked up 'the habit' since its foetal life. I shall have more to say later about speaking and hearing without formal training and education as well as writing and reading with formal training in a later book, *Language Disorders: A Critical Perspective.*

In the meantime, I will state that the orientation prior to formal schooling for a child *and* the pre-natal orientation during the foetal life are far more powerful and vigorous, as far as language development is concerned, than formal training. That is why anthropologists call the orientation prior to formal schooling Primary Orientation; formal schooling is called Secondary Orientation. In hunting and gathering societies, where there is no secondary orientation, primary orientation continues for a child (boy or girl) until the child becomes an adult who can then pass on to the next generation the continuation of language orientation, that is, primary orientation.

11 Structural Divisions of the Nervous System

Having described briefly the nervous system and the vocal apparatus from the cellular, pre-natal and functional anatomical point of view, it is important that I also follow the medical tradition to include the structural divisions of the nervous system to some extent. However, I should remind the reader that it is in such divisions, coupled with the functional and pre-natal divisions, that terminological differences arise. I was at first rather 'confused' when I learned neuroanatomy at SUNY, Buffalo, but became used to the differences. Be that as it may, there are physicians in different countries who are not aware of the differences, and yet they would insist that what they learned from their own medical schools was the only correct terminology; hence, the designation by the terminology they had learned was the absolute answer. In linguistics, the terminological situation for formulaic differences is not any better, perhaps even worse.

1. The Cerebrum

The cerebrum developmentally comes from the forebrain (prosencephalon). However, for some peculiar reason many neurologists and neurosurgeons, especially in countries where English is not the native tongue, learned from their respective medical schools that the cerebrum and the forebrain were the same thing. Recall that the forebrain (prosencephalon, its Greek origin) divides into telencephalon (end brain) and diencephalon (between brain). If the brain had only this division to be concerned with, there might not be any terminological difference. The fact is that there are other divisions, thereby giving rise to structural differences.

One major difference is that the cerebrum, in one terminology, does not include diencephalon but only includes telencephalon, which gives rise to the cerebral cortex, and one of the innermost layers of the forebrain, that is, the basal ganglia. In another terminology, the cerebrum includes the cerebral cortex, the basal ganglia and the limbic system, which is the other innermost layer of the forebrain; in this terminology, some structures of the limbic system, that is, the thalamus and the hypothalamus, the pituitary gland (the master gland), and the pineal gland, come from diencephalon. In still another

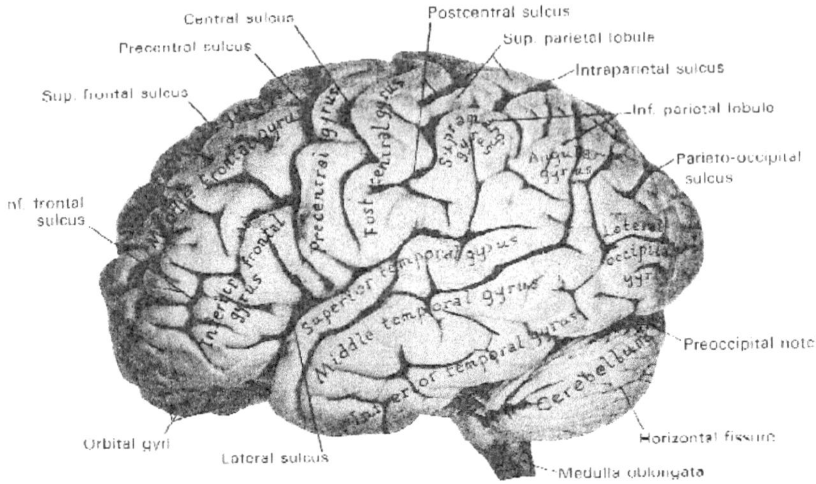

Figure 11.1 *Human left neocortex* (From Malcolm C. Carpenter, *Human Neuroanatomy*, 7th Edition, copyright © Lippincott Williams and Wilkins, 1976. Used by permission of Lippincott Williams and Wilkins.)

terminology, the cerebrum includes only a part of telencephalon, leaving out the basal ganglia and some of the limbic system; namely, the fornix, the thalamus, the hypothalamus, the pituitary gland, the pineal gland and the amygdala.

The cerebrum itself, nevertheless, has two hemispsheres, each one of which is covered by a mantle of billions of neurons referred to as the cerebral cortex ('bark'); the two hemispheres are divided by a deep fissure called sagittal fissure (cf. Figure 9.4). The cortex is the concentration of neuronal cell bodies, but they are not equally 'old', that is, phylogenetically homogenous. The convex surface (or lateral cortex, cf. Figure 11.1) is phylogenetically younger and, therefore, is often referred to as the neocortex ('new bark'). In contrast, the medial cortex (and the concave surface) are phylogenetically older; so, they are referred to as paleocortex or paleopallium (cf. Figure 11.3).

The cerebral cortex is made up of the thin layer of grey matter on the surface of the cerebral hemisphere. As the term implies, 'cortex' is not limited to the cerebrum; it is used in connection with the kidneys or the cerebellum or the like, as in adrenal cortex or cerebellar cortex, etc. The grey matter consists of neuronal cell bodies in the brain and the spinal cord; their axons, which are the myelinated nerve fibres, and their dendrites constitute the white matter for the conducting portion of the brain below the cerebral cortex and of the spinal cord.

The two hemispheres are connected by a thick bundle of fibres called the corpus callosum (cf. Figure 11.3). Each hemisphere has four lobes: frontal lobe, parietal lobe, temporal lobe and occipital lobe. Each lobe has gyri which

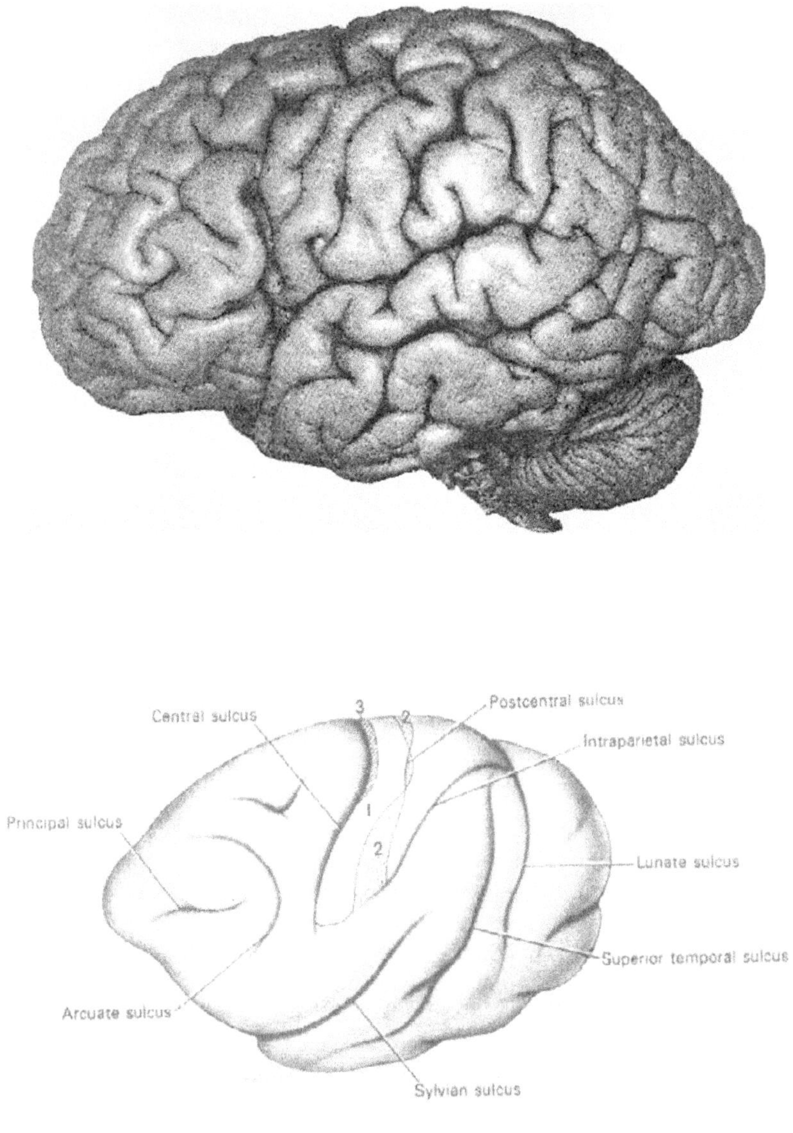

Figure 11.2 *Comparison of a human's and monkey's cerebral left hemispheres* (From Malcolm C. Carpenter, *Human Neuroanatomy*, 7th Edition, copyright © Lippincott Williams and Wilkins, 1976. Used by permission of Lippincott Williams and Wilkins.)

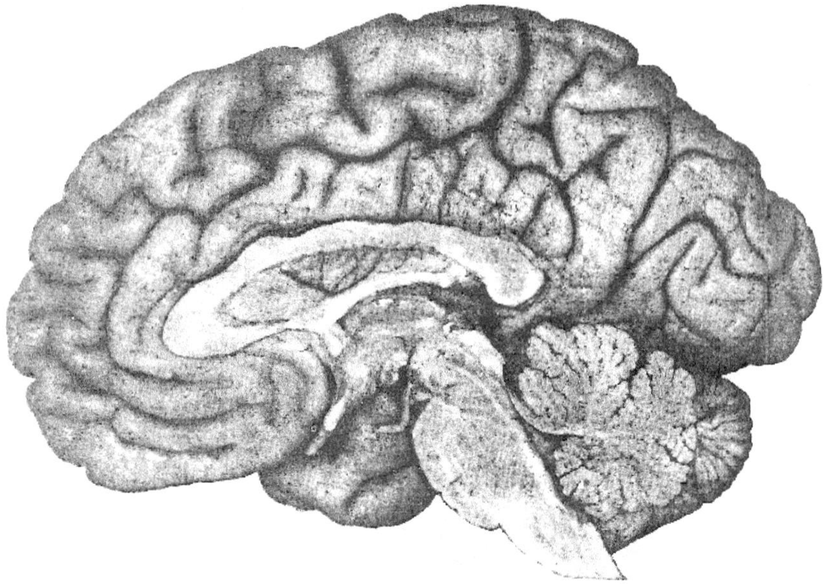

Figure 11.3 *Cingulate gyrus, corpus callosum, pons and other medial structures in the right hemisphere* (From *Structure of the Human Brain: A Photographic Atlas*, 3rd edition, by S. J. DeArmond and M. M. Fusco and M. M. Dewey, copyright © 1974, 1976, 1989 by Oxford University Press, Inc. Used by permission of Oxford University Press, Inc.)

are bundles of neurons; some of them have similar brain functions, but some others have different functions even within each gyrus. It is these specialized brain functions in the gyri that have led to the speculations (or even assertions) of regional differences of brain functions and the lateralization (or laterality) of higher brain functions often referred to as cerebral dominance or cerebral laterality. However, these assertions have now drawn fire. Structurally, nevertheless, there are markers for regional differences.

Between the frontal lobe and the parietal lobe there is a deep furrow, called the central (or Rolandic) sulcus (cf. Figure 11.1); between the temporal lobe and the parietal lobe there is another furrow, called the lateral (or Sylvian) sulcus (cf. Figure 11.1). Inside the lateral sulcus there are several short, oblique convolutions; they are known as the transverse gyri of Heschl; the two anterior transverse gyri constitute in humans the primary auditory cortex and are situated on the dorsal surface of the superior temporal gyrus. Anterior to the transverse gyri of Heschl are two strips of grey matter collectively called the insula 'island', which is the secondary auditory cortex.

The terms 'fissure' and 'sulcus' are not kept strictly; some neuroscientists prefer fissure to the exclusion of sulcus. The demarcation between the parietal lobe and the occipital lobe is not very clear, nor is that between the temporal lobe and the occipital lobe.

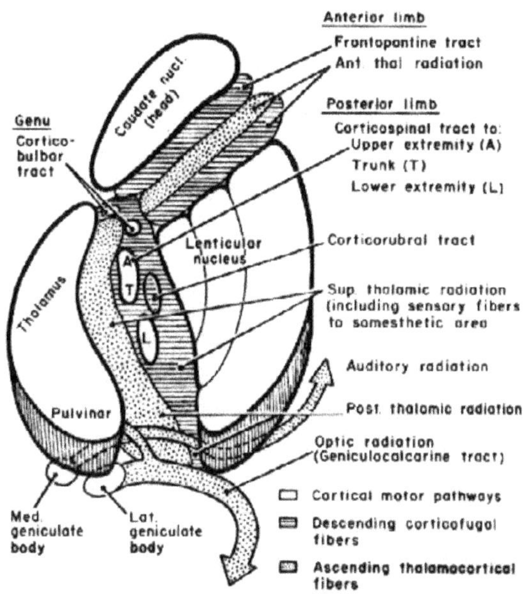

Figure 11.4 *Internal capsule, thalamus, medial and lateral geniculate bodies, and basal ganglia* (From Malcolm C. Carpenter, *Human Neuroanatomy*, 7th Edition, copyright © Lippincott Williams and Wilkins, 1976. Used by permission of Lippincott Williams and Wilkins.)

The convergent area of these three lobes is referred to as the posterior association area – sometimes also called the parieto-occipito-temporal region – in contradistinction to the anterior association area, which is located in the frontal lobe, receiving fibres from the occipital lobe and the parietal lobe. Association areas exclude the primary areas of the cerebral cortex, such as the primary and secondary auditory areas in connection with the temporal lobe and the primary and secondary visual areas in the occipital lobe. These association areas are connected with each other and with the thalamus, especially the neothalamus, the part connected to the neocortex, by numerous fibres passing through the corpus callosum and the white matter of the two hemispheres. They are thought to be responsible for the higher mental and emotional processes, including memory and learning and the like.

The gyrus immediately anterior to the central sulcus is called the pre-central gyrus (Figure 11.1) the functions of which are motoric, governing the contralateral parts of the body. The posterior third of the inferior gyrus of the left frontal lobe has been considered one of the so-called 'language centres'; namely, Broca's area (also called the *pars triangularis* and *opercularis*). However, Broca's area is the 'exit' of motoric impulses which have already passed the extra-pyramidal (i.e., basal ganglionic) loop on their way out, and not a language centre that controls expressive language. I shall have more to say about Broca's area in Chapter 17.

The gyrus immediately posterior to the central sulcus is called the post-central gyrus (Figure 11.1), the functions of which are somatosensory, receiving stimuli from the contralateral parts of the body. However, the fibres in these two gyri are mixed; that is, there are some somatosensory fibres in the pre-central gyrus and more motoric fibres in the post-central gyrus. Between the two on the medial side there is the supplementary motor area; it is considered a third so-called 'language centre'. Damage to this area may produce mirror writing (cf. Chan and Ross, 1988).

There are three gyri in the temporal lobe: superior, middle and inferior (Figure 11.1). The posterior one-third of the superior gyrus in the left temporal lobe is referred to as Wernicke's area, another so-called 'language centre'. However, this area varies from person to person; the location indicated is not meant to be an exact site. In my opinion, Wernicke's area is the 'entrance' of auditory stimuli, some of which also go to the opposite hemisphere and not a languge centre that controls comprehension. Thus, it has become a target of controversy.

Medially, there is a long curved gyrus, coursing along the corpus callosum from the anterior to the posterior region. It is called the cingulate ('girdling) gyrus; it is also called supracallosal gyrus. Lying within it is a long curved bundle of association fibres, called cingulum which connects the cingulate gyrus with the hypothalamus and the hippocampus (cf. Figure 11.3).

2. The Brainstem

Because of the aforementioned terminological differences, components of the brainstem also differ from one terminology to another. In one terminology, the brainstem includes the basal ganglia, mesencephalon, one part of metencephalon (i.e., the pons), and myelencephalon (which becomes the medulla).

In this terminology, the structure of the brainstem is detachable from the cerebrum, which is shown in Figures 11.5 and 11.6 from the dorsal and the ventral view.

In another terminology, however, the brainstem stops at mesencephalon, thereby excluding diencephalon. Since mesencephalon cannot be detached from prosencephalon, because developmentally it is connected to diencephalon, this version of the brainstem cannot be shown here. Perhaps, for this reason, most textbooks show the brainstem in the first sense.

It is of some interest to note that in 1999 the chief neurologist of a department of neurology at a major hospital in Taichung argued with me about the brainstem; he had published a case report about a disorder in the thalamus, on which I commented, because the thalamus is a very complex component of the brainstem in connection with the cerebellum. He told me to re-study neuroanatomy on the ground that the thalamus belongs to

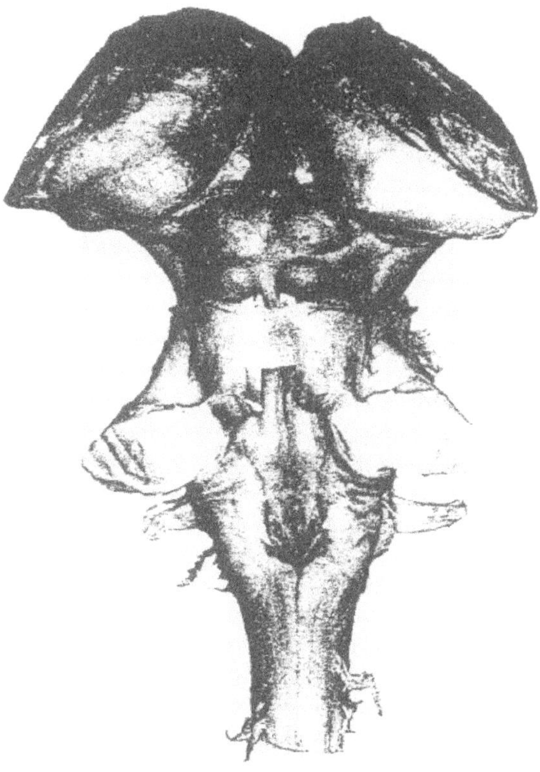

Figure 11.5 *Dorsal view of the brainstem* (From *Structure of the Human Brain: A Photographic Atlas,* 3rd edition, by S. J. DeArmond and M. M. Fusco and M. M. Dewey, copyright © 1974, 1976, 1989 by Oxford University Press, Inc. Used by permission of Oxford University Press, Inc.)

diencephalon and is not a part of the brainstem. I then showed him the textbook of neuroanatomy by Carpenter and told him that there are two views, one of which includes the thalamus and the basal ganglia and that he knew only one view and not the other; in fact, his paper was weakened by not taking into account several previous publications which had already talked about the thalamic symptoms he described.

It is quite obvious from the developmental point of view that the cerebrum and the brainstem must have neural connections, since they all started from one conceived cell which developed into the neural plate. In fact, within the cerebrum there are long and short connections: the long ones, which are heavily myelinated for transducing and transmitting impulses at high speed, connect the anterior portion with the posterior portion of the brain as well as between the two hemispheres and between the cortex and the subcortical structures and the spinal cord; the short ones, which are not as heavily

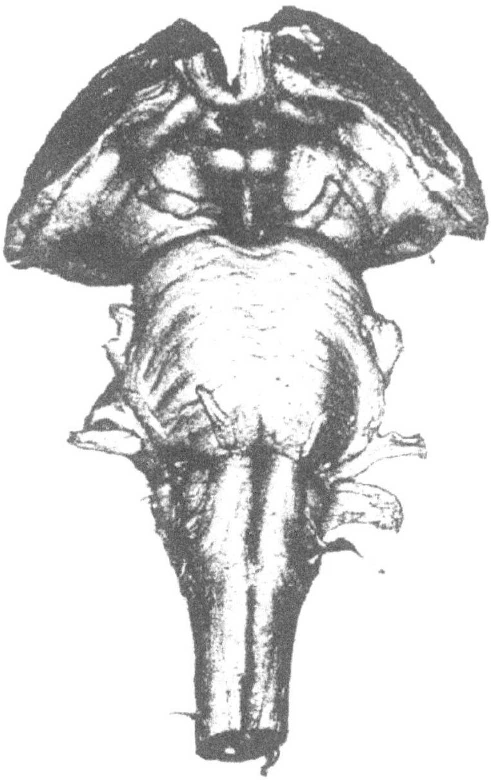

Figure 11.6 *Ventral view of the brainstem* (From *Structure of the Human Brain: A Photographic Atlas,* 3rd edition, by S. J. DeArmond and M. M. Fusco and M. M. Dewey, copyright © 1974, 1976, 1989 by Oxford University Press, Inc. Used by permission of Oxford University Press, Inc.)

myelinated, because high speed of signal transduction is not required, connect one ipsilateral gyrus to another.

The connections are called pathways. Those which terminate in the brainstem, because its shape looks like a bulb, are called cortico-bulbar pathways for production; they transduce motoric impulses to the eyes, the face, the vocal apparatus and the neck. Those which continue to the spinal cord are called cortico-spinal pathways for production; they transduce motoric impulses to the limbs (legs and arms) and trunk.

Cortico-bulbar pathways arise mainly from the pre-central and post-central gyri (i.e., the motor, premotor and somesthetic areas) and are distributed to sensory relay nuclei, parts of the reticular formation, and certain motor cranial nerve nuclei in man and primates (cf. Carpenter, 1976: 313–14). These fibres take the medial routes in the brainstem in association with the cortico-spinal fibres which take the lateral routes up to the pontine level and then move to the anterior routes in the medulla just before the pyramidal decussation. The distributions to the motor cranial nerve nuclei are highly relevant to expression plane in oral language, which are totally overlooked by linguists and phoneticians, although speech pathologists are concerned with them. There are two sets of cortico-bulbar fibres, one in each hemisphere.

Since there are two hemispheres, there are also two sets of cortico-spinal pathways, one in each hemisphere. These pathways consist of fibres that originate in the cerebral cortex, and take the lateral routes in association with the cortico-bulbar fibres. About 75 to 90 per cent of the cortico-spinal fibres cross in the medulla oblongata below the pyramid. The cross-over is called the motor or pyramidal decussation; hence, the crossed pathways are collectively called the pyramidal tract, for motoric behaviour conducted below the neck. The pyramidal decussation is at the anterior part of the lower medulla oblongata (the junction of the medulla oblongata and the spinal cord), so that the motoric impulses from the right hemisphere manipulates the left side of the body and the motoric impulses from the left hemisphere manipulates the right side of the body. A small anterior cortico-spinal tract, however, remains uncrossed.

In reception, the topographical arrangement of the neuronal fibres is somewhat more involved; pathways from receptor endings to the cerebral cortex, excluding those cranial nerves which receive stimuli from the external environment, typically through the five senses, require a minimum of three neurons (Everett, 1971: 45–6). The reason is the difference between spino-cortical pathways and bulbo-cortical pathways; the cranial nerves in the bulbo-cortical pathways have their own decussations in the brainstem.

In the spino-cortical pathways, the first neuron (also called primary neuron) has its cell body in a peripheral ganglion. The second neuron (also called secondary neuron) has its cell body in the posterior grey column of the spinal cord or in the brainstem (ibid.: 46). It is this secondary neuron that is a decussating neuron; that is, its axon crosses to the opposite side (ibid.: 46). The cell body of the third neuron (also called tertiary neuron) is in the thalamus and its axon courses upward to terminate in the cerebral cortex (ibid.: 46–7). The decussation in reception, formed by the fibres from both sides, is known as the sensory decussation, or as the decussation of the medial lemniscus in contrast to the motor (or pyramidal) decussation which is anterior and caudal to the sensory decussation.

As the decussating fibres from the nucleus gracilis (which is a collection of secondary neurons) and the nucleus cuneatus (which is also a collection of secondary neurons) have an arched course, when these fibres cross, they are known as internal arcuate fibres.

The involvement of the sensory decussation can be fully appreciated as follows. Up to the secondary neuron, the neuronal fibres ascend dorsally in the spinal cord as an ipsilateral pathway. But when they cross to the opposite side, in the medulla oblongata, they course medially (in the medial lemniscus, which is a bundle of neural fibres) and rostrally, in preparation for synapses with the tertiary neurons in the thalamus. Because the decussating fibres from the dorsal nuclei (the nucleus gracilis and the nucleus cuneatus) transduce impulses to the various nuclei in the brainstem, including the thalamus where the tertiary neuron is located before reaching the cortex, for relay and changes in the patterns and functions, the impulses are for discriminative touch, proprioception and vibratory sense.

The resultant impulses are transduced from the thalamus to the cerebral cortex, because they are sensory impulses, and the pathways are called spino-cortical (or more accurately, spino-thalamo-cortical) pathways. The fasculus gracilis is concerned with those sensations for the leg and lower trunk, while impulses from the upper trunk, arm and neck are transduced in the fasciculus cuneatus for the same sensations (Barr, 1974). Stimuli coming from the body parts above the neck, utilizing the appropriate cranial nerves, make use of the bulbo-cortical pathways, some of which cross in the midbrain.

Those neuronal fibres coming from the sensory nerves in the body through the posterior grey column of the spinal cord – for example, heat, pain, light touch, and coldness, in addition to the two fasciculi just mentioned – also belong to the spino-cortical pathways. There are two sets of such pathways. However, because of the sensory decussation, those impulses coming from the left side of the body go through the contralateral thalamus to terminate in the right cerebral hemisphere and those impulses coming from the right side of the body go through the contralateral thalamus to terminate in the left cerebral hemisphere. Figure 11.7 shows a simplified schematic representation of the spino-cortical pathways.

In the bulbo-cortical pathways, however, with the exception of the two olfactory nerves which do not cross in the brainstem, the cross-over is partial: some pathways cross over but others do not; that is, some are contralateral and others are ipsilateral pathways. Examples are optic and auditory pathways

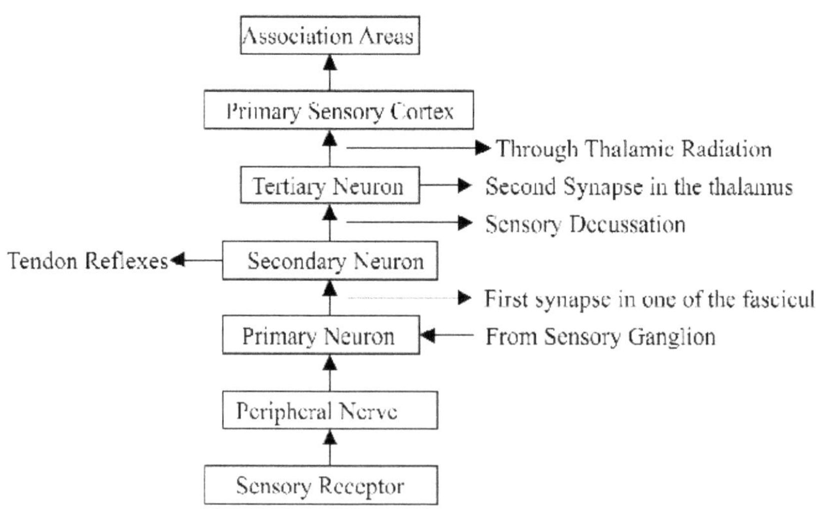

Figure 11.7 *Schematic representation of the spino-cortical pathways*

(including the lateral and medial geniculate bodies and the inferior and superior colliculi). Thus, like handedness, some people have right-eye and right-ear dominance. These dominances do not always coincide with handedness. That is, left handers may have right-eye and/or right-ear dominance and right handers may have left-eye and/or left-ear dominance.

Either cortico-bulbar or cortico-spinal, moreover, the pathways are *not* direct; for production, neuroscientists used to think that motoric impulses come down from the cerebral cortex directly to their muscular targets (i.e., innervated muscles) via the pyramidal tract, one in each side of the brain. But, because of recent studies on the diseases involving the basal ganglia, such as PD and HD or dystonia, an extra set of pathways, called the extra-pyramidal tract, has been established (Alexander *et al.*, 1986; Mink, 1996).

It comprises a loop, called the cortico-striato-pallido-thalamo-cortical loop. The motoric impulses going to the pyramidal tract must first go through this loop; even reflexes and eye movements, with the exception of tendon reflex and knee jerks, go through the loop. Since there are also two sides, there exist two extra-pyramidal tracts (or loops).

It should be kept in mind that these pathways, long or short, are not like hoses, an unobstructed conduit for water; rather, they are important neural structures which transduce chemical substances into electrical currents to become impulses. These structures are connected by important relay 'stations' whose function it is to change the patterns and rhythms of the impulses going through when such impulses from different regions interact therein by means of excitation, inhibition and disinhibition. These impulses and the changes of the patterns and rhythms of such impulses in the 'relay stations' are integrated as part of the brain activities that can become active behaviour, when expressed, or remain as passive behaviour, when not expressed.

Be that as it may, language in the brain in the form of impulses as behaviour is still *not* considered by neuroscientists or language/speech pathologists as passing through the extra-pyramidal tract for production, although movement disorders neurologists have agreed that speech may come through the extra-pyramidal tract. Those linguists who use 'pathways of the brain', though the term may seem to be metaphorical, to describe their 'rules' of language do not know what the real pathways of the brain are and are unaware of the functions of such pathways in the brain.

I have pushed this line of reasoning further by saying that since language in the brain consists of two planes (content plane and expression plane), it must utilize the extra-pyramidal tract for not only production in learning but also in thinking which, in conjunction with learning, is also relevant to reception. I shall explain my theory in greater detail in the next section when I have described the basal ganglia.

In the meantime, I shall explain a few structures in the brainstem which are more pertinent to language in the brain. In so doing, I shall include diencephalon in the brainstem. Typically, these structures are: the thalamus, the subthalamus, the hypothalamus, the lateral and medial geniculate bodies, the superior and inferior colliculi, the pituitary gland (or hypophysis),

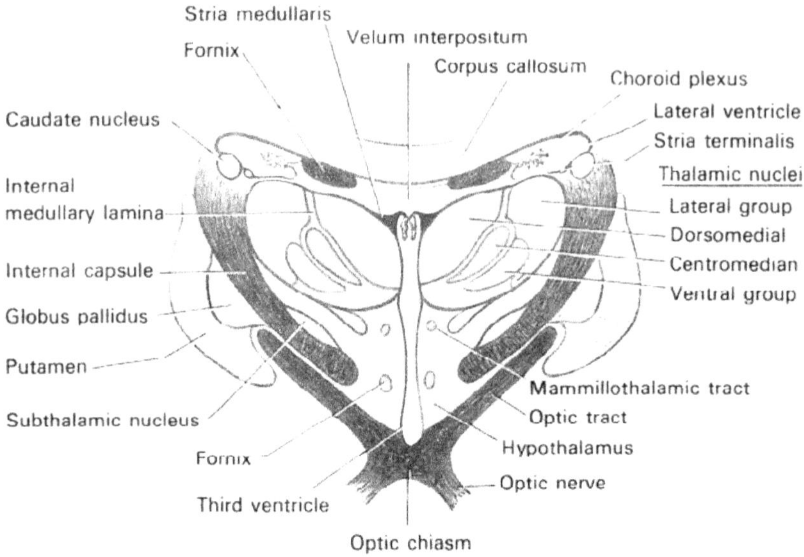

Figure 11.8 *Thalamus, hypothalamus, subthalamic nucleus, globus pallidus, internal capsule and third ventricle* (From Malcolm C. Carpenter, *Human Neuroanatomy*, 7th Edition, copyright © Lippincott Williams and Wilkins, 1976. Used by permission of Lippincott Williams and Wilkins.)

the cerebellar peduncles (superior, middle, and inferior), the pons, and the medulla oblongata.

Since in an adult human brain the basal ganglia are next to the thalamus and subthalamus, divided by the internal capsule (cf. Figures 11.4, 11.8 and 11.11), and functionally related to these two structures, the thalamus and the subthalamus in one terminology are functionally included in the basal ganglia. But as the basal ganglia, from telencephalon, and the thalamus, the subthalamus, and the hypothalamus, from diencephalon, are detachable from the two cerebral hemispheres, those structures may also in one terminology be regarded as part of the brainstem.

2.1 The Thalamus

The thalamus is the middle and larger portion of diencephalon, thereby forming part of the lateral wall of the third ventricle. There are two thalami in the brain, each one of which is shaped like an American football or an olive. Each thalamus has ten major subdivisions (or nuclei) which send afferent fibres to most cerebral areas that project fibres back indirectly via the corpus straitum to the thalamic nuclei from which fibres are received. In other words, there are close cortico-thalamic and thalamo-cortical interactions. Of these nuclei, two deserve some mention; namely, ventroanterior (VA) nucleus and ventrolateral (VL) nucleus.

The VA thalamic nucleus projects fibres back to pre-central gyrus (Area 4) and the VL thalamic nucleus projects fibres back to pre-motor gyrus (Area 6); but these nuclei also receive fibres from the basal ganglia, thereby completing the cortico-striato-pallido-thalamo-cortical loop.

For these reasons, there is a neurosurgical procedure, a form of functional neurosurgery, called thalamotomy, to treat resting tremor, gait disturbances and rigidity in PD; however, little attention is paid to the cause of the patient's language disorders, because neurologists and neurosurgeons tend to be more interested in the patient's other neurological signs than his/her language disorder.

Unfortunately, the treatment is only cosmetic. Some PD patients travelled from Taiwan to Japan for thalamotomy. When the surgery was done, the patients could walk easily and the tremor seemed to have disappeared; but as they left the airport to return to Taiwan, all symptoms of PD, including language disorder, reappeared. Of course, the patients' language disorders either remained the same or, in some cases, became worse, for the patients had had language disorders from the onset of the disease, albeit subtle at first.

Notwithstanding, the thalamus is also the main relay centre as it receives projections from the cerebellum through the superior cerebellar peduncle in the midbrain and the middle cerebellar peduncle in the pons (the cerebello-pontine tract) for the cerebello-cortical connections. These connections regulate voluntary movements, the brain functions of memory, and cognitive functions as well as all sensory impulses from the inferior cerebellar peduncle in the medulla oblongata that connects the spinal cord.

Recently, however, the thalamo-cerebellar and cerebello-thalamic interactions have become the focus of attention for modulating and facilitating thinking that takes place in the extra-pyramidal looping. Thus, if bilateral thalamotomy is performed, the patient's language disorders will detrimentally become quite obvious.

2.2 The Subthalamus

The subthalamic nucleus (or subthalamus) is the portion of diencephalon that lies between the thalamus and the tegmentum of mesencephalon. It is coffee coloured and has a rich blood supply, but is missing in reptiles and birds although all mammals have it; it is especially well developed in primates. It has no direct reciprocal connections with the cerebral cortex nor has it any connections with the substantia nigra, although some neuroanatomists have claimed such connections; however, it projects fibres to the medial side of the globus pallidus and receives fibres from the lateral side of the globus pallidus; these connections are ipsilateral, but a small number of efferent fibres pass toward the contralateral globus pallidus.

In humans, the subthalamic nucleus is especially well developed and, therefore, any lesion, usually caused by haemorrhage because of the rich blood supply, will result in violent, forceful and persistent choroid movements, collectively called haemiballism, on the opposite side. The reason is that the impulses projecting from the globus pallidus back to the cerebral (motor) cortex via the thalamus come down through the cortico-spinal pathways which cross at the pyramidal decussation.

There are four varying types of abnormal involuntary movements associated with diseases of the corpus striatum (cf. the basal ganglia); namely, resting tremor, chorea, ballism and athetosis.

2.2.1 Resting Tremor

This is so-called because the patient has all limbs resting, not moving, and yet they tremor in a rhythmical, alternating, abnormal involuntary fashion, having a relatively regular frequency and amplitude. It is the first sign of parkinsonism (not PD) associated with lesions in the basal ganglia. It affects language in the brain, initially in the expression plane but gradually influences the content plane, if it is caused by PD, to result in dementia. In this case, the voice becomes attenuated and weak in volume, and writing has the signs of micrographia (i.e., written words becoming smaller and smaller).

If medication is administered – for example, L-Dopa – the patient will gradually develop on–off phenomena after a few years, that is, an on-phenomenon when medication is in effect, but an off-phenomenon when the efficacy of medication has worn out; during the off-period, the patient is mute and cannot walk as the whole body becomes stiff (i.e., freezes); but during the on-period, the patient resumes all activities like a 'normal' person. As the on–off cycles repeat, the patient's brain functions of memory will deteriorate. The final destination is mute and bedridden, which is common to all patients with dementia, as in AD, FD, HD, and Pick's disease, to mention just a few.

2.2.2 Chorea

This is a 'graceful' but brisk series of successive involuntary movements of the upper and/or lower limbs; the abnormal movements are not rhythmical but involve considerable complexity, resembling portions of purposefully choreographed movements. Its lesion site is in the caudet nucleus and the cause is genetic; it is transmitted as an autosomal dominant trait, not sex-linked, which is to say that either parent who has the disease can pass it to an offspring; if both parents have the disease, every child will be a gene-carrier.

The disease is known as Huntingon's disease (HD), named after George Huntington (1850–1916), an American physician, and is neurodegenerative. The patient invariably develops language disorder. It has a variable onset and will spread from the side of the onset to the other side, but occurs mostly in the fourth decade and quickly results in dementia within a short period of time; death follows within 15 years after the onset. It was made famous by the popular American folk song singer, Woody Guthrie, in the 1940s, who died of HD.

2.2.3 Ballism

By contrast ballism is a forceful and persistent (not 'graceful') abnormal, involuntary movement that occurs usually on the opposite of the lesion site. Unless it is complicated by a neurodegenerative disease in one or more of the other nuclei, as the subthalamic nucleus (STN) is not a part of telencephalon, developmentally, any disorder in the STN is not known to be neurodegenerative. The disorder will affect language in the brain just the same. To my knowledge, however, no documentation of ballism in association with language disorder has been made, partly because neurologists are more concerned with involuntary non-language movements than abnormal involuntary movement resulting in language disorder.

2.2.4 Athetosis

To many neurologists this is the same as dystonia but to some the two are different forms of dyskinesia. The differences are that athetosis is a derangement marked by a ceaseless occurrence of slow, sinuous, writhing movements which are usually severe in the hands and legs (or feet), but that dystonia is a form of disordered tonicity of muscle, which may be a result of a lesion in the lenticular nucleus (putamen and globus pallidus); however, drugs may induce dystonia, especially when treating PD with various kinds of medication. Dystonia, moreover, may affect tongue movement and eye movements, thereby grossly distorting the manifestations of expression plane. The similarity is that both produce irregular movements or contortions of the extremities, especially when walking in a grotesque manner; they both produce language disorders.

2.3 The Hypothalamus

This structure is located caudal to the thalamus and medial to the subthalamus. It has a rostro-caudal thickness of about 1cm. Since there are two, divided by the third ventrical, they form the inferior and lateral walls of the third ventricle, one on each side (cf Figure 11.8).

Structurally and developmentally the hypothalamus is a subdivision of diencephalon; it has several nuclei which are divided into the medial group and the lateral group by the fornix (cf. Figure 11.8). Functionally, however, these nuclear groups are concerned with visceral activity, endocrine and metabolic activity (for secretion of hormones in sexual arousal), temperature control, and sleep and emotion (including aggression and sexual drive control). Thus, the hypothalamus is a part of the limbic system.

2.4 The Lateral and Medial Geniculate Bodies

These are part of the thalamus, often collectively called the metathalamus. Thus, they develop from diencephalon, but have close relationships with the superior and the inferior colliculi, even though the superior and the inferior colliculi develop from mesencephalon. However, the lateral and the medial geniculate bodies have different functions in respect to language in the brain.

The lateral geniculate bodies are particularly important for visual functions, because of their direct connections with the optic nerve and the striate cortex (i.e., visual cortex on the medial side of the occipital lobe) through the optic radiation (geniculo-calcarine tract) (see Figure 11.4). But the medial geniculate bodies are particularly important for auditory functions, because of their principal projections to the primary auditory centre (transverse gyri of Heschl) through the auditory radiation (i.e., geniculo-temporal tract).

When visual stimuli are received by the eyes, the stimuli project to the retinae upside down and the retinae, which are part of the brain and consist of bipolar cells, transduce the impulses to the lateral geniculate bodies through the optic nerve. At the same time, part of the impulses also go to the superior colliculi where the upside down images are partially corrected, so that the visual cortex after receiving the partially corrected images from the optic radiation will have the images right side up, corresponding to the objects in the visual fields.

The medial geniculate bodies do not project auditory impulses *en bloc* to the primary auditory cortex; rather, they have to coordinate with the inferior-colliculi for frequency (i.e., pitch) adjustment, because impulses of different pitches project to different parts in the inferior colliculi for adjustment in relation to the medial geniculate bodies.

2.5 The Superior and Inferior Colliculi

How the corrections take place and how the adjustments are made will be the main concerns of this subsection, because these corrections are of major importance in the brain functions of language, especially the individual aspect of *langue*, which will be explicated at length in Part IV.

First, the corrections take place in the interplays of the two retinae, the two superior colliculi, and the visual cortex. It should be mentioned that each superior colliculus receives projections from four sources; namely, the retina through the optic nerve, the cerebral cortex, the spinal cord, and the inferior colliculus (Carpenter, 1976: 372–3). Projections from the retina and the visual cortex (in the occipital lobe) will be the focus here, because the visual cortex has the most substantial and highly organized projections to the superior colliculus, even though portions of the frontal lobe, the temporal lobe, and the occipital lobe all project fibres to the superior colliculus. I believe it is the interplays of these projections that are pertinent to the corrections of upside down images.

The visual fields are not represented 'faithfully' in the superior colliculi before the impulses via each ipsilateral geniculate body go to the visual cortex, although the projections of stimuli from the visual fields to the superior colliculi are quite orderly: homonymous half fields to the contralateral superior colliculus; the central 30 degrees of the visual field occupying the rostral three-fourths of the superior colliculi which also represent the macular area of the retina; and the remaining 70 degrees crowded into the caudal quarter of the superior colliculus (ibid.: 373).

Under these circumstances, superior portions of the retina, or inferior half of the visual field (i.e., upside down projections because of the lenses), would be represented superiorly in the visual cortex if not corrected (i.e., as upside down images which must be corrected) but laterally in the superior colliculi; at one and the same time, inferior portions of the retina, or superior half of the visual field (i.e., upside down projections because of the lenses), would be represented inferiorly in the visual cortex (i.e., as upside down images which must be corrected) but medially in the superior colliculus (adapted and modified from Carpenter, 1976: 373). I then reason that the direct connections of the lateral geniculate bodies and the visual cortex, through the optic radiation, and the close relationships of the lateral geniculate bodies and the superior colliculi somehow interplay to change the upside down images to right side up images in the visual cortex, so that superior half of the visual field can correspond superiorly and inferior half of the visual field can correspond inferiorly in the visual cortex, that is, the whole visual field can be viewed right side up.

The inferior colliculus, like the superior colliculus, also receives fibres from different sources: the lateral leminiscus (which consists of the longitudinal ascending fibres from the pons and the medulla oblongata; the opposite inferior colliculus (i.e., crossing fibre); ipsimedial geniculate body; and the auditory cortex (see Carpenter (1976)).

Functionally, neurons in the inferior colliculi are arranged orderly in respect to frequencies. For instance, pitches from low to high or from high to low have different tonotopic localizations in the inferior colliculi; there are also neurons in the inferior colliculus that respond sensitively to interaural time relationships. Since it has been known that the localizations of sound sources depend on time and sound intensity, one significant role of the inferior colliculus may include just this kind of function. I may add that the distinction of different voice qualities – for example, age differences, hoarseness, and timbre in human voice or musical instrument – probably depend on the functions of the inferior colliculus.

2.6 The Pituitary Gland (or Hypophysis)

This stalk-like bundle of important nuclei is also known as infundibulum. It is a part of the hypothalamus, and therefore a part of the limbic system; developmentally, it comes from diencephalon. (See Figures. 9.6, 10.1, 11.6 and 11.10.)

Because of the importance in the secretion of a hormone pertinent not only to sexuality, ovulation and spermatogenesis in relation to reproduction but also to growth in relation to mitosis, hyperplasia and hypertrophy, it is often called clinically the master gland. If it is underdeveloped, during infancy, the child will become a dwarf in adulthood; on the other hand, if it is overdeveloped, during childhood, the child at the age of, say, seven, will weigh around 60 to 70 kilograms and will become a giant in adulthood. Goliath whom King David as a child killed, as described in the Bible, probably had an overdeveloped pituitary gland during his childhood or even infancy.

If an adult male has a tumour in the master gland, it must be removed through surgery, in which case, he will not grow or shrink in size but will lose sexuality, and reproductive ability, as well as his beard. If an adult has a disease in the hypophysis to cause it to mulfuction, he/she will not grow larger in size but the face will become enlongated. A face that looks like a horse's face clinically is known as 'horse face'. If an adult woman cannot conceive, because she does not ovulate, there is a medication to stimulate her infundibulum, so that she will ovulate and, hence, can become pregnant.

2.7 The Cerebellar Peduncles

As will be mentioned again later, with regard to the cerebellum, there are three bundles of fibres attached to the cerebellum for connection with the

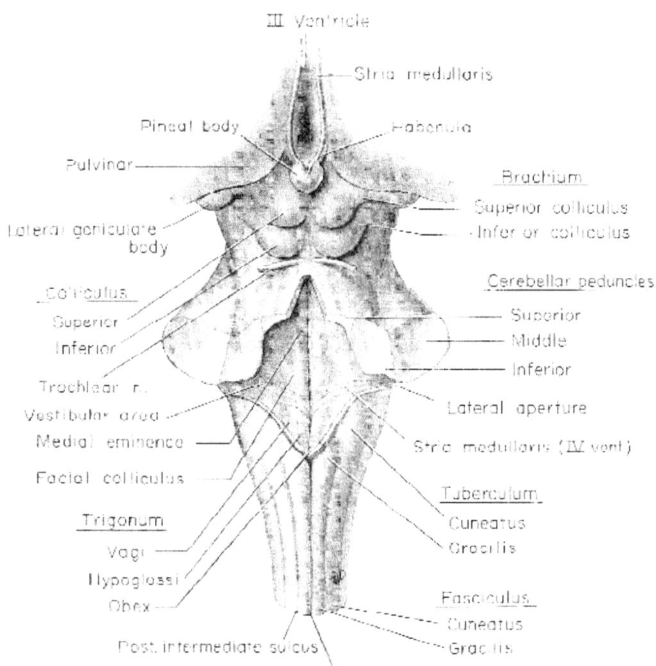

***Figure 11.9** Superior, middle and inferior cerebellar peduncles, fourth ventricle, superior and inferior colliculi, pineal gland, lateral geniculate bodies* (From Malcolm C. Carpenter, *Human Neuroanatomy*, 7th Edition, copyright © Lippincott Williams and Wilkins, 1976. Used by permission of Lippincott Williams and Wilkins.)

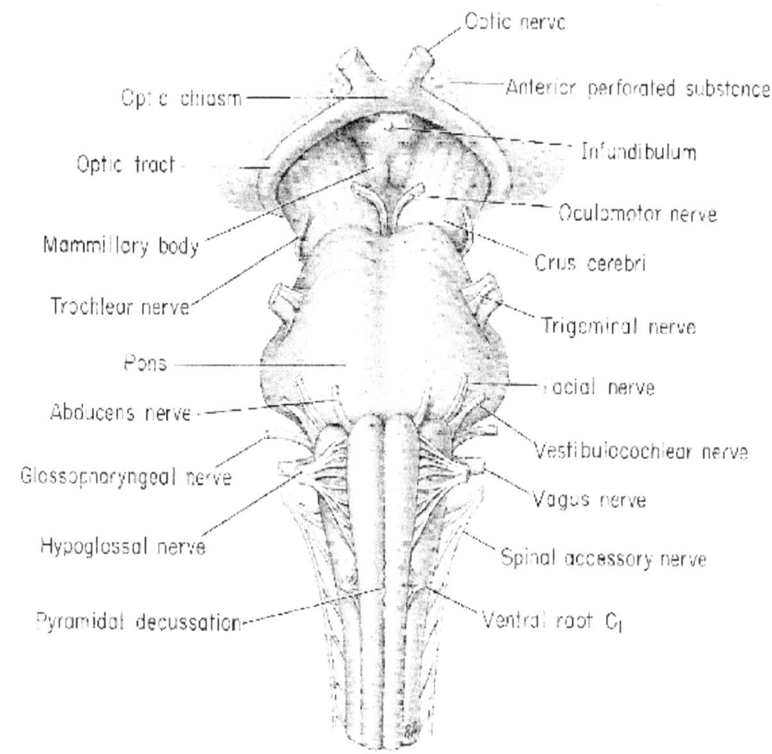

Figure 11.10 *Pons, medulla, infundibulum, mammilary body, optic chiasm and cranial nerves* (From Malcolm C. Carpenter, *Human Neuroanatomy*, 7th Edition, copyright © Lippincott Williams and Wilkins, 1976. Used by permission of Lippincott Williams and Wilkins.)

brainstem and the spinal cord. First, the superior cerebellar peduncle forms the most important efferent fibre system of the cerebellum that connects with the midbrain (Carpenter, 1976). Note that there are no afferent fibres to the cerebellum from the midbrain in the superior cerebellar peduncle; that is to say, the superior cerebellar peduncle contains only outputs from the Purkinje cells in the cerebellum, each one of which, however, may have 150,000 to 200,000 inputs from other cells within the cerebellum as well as from cells outside the midbrain; the outputs go through the thalamus to reach the cerebral cortex. Second, the middle cerebellar peduncle has efferent and afferent connections with the pons, and contains the ponto-cerebellar fibres which convey impulses from the cerebral cortex to the cerebellum; in other words, the cerebro-cerebellar connection are indirect, via the ponto-cerebellar fibres, and the outputs also go through the thalamus via the ponto-thalamic tract to reach the cerebral cortex; put differently, the cerebello-cerebral connections are abundant, albeit indirect via both the midbrain and the pons. Third, the inferior cerebellar peduncle has efferent and afferent connections with the spinal cord through the medulla oblongata; such reciprocal connections are not limited to motoric fibres; for this reason, the cerebellum responds to sensory stimulations.

I should add that it is through these peduncles for connections with many other parts of the central nervous system that the brain functions of memory and cognition of the cerebellum have increasingly gained better recognition in neuroscience. However, this is not tantamount to saying that the cerebellum has to depend on other brain structures for its functions of memory and cognition. The cerebellum, more likely, has its own internal cellular organization that contributes to its functions of memory and cognition.

2.8 The Pons and the Medulla Oblongata

These two structures belong to the brainstem but developmentally come from metencephalon and myelencephalon, respectively. They are important to language in the brain for three reasons. First, the pons literally 'bridges' structurally and functionally the midbrain, the basal ganglia, the cerebellum and the medulla. Both structures contain a central core of the reticular formation, which is the structure that subserves consciousness. The remaining reticular formation is in the midbrain. Second, eight out of the twelve cranial nerves are divided equally by the two structures, that is, V, VI, VII, and VIII cranial nerves are attached to the pons and IX, X, XI, and XII cranial nerves are attached to the medulla. These cranial nerves are more relevant to oral language than to sign language, however. Third, the centre of heart beat and pulmonary function (i.e., breathing) is in the floor of the fourth ventricle which also contains many important nuclei that are not described here.

3. The Basal Ganglia

The basal ganglia, structurally speaking, are made up of three nuclei as a unified group, which come from telencephalon; the three nuclei are often collectively referred to as corpus striatum (or corpora striata, since there are two sets): the globus pallidus ('pale ball'); the putamen ('that which drops when a tree is pruned'); the caudet nucleus ('tail-shaped' nucleus) which has a head and a tail; the tail ends in the amygdala. The first two may be grouped together as the lentiform or lenticular ('lens-shaped') nucleus. The caudet nucleus wraps around the lentiform nucleus with the tail. The first nucleus is said to be phylogenetically older and, therefore, may be referred to as palaeostriatum in contradistinction to the latter two nuclei which are phylogenetically younger and, therefore, may be collectively referred to as neostriatum or striatum because they have a common origin and structure.

The globus pallidus, moreover, is subdivided into internal (or medial) globus pallidus (Pi for abbreviation) and external (or lateral globus pallidus (Pe for abbreviation). Pi receives fibres from the subthalamic nucleus and Pe projects fibres to the subthalamic nucleus. When neurosurgery, called

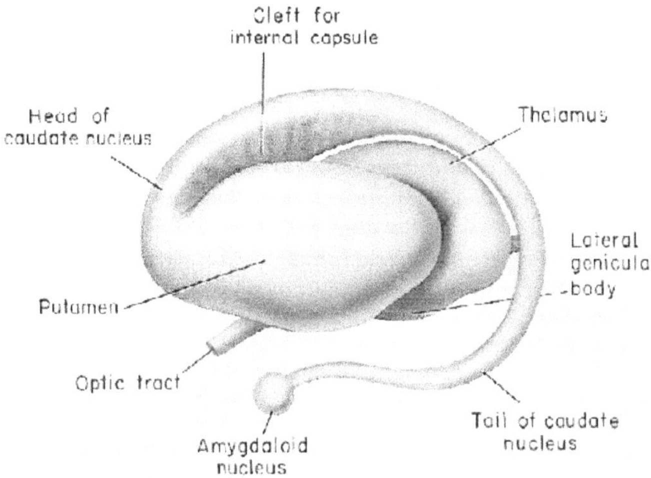

Figure 11.11 *Left basal ganglia and left thalamus* (From Malcolm C. Carpenter, *Human Neuroanatomy*, 7th Edition, copyright © Lippincott Williams and Wilkins, 1976. Used by permission of Lippincott Williams and Wilkins.)

functional neurosurgery, is performed on PD patients, in addition to thalamotoy, to treat their resting tremor or rigidity, it is called pallidotomy, which is to destroy the tissues in Pi. When foetal neural tissues are used in grafting (transplantation), it is the putamen where the foetal neural tissues are grafted.

Functionally, however, the basal ganglia constitute a system that is so important to not only motor functions for non-language behaviour but also the brain functions of language as behaviour. As such, it has two more components; namely, the substantia nigra, the black substance consisting of a layer of grey substance that comes from mesencephalon to separate the tegmentum of the midbrain from the crus cerebri (leg of the cerebrum); and the subthalamic nucleus (or simply subthalamus) which comes from diencephalon. Some neurologists would also include the red nucleus in the basal ganglia as a part of the functional system.

The substantia nigra is included in the basal ganglia as a system because it is dopaminergic (i.e., produces dopamine which is an excitatory neurotransmitter). In other words, the substantia nigra is a 'manufacturer' of the neurotransmitter called dopamine needed by the corpora striata as 'consumers'. The two subthalamic nuclei are relay stations that help facilitate the looping of impulses in the corpora striata (especially the lenticular nucleus).

It has been known that PD is caused by an insufficiency of dopamine; that is, the substantia nigra fails to produce the needed neurotransmitter to supply its consumption in the putamen. When the supply is disrupted or depleted, the basal ganglia become erratic, resulting in resting tremor, gait disturbances, muscle rigidity, mask face and, most important of all, language disorder (first in expression plane and then in content plane to show symptoms of dementia).

The patient gradually loses his/her brain functions, because the disease is neurodegenerative, with Lewy bodies building up to cause neuronal deaths; recently, however, it has been found that Lewy bodies are not the necessary markers of PD, so long as the substantia nigra has failed to produce dopamine. Maybe Lewy bodies are the 'by-products' of the failure in producing dopamine from the substantia nigra and the red nucleus, a by-product that may or may not appear in the patient's brain, rather than the cause of PD, because they may also be found in cortical diseases.

The disease starting from one side gradually spreads to the other side, as neuronal deaths aggravate, and eventually to the cerebral cortex. The patient with PD eventually becomes bedridden and mute, as do patients with AD (including only neurofibrillary tangles), or Fischer's disease (FD) which, as I have proposed, includes only senile plaques, now called amyloid plaques, because both neurofibrillary tangles and senile plaques may co-exit in a patient's brain, in which case, the severity of dementia may be worse; the patient gets a 'double-dose' of apoptosis. Any other neurodegenerative diseases, such as Pick's disease, HD, and SCA (Spino-Cerebellar Ataxia), will also lead to the same end result.

I have called this neurodegeneration of PD, or any other subcortical disease, such as HD and SCA, the bottom-up course of neurodegeneration, in contrast to the neurodegeneration of AD, or any other cortical disease that results in dementia, such as Pick's disease and FD, as it takes the top-down course of neurodegeneration, because the end result of both kinds of neurodegeneration is the same: bedridden and mute.

First line medication employed to treat PD is L-Dopa which, among others, supplies dopamine to the brain; its efficacy, however, lasts only five years; after that, the patient's condition continues to deteriorate until the patient becomes bedridden and mute before expiration. Research is going on in many centres to find out what causes the substantia nigra to stop manufacturing dopamine. Until the cause is found, the 'stop-gap' medications are the only measures available.

The looping of impulses from expression plane within the basal ganglia, however, is not self-contained; it involves the thalamus which used to be thought of as a mere relay station; it is now believed to be a very important structure for regulating and integrating brain functions of memory and cognition. I may venture to say that the interplay between the superior colliculi and the visual cortex for the corrections of visual images is mediated by the thalamus (in the lateral geniculate bodies) and the superior colliculi in the midbrain. The same is true of the interplay between the inferior colliculi and the auditory cortex for the modulation of acoustic images (in the medial geniculate bodies).

The looping is understood to be cortico-striato-pallido-thalamo-cortical, with the STN assisting, as it were, the globus pallidus; that is, it starts from the cerebral cortex and goes back to the cerebral (motor) cortex before any impulse from the expression plane will come down through the pyramidal tract for behavioural manifestations. The looping wherein thinking takes place is also modulated by the cerebello-cerebral circuit (Schmahmann, 2003) and the Papez Circuit (Snider, 1976) (see Figures 11.12, 11.13 and 11.14). I am inclined to suggest that the limbic system in the Papez Circuit plays a more important role in the 'trigger' or 'drive' of the manifestation of behaviour, as may be evidenced by the choice of words in anger or schizophrenic behaviour or suicidal attempts.

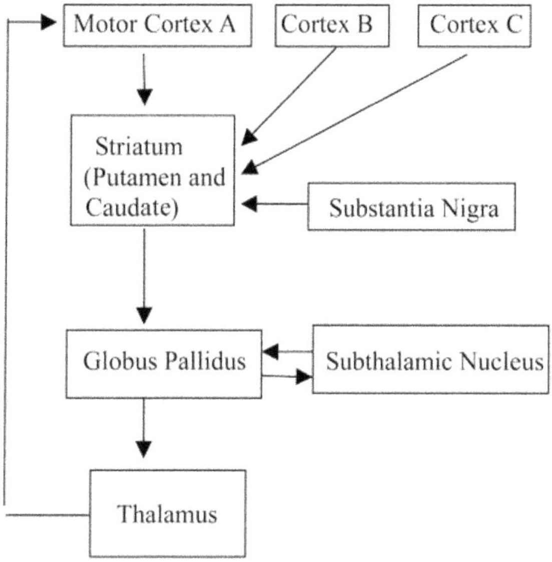

Figure 11.12 Schematic representation of the oversimplified extra-pyramidal loop

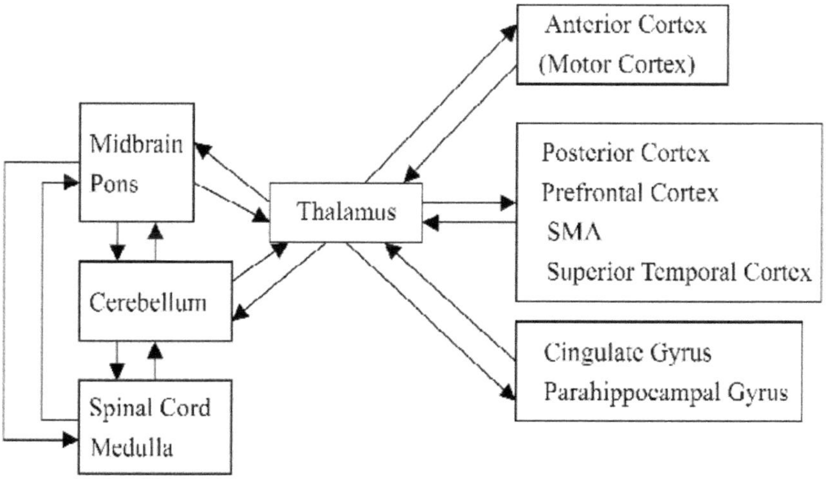

Figure 11.13 Diagram of the oversimplified cerebello-cerebral circuit

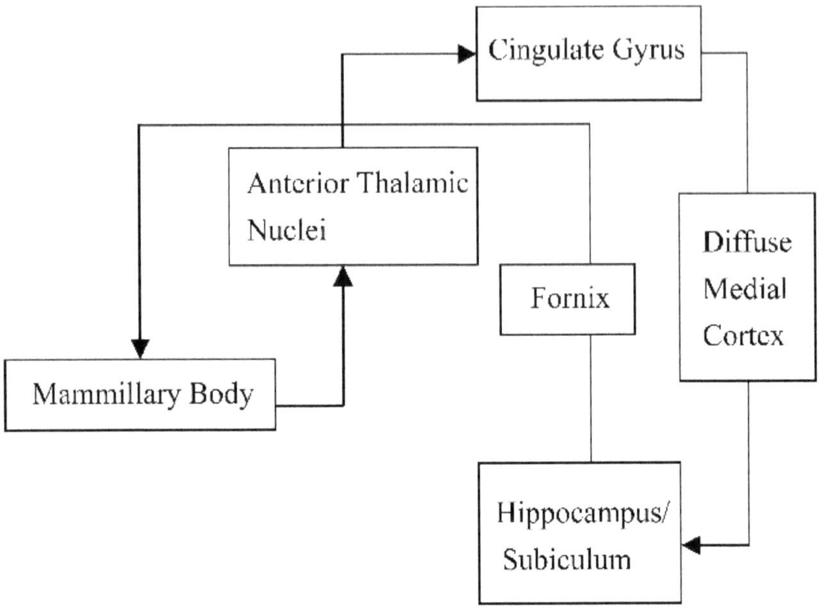

Figure 11.14 *Diagram of the Papez Circuit*

As briefly mentioned above, the basal ganglia as a system regulate not only motoric impulses but also thinking; I have suggested that it is in the looping where thinking takes place, because the cerebral cortex is involved at least twice, before and after the looping, for any motoric impulse that is destined to come out. However, thinking itself is not expressive, which is known in the literature of linguistics as inner speech; that is, unless an individual says, does, or writes something for expression as behaviour, there is absolutely no way in which another person can understand, know, or detect what the individual is thinking about; the best the other person can do is to 'guess', a counter-behaviour which may or may not be correct. When the looping runs its course, after a mental state which I have called language potentiation, or when the individual decides to say, do, or write something, the extra-pyramidal tract must pass on the impulses to the pyramidal tract for expression, which unfortunately is often misunderstood. One misunderstanding is that expression plane is equated with speech which is then separated from language; another misunderstanding is that it is taken to be motor function having nothing to do with language. The truth is that expression plane (or speech, if you will) and content plane must be put together to constitute language in the brain as behaviour; both planes are brain functions that pertain to behaviour as defined earlier. Moreover, as sign language is now considered language, the term 'speech' is no longer sufficient to represent expression plane which must, therefore, be multifaceted to include not only oral language but also sign language, written language, or the use of Braille.

Having briefly described some structures of the brainstem, I should now allude to the fourth ventricle which has the cerebellum as its 'roof'. The reason is that there are nuclei in the floor of the fourth ventricle, which are vital to the expression of language in the brain; these nuclei control the heartbeat and pulmonary function (cf. Figures. 11.5 and 11.9).

In cardiology, the heart and the lungs are often treated together because of these vital functions. When something goes wrong in the fourth ventricle, the heartbeat stops and the individual stops breathing at the same time. (In Chinese medicine, interestingly, the heart and the lungs are considered belonging to the same functional unit.)

Thus, when a person is dying of cancer the cells of which have spread to the intestine, the person's heartbeat gradually increases to pump blood into the brain from the normal rate of 70 or so per minute to 180 or so, because the brain has the top priority of blood supply. At the same time, the person has grave difficulty breathing. At that time, up to a point, the heartbeat will then decrease, because the brain is no longer in need of blood, thereby 'telling the nuclei in the fourth ventricle not to supply any more blood'; the heartbeat quickly drops, and when the heart stops beating, the person's breathing also stops and he/she is said to 'expire'. Before the expiration, there is of course no more brain function of language as behaviour for that person, as the brain has ceased to function properly to enable that person to make any adjustment whatsoever to the internal and the external environments.

Here are some philosophical or even theological questions which may be of interest to linguists and semioticians: What is life? Or where and when does what Christians call the 'soul' leave the body as a person 'expires'? Or is life the same as the heartbeat and breathing? Or is the soul the same as breathing? Before these questions can be properly answered, clinicians have to grapple with the notion of brain death, when the person's heart may still be beating weakly, their breathing is slight, and some reflexes of the limbs may be intact.

4. The Limbic System

The limbic system consists of the following structures:

1. the cingulate gyrus;
2. the cingulum;
3. the corpus callosum;
4. the fornix (which is an extension of the hippocampus);
5. the thalamus;
6. the hypothalamus;
7. the mammillary body (which is the anteroinferior end of the fornix, the two fornices forming a structure that looks like a 'wishbone');
8. the hippocampus;
9. the amygdala (which is the terminal of the tail of the caudet nucleus);
10. the olfactory bulb.

The olfactory bulb is an important part of the limbic system because it arouses sexual desire in mammals, including humans. For instance, when a female dog is in heat, it attracts many male dogs from miles away. Perfume worn by women has the same end result in men, although the human olfactory bulb has lost much of its instinctive, phylogenetic functions.

A dog's olfactory bulb is 10,000 times more powerful in function than a human's. For this reason, dogs are trained to sniff drugs, gun power, human scent, for instance, and other substances in order to detect illegal smuggling at many airports or the presence of humans buried in the debris after an earthquake.

Recall that the caudet nucleus is an important part of the basal ganglia, disorders of which result in Huntington's disease; the patient has abnormal chorea-like involuntary movements, a pathological behaviour that gives it a nickname 'Huntington's chorea'. But the amygdala belongs to the limbic system, bilateral disorders of which result in the failure to differentiate edible things and not edible things; the patient may eat a shoe sole as if it were a piece of meat.

The limbic system is, therefore, an important system as the source of emotional impulses (e.g., joy, sorrow, love, sex, pleasure and hate), among other things, to become proto-meanings, as part of the brain functions of meanings, not only for humans but also for other mammals, albeit not with the same degrees of functions. Structurally, it encircles or is tucked in around the brainstem with the 'wishbone', bounds the neck between diencephalon and telencephalon. Since functionally it handles emotions and is involved in the brain functions of memory, albeit not the only place that controls memory, it is regarded as a mini brain.

Indeed, the human limbic system shows very little difference, like the brainstem, from that of lower mammals; it is nicknamed the 'old mammalian brain'. Its functional importance in terms of behaviour has recently been emphasized not only for affect but also for thinking which is essential to both cognition and memory. Recall the important role played by the thalamus in the looping of impulses of the extra-pyramidal tract before such impulses exit through the pyramidal tract. It is for this reason that I have advocated that cognition and memory are two sides (i.e., heads and tails) of the same coin, a theoretical construct that will be illustrated in Part IV and elaborated upon further in a later book *Language Disorders: A Critical Perspective*. A precursor of this elaboration, entitled 'Memory and cognition: what are they?', was presented as a keynote lecture on 16 June 2003 during the 84th Annual Meeting of the AAAS, Pacific Division, in San Francisco. It is incorporated in Chapter 12.

5. The Cerebellum

The cerebellum comes from mesencephalon but is not a part of the brainstem. Its functions used to be regarded as pertaining only to voluntary movements.

However, recently, because of several cerebellar disorders which impair language behaviour, memory, and cognition, its importance in respect to intellectual functions has been gradually recognized.

One such disorder is known as Olivo-ponto-cerebellar atrophy (now called spinocerebellar ataxia, SCA for short), the characteristic of which is the atrophy of the cerebellum. The symptoms are neurodegenerative. The patient falls occasionally but the frequency of this gradually increases; hand movements are severely compromised, to the extent that if he/she knows how to write, the written words are illegible; for this reason, patients in an advanced stage of SCA often refuse to write. Since the disorder is neurodegenerative, the patient gradually becomes demented, suggesting that either the cerebellum itself has the functions pertinent to language behaviour or the disorder is 'contagious' and, therefore, can spread to the cerebral cortex. The prominent symptoms of dementia are language disorders. There are now 25 types of SCA, most of which, with the exception of SCA8, SCA10, and SCA12, are caused by CAG trinucleotide repeat expansions on different chromosomal loci; all SCAs are autosomally dominant, which is to say that either parent can pass the disease genetically to the offspring.

Recall that a nucleotide consists of a special kind of complex sugar (deoxyribose), a phosphate and one of four nitrogen-containing bases, that is, A (adenine), T (thymine), G (guanine) and C (cytosine). Each one of these bases is a molecule. It is each sugar-phosphate linkage that is tied to a base. However, as the linkage of sugar-phosphate is usually skipped, and there are two chains in the helix, both bases in the two chains follow a specific correspondence. That is, every T base in one chain must correspond to an A base in the other chain; likewise, every G base in one chain must be paired with a C base in the other chain.

These correspondences may repeat, expanding to a certain range for a normal person. For instance, the TA correspondence (i.e., T in one chain and A in the other chain) may repeat within a certain range without causing any abnormality, which is called the normal range. When a mutation occurs, that range may be expanded to result in abnormality.

When the correspondences do not obey the two restrictions just mentioned, for instance, instead of a G corresponding to a C and a T corresponding to an A, a patient may have a C corresponding also to a C within a nucleotide, an A corresponding also to an A in the next nucleotide, and a G corresponding also to a G in still the next nucleotide in a DNA allele, a mutation is said to have occurred and such abnormal correspondences are called homozygosity in a trinucleotide sequence written as CAG, because they come from both parents. If this abnormal trinucleotide sequence repeats and expands beyond the normal range on chromosome 8 written as 8q23, the abnormalities are identified as homozygotic SCA16, which causes cerebellar atrophy in the patient's brain. The patient's brain functions will deteriorate, leading eventually to dementia. If the repeats appear in only one chain of DNA in the allele, failing to observe the strict correspondences required, the resultant SCA is called heterozygotic; for example, SCA1, identified on chromosome 6 and written as

6p23, because the abnormal trinucleotide repeat expansion, CAG, comes from one parent.

On the other hand, the neurodegenerative disorder may also affect the limbic system, creating an emotional deterioration that manifests itself in the patient's behaviour. I have mentioned the functional connections of the Papez circuit and the brain functions of memory, which suggest that the brain functions of emotion play an important role in relation to the brain functions of memory. There now exist several studies pertinent to contributions of the cerebellum to the brain functions of memory and to linguistic production (Snider, 1976; Silveri, 1998; Silveri and Leggio, 1994).

I have examined several patients with SCA, who have varying degrees of language impairment. The most serious case was a woman in her late fifties, who was confined to a wheelchair; she could still talk but her language disorder was quite obvious. The disorder was genetically transmitted. If at all possible, a cross-linguistic and cross-cultural assessment of language disorders in patients with SCA would be extremely interesting, for most neurologists and aphasiologists are not aware that the genetic disorder causes not only language disorder but also dementia, which is the consequence of differential manifestation of degenerative language disorder over time and not a disease. This awareness, however, is not tantamount to saying that when the defective (or mutant) gene was intact, it controlled or was exclusively responsible for the brain functions of language.

In contrast to basal ganglionic diseases which produce involuntary movement disorders of the limbs, cerebellar diseases, including SCA, impair voluntary movements. That is, if the patient does not do anything with the limbs or the vocal apparatus, the symptoms are not obvious; but the moment the patient intends to do something with any of those body parts, the irregular movements appear. However, such impaired voluntary movements are not considered movement disorders.

The role of the cerebellum in the brain functions of memory is only beginning to draw attention from neuroscientists. I will add that when a congenital deaf signer has SCA of any type, will the speech pathologist consider his/her voluntary disorders of the limbs a form of language disorders or of 'speech' disorders or of something else?

Structurally, the cerebellum has three parts; the median portion (called also vermis 'worm') and two lateral lobes (the hemispheres). These structures are connected with the brainstem by three bundles of fibres: superior cerebellar peduncle connecting the midbrain; middle cerebellar peduncle connecting the pons; and inferior cerebellar peduncle connecting the medulla oblongata and, by extension, the spinal cord. If the cerebellum is flattened and spread out, it can cover half of an open newspaper; in comparison, if the cerebrum is also flattened and spread out, it can cover the whole of an open newspaper.

The comparison suggests that the cerebellum, when flattened, occupies more or less the same space area as a cerebral hemisphere but, when folded up, it is smaller. That is to say, the cerebellum is more neatly packed in the cranium, suggesting that there are more intricate neuronal interconnections

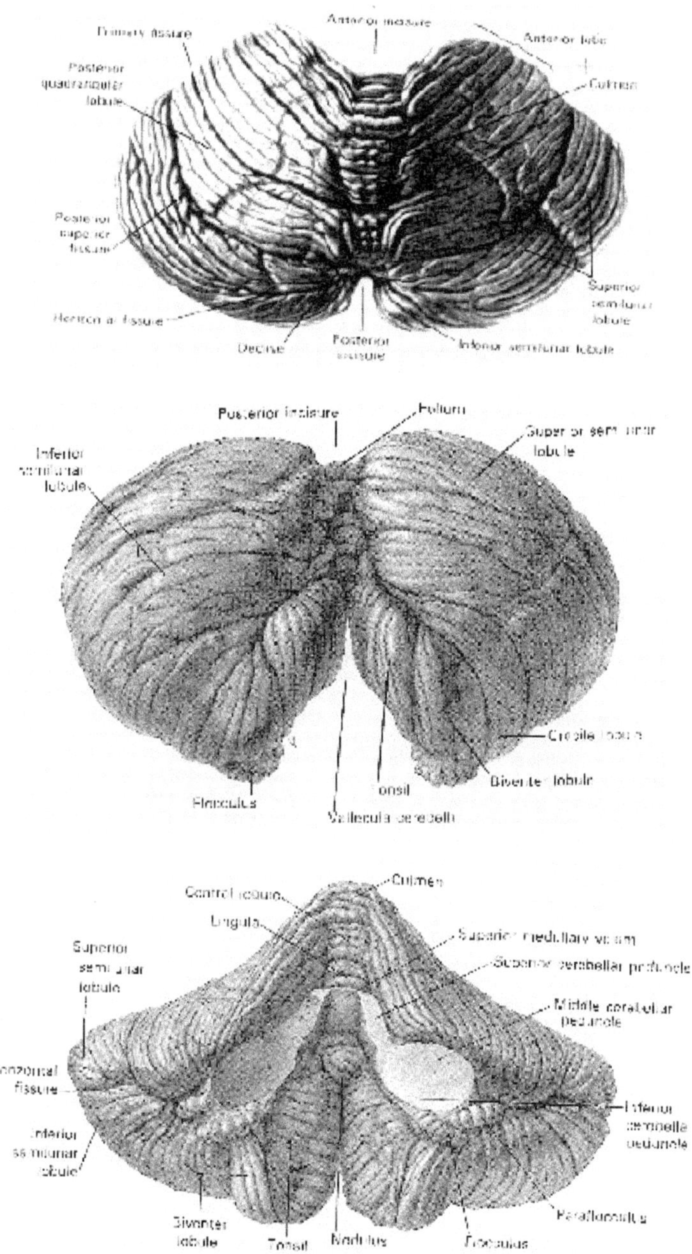

Figure 11.15 *Superior, posteroinferior, and inferior views of the cerebellum* (From Malcolm C. Carpenter, *Human Neuroanatomy*, 7th Edition, copyright © Lippincott Williams and Wilkins, 1976. Used by permission of Lippincott Williams and Wilkins.)

in the cerebellum than in a cerebral hemisphere. For instance, there are five kinds of cells in the cerebellum:

1. Purkinje cells (the largest cells with more dendrites than any other neurons in the brain);
2. granule cells (the smallest cells but most numerous in the brain, with 6 million packed together per square millimetre in the cerebellum);
3. stellate cells;
4. Golgi cells (next to Purkinje cells in size);
5. Basket cells.

In addition, there are neuroglias which support the dendritic processes of the Purkinje cells.

One amazing feature of the interconnections within the cerebellum is the fact that one Purkinje cell alone receives up to 200,000 inputs: these inputs are from granule cells mostly, and also from cells outside the cerebellum; however, the axon of the Purkinje cell provides the sole output of the cerebellar cortex, through each of the peduncles.

Another intriguing feature is the role played by the granule cells in their interconnections with the Purkinje cells and the other types of neurons. The axon of every granule cell rises vertically out of the granule cell layer, making multiple inputs with its overlying Purkinje cell; the axon then splits into two segments that stretch in opposite directions, each aligning into parallel fibres that run through the dendrites of a Purkinje cell like wires through an electric pole, providing a single input to many hundreds of Purkinje cells (Bower and Parsons, 2003: 43). In so doing, the granule cells also communicate with the three other types of neurons which help modulate the signals emitted by both the granule cells and the Purkinje cells (ibid.: 43). It is the interconnections of such synaptic features that have increasingly drawn attention from neuroscientists for a better scrutiny of the cerebellar participation of brain functions in memory and cogntion in relation to language in the brain.

When there is a lesion in the cerebellum, it affects the expression plane in a way different from the impairment caused by a lesion in any other part of the brain, such as the cerebrum as a whole or the basal ganglia. The cerebellar impairment of language is most noticeable in what is known as 'cerebellar speech'; in the case of sign language, the patient will have great difficulty signing, just as he/she will have great difficulty drinking tea from a cup or soup from a spoon without spilling it. The content plane may also be impaired by a lesion in the cerebellum, especially when it is a right side lesion, or atrophy as in SCA, with respect to memory that also pertains to linguistic production and emotions. But as far as I know no study is available in the literature concerning such impairments; I am probably the first and only neuroscientist beginning to study language disorders in cerebellar damage, including different types of SCA.

6. The Spinal Cord

The spinal cord, although it is a significant part of the central nervous system, has been avoided by researchers as irrelevant to language, in particular, the individual aspect of language; I am almost certainly the only one in neuroscience who takes the spinal cord seriously as relevant to the individual aspect of language, in respect to not only sign language but also oral language. One reason for this is that language had been regarded as only oral (until 1962) without due consideration to sign language and the awareness of dementia in SCA in relation to memory impairment.

But even with sign language being regarded as language there are still some sign language experts who have claimed that sign language, like oral language, is manipulated by the left hemisphere of the cerebrum, without realizing that even oral language is not manipulated by the left cerebral hemisphere. Such a claim will be dealt with seriously and refuted in Part IV. In the meantime, I will describe briefly the structure of the spinal cord and the nerves attached to it.

The spinal cord, as the extension of the medulla oblongata, is a continuous unsegmented structure; thus, the spinal cord belongs to the central nervous system. It goes all the way from the cervix (the neck) to the lower border of the first lumbar vertebra (Carpenter, 1976: 213). In between there are many nerves attached to it, which are divided into five regions: cervical nerves; thoracic nerves; lumbar nerves; sacral nerves; and coccygeal nerve.

These nerves, together with the autonomic system and the cranial nerves, belong to the peripheral nervous system. It is this peripheral nervous system that enables the individual to maintain contact with the external and the internal environments (which include the uterus for the foetus before birth). The contact is important to language in the brain as behaviour for not only the expression plane but also the content plane; the latter may surprise many neuroscientists. I shall explain below the important relevance of the peripheral nervous system to both the expression plane and the content plane, in respect to memory, through the varying interplays of the spinal cord and the brain in connection with the peripheral system, because without the peripheral nervous system, the individual simply cannot conduct human interactions; hence, the individual aspect of language is multifaceted. The reason is that the patterning of such human interactions through the expression plane constitutes the social aspect of language.

6.1 The Spinal Cord and Dementia

In the section on the cerebellum, I mentioned the genetically transmitted disease Olivo-ponto-cerebellar atrophy, a term that was first introduced by Déjérine and Thomas (1900). This was first thought to be a disease involving only the brainstem (the olivar nucleus and the pons) and the cerebellum (Critchley and Greenfield, 1948). It was later further elaborated by Machado and Joseph, for whom the disease was given an eponym called Machado–Joseph disease. However, as more and more different types of SCA have been described in the literature through clinical and genetic examinations, in connection with the spinal cord, the old term was abandoned and the new term, Spino-Cerebellar Ataxia (SCA) was introduced; as a result, the Machado–Joseph disease (MJD) was designated as SCA3.

There are now at least 25 types of SCA, all of which are autosomally dominant with different chromosomal loci. The symptoms of behavioural degeneration and the progressive course of dementia resulting from SCA are language disorders first in expression plane and then involving content plane; the patient will be confined to a wheelchair, with little mobility, and later become bedridden and mute with severe memory impairment, just like other demented patients in AD, FD, HD, PD, or the like, suggesting the relevance of the spinal cord to the brain functions of memory.

These different types of SCA, with the exception of SCA8, SCA10 and SCA12, are caused by a CAG trinucleotide repeat expansion in the coding region of the respective genes, resulting in an expanded glutamine repeat. The three other types are caused by untranslated (CTA)n/(CTG)n for SCA8, (ATTCT)n for SCA10, and (CAG)n for SCA12. Most of these types are homozygotic, whereas some (SCA1, SCA2, SCA3, SCA6, SCA7, SCA8, SCA12) are heterozygotic, which is to say that the repeats are found in only one chain of DNA in the allele, which do not follow the restrictions of correspondences of the bases in the other chain of the allele.

In this connection, I should mention the brain functions of memory in relation to phantom limbs which are discussed in an interesting article by Ronald Melzack (1992); there are other publications before and after 1992 by Melzack and/or others concerning phantom limbs and pain sensations associated with phantom limbs as a result of amputation or spinal cord injury. Even phantom seeing and phantom hearing have also been reported. So, I will describe briefly the literature and my own clinical experiences with epileptic patients.

6.2 Interplay of the Spinal Cord and the Brain

To explain phantom limbs, Melzack postulates the idea of a neuromatrix, a network of neurons, that, in addition to responding to sensory stimulation, continuously generates a characteristic pattern of impulses, which he calls a neurosignature, indicating that the body is intact and unequivocally one's own (1992: 123). According to Melzack, such a neuromatrix involves three major neural circuits in the brain:

1. the classical sensory pathways passing through the thalalmus to the somatosensory cortex;
2. the pathways leading through the reticular formation of the brainstem to the limbic system, which is critical for emotion and motivations;
3. cortical regions important to recognition of the self and to the

evaluation of sensory signals, especially the parietal lobe which has been shown to be essential to the sense of self.

Melzack's idea of a neuromatrix has been modified by Gallagher (1995) as 'body schema', which he uses interchangeably with 'body knowledge'. However, there is no discussion of phantom perception, such as phantom seeing and phantom hearing. I suspect that, in keeping with this line of observation, phantom smell may also happen, if looked into, or even phantom taste, as will be shown later.

In 2003, at the 55th Annual Meeting of the American Academy of Neurology, H. Branch Coslett expands Gallagher's idea by distinguishing three types of body representation; namely, 'body schema', 'body image' and 'body structural description'. His definitions of the three terms, in his presentation 'Body Schema Representation (Patients and Function MRI)', are as follows (see Coslett, 2003): 'The term *body schema* refers to an on-line, real-time representation of one's own body in space that is derived from sensory input (including muscle, proprioceptive, cutaneous, vestibular, tactile, visual and auditory). The body schema provides a three dimensional, dynamic representation of the body in space that articulates with motor systems in the genesis of action' (Gallagher, 1995).

Coslett then goes on to say that 'the *body image* refers to conceptual knowledge about the body in general as well as knowledge of the role and function of body components. This representation is thought to be primarily propositional in nature, and is **thought to be linked to the verbal system** (emphasis mine). Finally, as the body image consists of a set of beliefs about the body as well as one's conceptual understanding of the body in general, it is readily accessible to consciousness.'

In contrast, the *body structural description* is said to 'refer to a representation of the shape and contours of the human body in general and one's own body in particular. This representation defines a detailed plan of the body surface on which the location of body parts and boundaries between body parts are encoded; additionally, the relative positions of body parts are defined in this representation. Like structural descriptions for familiar objects, the body structural description is assumed to be viewpoint independent.'

All this actually points to the interplay of the spinal cord and the brain in terms of the brain functions of memory. That phantom limbs have been reported, but not 'phantom ear' (albeit phantom hearing) or 'phantom nose' or 'phantom eye' (albeit phantom seeing) or even 'phantom tongue' may be because limbs are motor-controlled, that is, movable, body parts, although eyes and tongue are also movable, while ears and nose are not. Therefore, I have speculated that sensory input alone, as suggested by Melzack, may not enable the brain, in spite of the involvement of the limbic system and the parietal lobe as Melzack has suggested, to retain the images (i.e., impulses) of those body parts after they have been detached from the main body. Perceptions through the five senses seem to be quite a different matter to which I shall return.

Images of the body parts will remain in the brain if and only if these body parts were originally also involved in body movements.

To support this explanation, I refer to an article, published in 1994, by Aglioti, Bonazzi and Cortese. But, in the same year, Aglioti, Cortese and Franchini also published an article, entitled 'Rapid sensory remapping in the adult human brain as inferred from phantom breast perception' which seems to counter my explanation. However, I must hasten to add that while the chest muscles can move one breast or both up and down, before the mastectomy, the facial muscles cannot move ears or nose in any direcion. Since the tongue is the most movable body part, if a person has his/her tongue cut off, I am willing to further speculate that he/she may experience 'phantom tongue'. It follows that my explanation still stands, upholding the relevance of the motoric interplay between the spinal cord, the cranial nerves involved in motor functions, and the brain to the brain functions of memory.

There is also plenty of clinical evidence in the literature from patients with stroke, which will support the idea of body schemata in each individual's brain formed by that individual's brain functions of memory. Examples are neglect, inattention (or attention deficit), denial, prosopagnosia and the like. In the paramedical literature, for instance, neglect is regarded as 'a syndrome in which a patient fails to recognize one side of the body and the environmental space surrounding that side' (Love and Webb, 1996: 242–4). Put differently, the patient had had the body schemata intact in the brain prior to the stroke which then partially destroyed the schemata, leaving him/her to deny or neglect that part of the body even though it is free of paralysis. Thus, rather than calling neglect a syndrome, it is better explained as a form of memory impairment involving the partial destruction of body schemata.

Despite my explanation, I am willing to accept another explanation; that is, nobody has asked those patients who lost an ear or the nose as to whether they felt or perceived as if those body parts still existed. Even if there are such reports, the involvement of the spinal cord, the brainstem, through the sensory input, in the retention of images of body parts in the brain as part of the brain functions of memory cannot be disputed. In support of this statement, see Berlucchi and Aglioti (1997) and Aglioti *et al.*, (1997).

On the other hand, the lack of such information may also arise from the use of different terminologies in medical practice. For instance, I have interviewed many epileptic patients who told me that they had experienced tinnitus (ringing or buzzing in the ears) pre- and/or post-operatively. It is also known in epileptology that epileptic patients, especially patients with TLE (temporal lobe epilepsy), often experience an aura minutes or even seconds before a seizure attack; an aura is a warning sensation (strange smell or taste or a stream of 'air' (*Chi* in Chinese) coming from the abdomen). I am willing to speculate that tinnitus is phantom hearing, and that an epileptic aura could be phantom smell or phantom taste.

7. The Autonomic System

There are two subsystems in the autonomic system: the Sympathetic Subsystem and the Parasympathetic Subsystem. They regulate functions of the viscera, including sweating, heartbeat, breathing (i.e., pulmonary ventilation), sexual activities (such as secretion for erection, ejaculation, ovulation, menstruation), and excretion for urination and bowel movement, and the like.

The autonomic system is important because it tells the brain the goings-on of the internal environment; anything that goes wrong in such an environment must be conveyed to the central nervous system via impulses; the central nervous system, the brain in particular, must decide to do something as behaviour which may be verbal (i.e., through oral language) or non-verbal (i.e., through sign language or gesticulation). It is these impulses from the autonomic system that enable the individual to seek help, medical or otherwise, or choose the right words about the feelings (i.e., the meanings of his/her body conditions) when speaking to a physician if the individual feels sick. The physician can then reconstruct his/her own meanings, on the basis of the sounds heard or gestures seen, for a diagnosis in order to prescribe medicine.

Recently, many biomechanical experts have tried to build artificial hearts for transplantation to patients who have incurable cardiac diseases. It should be emphasized that the heart is not just a pump to push blood into the brain and other body parts for nutrition. It is regulated by the autonomic system in order to respond to the central nervous system, particularly to the brain, in case of startle, shock, or other unexpected external environmental disasters. For instance, when startled, the individual's heartbeat has to increase several times in order to supply more blood to the brain which has the top priority for blood, or else the individual may pass out. An artificial heart is a pump which cannot respond to the brain in this way. Thus, any individual wearing an artificial heart cannot face extremely startling shock or stress. Likewise, any person wearing a pace-maker for his/her heart has to be excluded from any magnetic field, such as MRI (magnetic resonance imaging) which emits a powerful magnetic field, or else that person's pace-maker, made of metal, will be displaced or may even be destroyed to his/her detriment.

PART IV THE INDIVIDUAL ASPECT OF *LANGUE*

General Remarks

Recall that Saussure's distinction of *langue* and *parole* is a methodological convenience for the sake of epistemology. Therefore, there was no need for him to be concerned with the brain functions of language. 'The object of study in linguistics is not the immediately given phenomenon' (Thibault, 1997: 14). But the distinction of the Social Aspect and the Individual Aspect I have proposed and introduced as 'A Mild Proposal' in Chapter 4 is no longer an epistemological issue; rather, it is an ontological issue that must be taken seriously. Hence, this individual aspect of *langue* is based on the individual aspect of *parole* previously described, and continues the elaboration of the mild proposal set forth above. That is, unless the individual aspect of *parole* is clearly understood and well kept in mind, the reader may have some difficulty comprehending the principles behind these chapters. However, these chapters are intended only to illustrate some fundamental features of the mild proposal, which is to say that they are not meant to be exhaustive in my exploration of the individual aspect of language.

Given such a distinction, there is no denying that while language has the social aspect, because no individual can live alone – for example, by him-/herself without recourse to social interactions which shape his/her reservoir of experiences in his/her memory – it also has the individual aspect. There have been reports about children deprived of such interactions and the consequences they faced; for example, the wild child of Aveyron in France (Itard, 1894), or *Wolf Child and Human Child* (Gesell, 1941) and, recently, Gennie in Los Angeles.

Without too much ado with their consequences, I shall now speak of the individual aspect of *langue* as a continuation or on the basis of the individual aspect of *parole* in order to pursue the general theme of 'What is language?'. In so doing, I shall concentrate on the brain functions of memory by first reviewing briefly the current theories on memory and cogntion, and then presenting my own theory as an alternative and more plausible (or realistic) view. Thus, this Part is divided into five chapters and aims to indicate what the individual aspect of language will look like.

12 Language in the Brain is Memory-Governed

The brain functions of memory and cognition have intrigued so many people in all walks of life for many centuries, and yet their relationships have remained the greatest enigma in neuroscience and the behavioural sciences. The enigma is compounded by different views regarding the neural substrates of these brain functions. Thus, dozens of theories of memory, on the one hand, and of cognition, on the other, have been offered in not only neuroscience but also psychology, each contradicting the other. For instance, some neuropsychologists regard memory as a part of cognition, consisting of learning, thinking and memory, while neurologists tend to feel comfortable with the idea that memory and cognition are subserved by different brain structures, that is, memory by the two hippocampi and cognition by the neocortex as a whole, especially the frontobasal systems. In keeping with this trend, memory and cognition have been the centrepiece in psychology, especially cognitive psychology and neuropsychology. Thus, different classificatory dichotomies have also been offered:

1. short-term vs. long-term memory;
2. episodic vs. semantic memory;
3. implicit vs. explicit memory;
4. procedural vs. declarative memory;
5. encoding, consolidation and retrieval.

However, linguists have always shunned memory, and even declared that memory has nothing to do with the ideal speaker/hearer's knowledge of its language, if that monster has language at all. Of course, the ideal speaker/hearer was a fictional monster created by Chomsky, and therefore it had no brain functions and no need for memory of any kind. Unfortunately, many linguists have followed that idea since the 1960s, although I am not sure whether semioticians have bought into this idea or not. To replace this ideal speaker/hearer, a new fiction is produced, called language template, which is claimed to be innate.

But a real human being's every move and act as behaviour, including language behaviour, depend entirely on his/her brain functions of memory. For this reason, I have objected strongly to neuroscientists' limitation/confinement of memory to the two hippocampi in the limbic system. I have advocated that not only the two hippocampi but also the cerebral cortex, the basal ganglia, the two thalami and the cerebellum are involved in the brain functions of memory for language behaviour.

Nevertheless, some linguists began to embrace cognition by parroting cognitive psychology probably because of the most unfortunate historical fact that in the 1960s someone started to call linguistics a branch of cognitive psychology. Thus, there has now appeared a brand of linguistics called Cognitive Linguistics which may be another offshoot of TG or just a 'bastard', without specifying what the brain functions of cognition are; they only take 'cognition' as a given, as if it is understood by everybody, when this is not the case.

Recently, however, a new theory called Working Memory has been proposed, which is claimed to be subserved by the prefrontal cortex. It is said to consist of a central executive and two slaves, which are phonological loop and visuo-spatial scratch pad: the latter is metaphorically likened to a 'blackboard of the brain'. Some neurologists, behavioural neurologists in particular, have adopted this framework in part by taking only the executive function for their interests in cognition while ignoring the two slaves which are too simplistic.

Such a framework further complicates the existing problem in the relationship of memory and cognition. It is asserted that working memory is a tripartite network for very brief short-term memory in the prefrontal cortex and is somehow used to manipulate other information and to draw on multiple parts of the brain; it is then claimed to be dedicated to other cognitive functions as well, such as object recognition, language production and comprehension, and mathematical reasoning or the like. The brain functions of memory do not work that way. But, for the possibility of making a distinction between long-term and short-term memory, Hebb in 1949 had long suggested that there might be two neurophysiologically separate storage systems within the brain: temporarily reverberating circuits, which are electrically based; and a permanent change based on a growth of links between nerve cells.

Whether Hebb was right or not, working memory has now replaced short-term memory, the theories of which had peaked in the 1950s. More incredible is the fact that short-term memory (hence, working memory) is, for all intents and purposes, equated with consciousness by some, a brain function that is usually attributed to the reticular formation in the brainstem, rather than to the prefrontal cortex.

In as much as a great deal of enthusiasm has been generated from working memory by its proponents and their followers, there exist plenty of epistemological problems on theoretical and empirical grounds, which fundamentally flaw the framework. For instance, every experiment conducted to uphold working memory allows subjects at least a couple of seconds to recall, or respond to, a task, without regard to the time during which the neurons supposedly controlled by stimulation and/or suppression have already interacted in milliseconds with millions of neurons in many other parts of the subject's brain.

There are thousands of instances of language behaviour in daily life that simply cannot be experimented, because the impulses in neuronal communication in the nervous system (central and peripheral) are transduced too fast (in milliseconds) to merit any artificial (and, I must add, simple) experiments, some of which will be illustrated later. Such daily instances of the brain functions of memory and cognition can be observed routinely but cannot be experimented.

Another major problem is that without first specifying what language is to the experimenters, the proponents of working memory simply take language for granted by asserting that it handles other cognitive functions such as language production and comprehension through the two slave systems (Goldman-Rakic, 1992) in the prefrontal lobe. Such problems have seldom been pointed out in the literature or have been largely overlooked by other neuroscientists until now.

Some psychologists or psycholinguists may even attempt to counter that language in the brain is attention-governed, instead of memory-governed, and that language disorders are a result of attention deficits. However, I shall repudiate such notions on the ground that while there are impulses as the brain functions of memory, modulated by CREB proteins, which many brain structures emit, such as the cerebral cortex, the hippocampus, the thalamus and the cerebellum, there are no impulses to be called the brain functions of attention from comparable brain structures. At best, attention is mediated by excitatory or inhibitory impulses in the course of neuronal interactions without any structural origins.

Whatever attention may be in neurophysiological and neuroanatomical terms, such mediation may result in one of three ways in respect to the brain functions of memory: improvement, no change and hindrance (see Peng, 2001). Therefore, attention can in no way govern any behaviour, human or otherwise, although it can influence behaviour, as in neglect. However, as I have already pointed out, neglect is better explained as a form of memory impairment, the loss of a body schema in the patient's brain. Such being the case, attention may and will be regarded as belonging to the brain functions of memory as mechanism.

1. Memory vs. Cognition

Whatever cognitive linguistics may be, practitioners of this brand of linguistics have never given much thought to the notion of cognition; that is, they do not know or have not defined what cognition is in behavioural neurology or neuroscience. Even Saussure himself uses the term *psychique* (which is translated as 'psychological' by Baskin) in relation to the speech circuit in a very vague way, as if it refers to something inexplicable in the mind of the individual, so much so that the term becomes a 'waste basket' for something that is not accountable in his framework. 'Psychological' is then changed to 'psychic' in Thibault (1997: 134).

To cognitive psychologists or neuropsychologists, on the other hand, e.g., Tulving who gave a keynote lecture at the 1996 Annual Meeting of the AAAS in

Seattle on the brain functions of memory, which I attended, memory is a part of or subsumed by cognition. I suspect that in his view, which is shared by most if not all psychologists dealing with memory, cognition consists of learning, thinking and memory.

In this chapter, I shall now offer my own framework as a part of the 'Mild Proposal', in terms of which the issues surrounding memory and cognition will be delineated in order to put them in the right theoretical perspective. The new framework will be advocated, with anatomical and neurophysiological evidence in the literature, to support the idea that memory and cognition cannot be two separate entities of the brain functions any more than memory can be a part of cognition in the brain or switched to working memory as short-term memory however brief it may be.

Presumably, this hierarchical relationship of memory and cognition is based on the traditional assumption in neuroscience that memory is subserved by the two hippocampi, which are two subcortical structures in the limbic system, whereas cognition is the function of the cerebral cortex as a whole. However, this assumption has now been criticized from many behavioural neuroscientists, especially from me, because of research resulting from epileptology on patients with epilepsy. I have found that all forms of epilepsy, symptomatic, idiopathic, or cryptogenic, cause the patient to have language disorders of various degrees, because language in the brain as behaviour is memory-governed.

To me, therefore, memory cannot be a part of or subsumed by cognition, because they are two sides (heads and tails) of the same coin and subserved by the same sets of brain functions. Memory deals with the past and the past in the present (never with the future, because it has yet to be experienced by any individual), whereas cognition refers to the handling of the goings-on of the here-and-now by the individual's brain.

That the future cannot be dealt with by the brain functions until it becomes a reality in the present can be vividly illustrated by the terrorists' multiple attacks on September 11 2001 in New York, Washington DC and Pittsburgh, and the subsequent attacks in Europe such as in London on July 7 2005 and what have followed since then or will follow for many years to come.

The United States government had been planning to build a missile shield, with nuclear weapons, to protect the US homeland against attack from a hostile or terrorist country. Nobody had thought of Pearl Harbour in the same way as the suicidal terrorist attacks on the World Trade Center and the Pentagon, because the attacks on September 11 2001 were a future terrorist behaviour to the government's planning based on the past in the present and the goings-on prior to that date, which could not have been dealt with or even anticipated until it happened; by then it was too late to handle the goings-on of the here-and-now, because the future, once it happens to become a reality, cannot be handled retroactively, as if the reality is still in the future. There are no such things as the goings-on of the here-and-now in the future. The fourth plane that went down in the suburb of Pittsburgh, as it was learned later, was targeted at the White House. Had it successfully carried out the attack, the goings-on of the cognitive handling would have been unthinkable.

However, all these terrorists' attacks have now become part of the memory, not only in the brains of the world leaders and the rest of their Cabinet members but also in the brains of all human beings who heard or watched the repeated news reports on TV. Such memories have also become the past in the present for these people to plan (and/or talk about) the prevention of similar attacks in the future on the basis of the daily handling of the goings-on of the here-and-now. As a result of such planning, a new department, called Department of Homeland Security, was established.

It is no exaggeration to say that Operation Iraqi Freedom, as the code name for the war that lasted less than a month to topple Saddam Hussein's regime, would not have taken place had the terrorrists' attacks on September 11 2001 not occurred. Now that Saddam Hussein's regime no longer exists in the present, which had been dealt with in the past, the memories of terrorists' attacks lingered on, especially during the presidential election year, because the Al Qaeda was deemed capable of launching a major attack during that period, as was alerted by the Department of Homeland Security.

Moreover, Operation Iraqi Freedom has become the past in the present to the extent that Syria was warned by President Bush and Secretary of State Colin Powell, as the new goings-on of the here-and-now, not to harbour Saddam Hussein and his henchmen as they apparently had crossed the border to seek a safe haven in Syria. The terrorist suicidal attacks of foreign residences in Saudi Arabia, in May 2003, when Secretary of State Colin Powell was visiting that country, also brought back many memories of the September 11 attacks in connection with the Al Qaeda. And the goings-on of the aftermath did confirm the involvement of the Al Qaeda.

Now that Operation Iraqi Freedom is over, new goings-on occur daily in Iraq *vis-à-vis* the domestic politics of the United States:

1. American forces suffered casualties daily as a result of guerrilla attacks, now called insurgency;
2. Saddam Hussein was captured, and his two sons had been killed, but their loyalists may be among the insurgents;
3. the American coalition forces handed over the sovereignty on 28 June 2004, two days ahead of schedule, to the Iraqi Interim Government;
4. the big question of re-building Iraq as a democracy has remained;
5. the Interim Prime Minister of Iraq declared a martial law to impose a curfew to crack down on the insurgents;
6. the impact on the American presidential election in November, 2004, was great, with fierce debates between the two candidates, because the Senate Intelligence Committee has now formally announced that the pre-war intelligence supplied by the CIA, which said that Iraq then had stock piles of WMD (weapons of mass destruction) and could produce nuclear weapons within a decade, was wrong.

As the Democratic ticket, Kerry–Edwards, for the presidential election was complete, each of these goings-on was brought back from the past to the past in the present in the memories of those concerned regarding Saddam

Hussein's 'Trial of the Century' and the justification of the war in Iraq on the issue of WMD. In other words, such daily goings-on became the constant present and the past in the present not only for the American and British troops but also for the troops from other countries in Iraq. More importantly, they would also become the constant present and the past in the present for Mr Bush, Secretary Powell (or his successor), and Secretary Rumsfeld, in the United States, and Mr Blair, in UK, for many years to come, irrespective of who succeed Mr Bush and Mr Blair. I should add that Mr Bush was re-elected for the second term and that one consequence of the re-election was that Secretary Powell resigned and was replaced by Ms Rice, a personnel change that had much to do with the past in the present regarding the Iraqi situations.

2. Brain Functions of Memory

In my view memory is experience-based and time-sensitive. It is experience-based because experiences belong to the content plane and are the source of meaning; it is time-sensitive because forgetting is an important component of memory, without which the individual either develops the clinical symptoms of perseveration in behaviour as a pathology or becomes bombarded daily by past events, as in people who cannot forget the past; these people cannot sleep well and must take sleeping pills every night. Neurodegenerative forgetting in pathology, however, is a different story, as in dementia due to AD, FD, PD, HD, or any other cortical or subcortical disease.

Incidently, dementia is not a disease; it refers to the phenomenon of the overall differences between varying states of the intellectual condition in an individual with neurodegenerative illness caused by gradual neuronal death as in AD, FD, PD, HD, or the like. Thus, there appear to be two brain functions of memory: Memory as Content and Memory as Process; the latter can be divided further into Memory as Capacity and Memory as Mechanism. The detailed discussions of this view will be presented in a future book entitled *Language and the Brain Functions of Memory*. A brief sketch, however, will be provided below.

In the meantime, I will say that the brain functions of memory simply cannot be confined to the two hippocampi in the limbic system (as have been so asserted traditionally by most neuroscientists) on the ground that the brain functions of memory change constantly in milliseconds by way of neuronal synapses across and throughout many parts/regions of the brain – cortical as well as subcortical – including the cerebellum. It is when memory as defined above is called upon to serve the present – for example, recollection of a past event, such as the terrorists' attacks, or for a reminiscence during a conversation or any other behaviour – that memory becomes or merges with cognition.

On the other hand, the brain functions of memory as capacity depends on the individual's experiences. When a person encounters a new situation, such as visiting a foreign country for the first time or President Bush's daily world-wide campaign against terrorism in Afghanistan, Iraq and elsewhere, his/her memory as capacity is greatly enhanced. This is because his/her brain functions of cognition meet with or depend on his/her brain functions of memory; he/she must rely on the past in the present (i.e., experiences in the home country or reports received at the White House, respectively) in order to handle the goings-on of the here-and-now for every event encountered in the foreign country or the day-to-day intelligence report received from the CIA or the military about the war in Afghanistan against the Taliban and Osama bin Laden or the reconstruction of Iraq in cooperation with the interim government.

The goings-on of the here-and-now increase the brain functions of memory as capacity because of familiarity. In the case of a visit to a foreign country, they include shopping, taking a tour, or asking for directions to get back to the hotel when the visitor is lost; so, next time the individual comes back to that foreign country, all these shops and tours, and hotels will become familiar territories in his/her brain functions of memory as capacity.

In the case of Mr Bush and his Cabinet members, especially Secretary Powell and Secretary Rumsfeld, they must have handled the goings-on during Operation Iraqi Freedom against Saddam Hussein's regime. But they must also handle the goings-on in the on-going tasks of the reconstruction of Iraq, coupled with the goings-on of the insurgency waged by Hussein's loyalists and the rival groups, now that Saddam Hussein's regime is gone for good: their goings-on of the here-and-now include the daily briefings from the Cabinet members and the military in Iraq and Afghanistan not only about the experience of each attack on the coalition forces by the insurgents but also on the interim government in Iraq and the new government in Afghanistan. Now that Secretary Rice has taken over Mr Powell's job, she will have to start not only handling the goings-on from where Mr Powell left off but also enhancing her brain functions of memory as capacity by bringing the content of what Mr Powell had had in the past to the present in order to handle the new cognitive goings-on that now keep coming to her office.

On the other hand, the insurgents also have their experiences of carrying out each attack which, on the basis of the previous attacks in their memories, they are likely to improve, modify and change in order to launch the next attack as the future for the American troops and the interim government in Iraq, and the new government in Afghanistan. In this respect, Mr Bush's experiences of the goings-on in the White House greatly increase his brain functions of memory as capacity and cannot be shared by the majority of not only Americans but also people throughout the world.

3. Prediction of the Future and Language Behaviour

In light of the aforementioned, it can be said that prediction of the future is actually only talked about on the basis of the present and the past in the present; it may be anticipated but the anticipation of the future is nine times out of ten a rhetorical proposition. In other words, the future cannot be dealt with or handled in any ontological way; at best, the present may reveal some signs which can lead to various speculations of what may or may not happen in the future. There is a new discipline that specializes in this kind of speculation called futurology; it is very popular in Japan. Many times, however, there is no sign for any ground on which to predict the future; or there may be signs but people pay no attention to or cannot read them. The attacks on September 11 2001 and July 7 2005 were the best examples.

What I am trying to emphasize here is that any prediction of the future, such as weather forecast, stock market, physician's prognosis, political election, or recurrences of the terrorists' attacks, is based solely on the past and/or what is happening in the present. The past and the present must be constantly modified and reviewed as time goes by or the present changes, that is, as new information comes in or new events take place to change the here-and-now. That is to say, the future may or may not come out as predicted or even anticipated in reality on the basis of the present and the past in the present.

A good example of such changes was the FBI's warnings of the terrorists' attacks on the major bridges in New York and California, in early November 2001, a warning that turned out later to be a false alarm; likewise, the accident of A-300 that belonged to the American Airlines, which went down on 12 November 2001 in New York City, had to be evaluated in the context of the previous terrorists' attacks; that is, the previous terrorists' attacks had to be 'retrieved' from the memories of the past in any discussion of the accident. If an individual does not have such memories of the past regarding the previous terrorists' attacks, someone else who does will have to fill in the gap or 'blank' by way of language behaviour for that individual, so that he/she will be able to conduct a decent conversation on the subject without looking 'stupid'.

Another example is the sad suicide report of the British scientist, Dr David Kelly, who had leaked the information to the BBC regarding his role in the fabrication of the intelligence about Iraq's purchase of a large quantity of uranium from Africa. His suicide was in the future when Baghdad fell on 29 April and Operation Iraqi Freedom ended as was publicly announced on 1 May 2003 by President Bush. Nobody could have anticipated that Dr Kelly would commit suicide; or, I should say, nobody could have read the 'signs' of his future behaviour; even Dr Kelly himself could not have predicted, at the time of the closure of Operation Iraqi Freedom or even prior to it as the British and the American governments had been busy gathering the needed intelligence regarding WMD in Iraq in order to go to war, that he would end up committing suicide.

Dr Kelly's apparent suicide was reported to Mr Blair in Japan, during an official state visit to Japan from 18 to 22 July 2003. He said in a TV interview (19 July) that he was shocked to have learned the news and asserted that all politicians and the mass media should show respect and restraint to refrain from further speculations until such time as an independent inquiry of the cause was completed. His reactions certainly became more signs of the present on which the opposition would base their attacks against Mr Blair, to predict the future, so to speak, as he returned to England. Their prediction was that Mr Blair would resign, on the basis of the past and the past in the present, and take the responsibility, but it did not come out the way the opposition wanted. Had Mr Blair resigned, as the opposition wanted him to, his resignation would have signalled the defeat of Operation Iraqi Freedom.

It follows that what Thibault calls mediation of the social-semiological system (= *langue*) and the instantiations of raw data (= *parole*) or what Saussure calls 'the dynamics of signs in social life' (1959: 33), which Thibault uses as the subtitle of his book, is none other than the functioning of the individual's memory about a particular language – English, Japanese, Chinese – or whatever language the individual happens to be capable of; without it, such an individual simply cannot speak and understand the language for social interactions with other individuals who can speak and understand that language. But, interestingly enough, Saussure regards 'a science that studies the dynamics of signs in social life' as a part of 'social psychology' and consequently of 'general psychology'; he quickly adds that 'I shall call it *semiology*' (1959: 33). It is for this reason that this monograph is entitled *Language in the Brain* so as to modify Saussure's view of language in order to tap the brain functions of memory.

One major issue in the study of the brain functions of memory is to unravel two 'tangles' which have traditionally plagued the medical sciences and psychology: the relationships of memory and cognition, which have been the greatest enigma in neuroscience; and the assertion that memory seems to be irrelevant to language behaviour, as may be evidenced by the warning signs of AD quoted from the *Honolulu Advertiser* (page 72). Hopefully, some progress will be made in a future book entitled *Language and the Brain Functions of Memory*. However, a preliminary work dealing with this subject was already presented on 16 June at the 84th Annual Meeting of the AAASPD in San Francisco, entitled 'Memory and cognition: what are they?'. Some highlights are recapitulated here.

4. Brain Functions of Memory as Content

Since the brain functions of memory are experience-based, all experiences that an individual encounters become brain impulses which are his/her memory as content. However, these experiences do not enter the brain through the five senses as icons. That is, they are not received by the brain *en bloc*; rather, these experiences are decomposed into impulses which roam around in the brain. Some if not all of these impulses will be 'erased' (i.e., forgotten) as time goes by but the rest remain in the brain as background noises which will form images, such as body schemata mentioned earlier in connection with phantom limbs, phantom breast, phantom pain, etc. Most neuroscientists regard such background noises as 'trash' or irrelevant to the brain functions of memory. To me, however, the background noises each individual has accumulated through his/her lifetime are precisely the 'treasure' wherein the brain functions of memory can be ascertained.

Before I proceed to elaborate on background noises, I should mention that while they are impulses, which may be excitatory or inhibitory, they are much more than the impulses constituting the brain functions of memory as content. In other words, there are background noises which are engaged in brain functions other than the brain functions of memory as content, as will be shown below.

Such images as background noises, which are considered the brain functions of memory as content, may be divided into two planes; namely, content plane and expression plane. Those in the content plane constitute Thought, which is an inchoate mass of impulses roaming around in the brain; they become concepts (or the signified) in active behaviour (i.e., when there is expression) or passive behaviour (i.e., when there is no expression). Those in the expression plane are equally indeterminate but somewhat complicated, as I shall have to separate the impulses for oral behaviour and the impulses for non-oral behaviour. Both oral and non-oral behaviours are based on body movements but they utilize different pathways: cortico-bulbar and bulbo-cortical pathways for oral behaviour and cortico-spinal and spino-cortical pathways for non-oral behaviour. The reason for this is that all behaviours, in production or reception, require the interactions of impulses from these two planes. So, I will now explain in some detail the impulses in the expression plane first as follows.

The impulses in the expression plane for oral behaviour include not only the impulses for oral language in both production and reception, but also the impulses for other oral noises, such as yawning, sneezing and coughing. To simplify the explanation, I shall concentrate on oral language here.

Those impulses in the expression plane for oral language constitute Sound, which is also equally indeterminate, consisting of numerous acoustic images, but those which have become sound-images (or the signifiers upon which concepts are mapped) in each individual's brain are no more in number than the individual's vocabulary items he/she has acquired in his/her lifetime. The same goes for sign language which is non-oral; its impulses in the expression plane, however, constitute Gesture, which consists of numerous visual images, but those which have become sign-images from visual images in each signer's brain are no more than the vocabulary items he/she has acquired in his/her lifetime.

The impulses in the expression plane for non-language behaviour, then, include all other behaviours, in both production and reception, such as daily body movements in motoric behaviours – for example, eating, walking, playing an instrument, swimming, or even sexual activities – and the perceptions of these motoric behaviours. The discussion of these non-language behaviours will be foregone at this time.

I have mentioned that body schemata or body images are formed through not only sensory stimuli (i.e., experiences) but also the interplay of motoric impulses and sensory stimuli. Such being the case, the events and sounds an individual has experienced and heard from foetal life through infancy and childhood to adulthood must also have become impulses in each individual's brain as part of the background noises. Through the interplay of motoric impulses of the tongue (which is the most movable body part) and the individual's experiences with auditory stimuli, in the case of oral language, or of motoric impulses of the upper limbs and the individual's experiences with visual stimuli, in the case of sign language, concepts and sound-images (or sign-images) are also formed in the individual's brain; they are to become linguistic signs (or coherent images) as part of the brain functions of memory as content, through mapping for production and coupling for reception, which are part of the background noises.

In Saussure's *CLG* (1959), he makes no distinction between acoustic image and sound-image, as these terms appear interchangeably. However, for my purpose, I shall make an ontological distinction between them. That is, the term 'acoustic image' will be used in relation to proto-meanings, whereas the term 'sound-image' will be used when an acoustic image is mapped onto a corresponding meaning from the content plane to become a part of the linguistic sign (or coherent unit which is in keeping with the notion of 'coherence' in electroneurophysiology) in connection with concept. In other words, sound-image is synonymous with *signifiant* and concept is synonymous with *signifié*, the two making up *le signe* in Saussure's terminology, except that it has been modified by me and is no longer in keeping with his original idea (see Peng, 1992b). Likewise, I shall use the term 'visual image' in line with acoustic image, and the term 'sign-image' in keeping with sound-image, when sign language is mentioned.

The two planes of brain functions just briefly described may thus be succinctly depicted in schematic form to illustrate their relationships in the brain as shown in Figure 12.1.

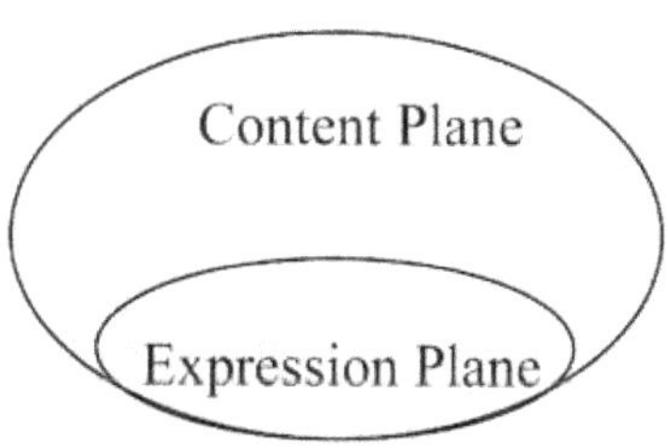

Figure 12.1

5. Brain Functions of Memory as Capacity

An increase of the sheer number of images through experiences, if retained, in both the content plane and the expression plane implies, albeit tacitly, that there is an enormous capacity in the brain functions of memory. However, such a capacity is not at all like a static container or book shelves in a library; rather, it is a dynamic process of familiarity that hinges on how experiences are received into the brain to become memory as content. Put differently, if experiences enter the brain *en bloc* each time, no matter how large the number of neurons there are in the brain, there is simply not enough room in the brain to accommodate all the experiences each individual will have encountered through his/her lifetime. I have posited five processes to account for this situation: decomposition, forgetting, replication (or copying), dreaming and maturation.

5.1 Decomposition

Since each event experienced by the individual is not registered *en bloc*, how is it received in the brain? Electroneurophysiologists have suggested binding and coherence for impulses that come from visual figures. For example, a blue square, whereby the impulse of 'blue' and the impulse of 'square' will bind together in the brain to become a coherent unit in the striat cortex visualized as BLUE SQUARE (Niedermeyer and Da Silva, 1999). In the course of binding and coherence, however, the impulses must be adjusted in the lateral geniculate bodies (probably involving other nuclei in the thalamus as well) in connection with the superior colliculus and the visual cortex, as was pointed out earlier.

Livingston and Hubel (1988), in their researches, have also demonstrated that the bipolar ganglion neurons in the retinae do not respond to a visual stimulus as a whole; rather, they respond to individual components, for example, lines, colour, movements and depth. I assume that this selectivity applies to all visual objects. Thus, I have called the process of such selective responses to any visual object decomposition, pertinent to the brain functions of memory as capacity.

Be that as it may, if this process of decomposition is limited to visual stimuli, the brain functions of memory as capacity will not be able to account for the enormous amount of stimuli that come from the other senses. Fortunately, in the perception of smell (olfactory functions), similar decomposition also takes place (Freeman, 1991; Skarda and Freeman, 1987).

Likewise, in auditory perception the process of similar decomposition plays an important role. For instance, in the inferior colliculi, the superior colliculi, and the medial geniculate bodies, different frequencies of sounds are received and processed, through their interplay with the cerebral cortices (the gyri of Heschl and the auditory association area) for combination or re-combination, before impulses can be understood as integrated percepts in the cerebral cortex.

In the same manner, in tactile perception, the two fasciculi (gracilis and cuneatus) for discriminative touch, proprioception and vibratory sense, and the posterior grey column for other senses, the stimuli are all decomposed presumably after the sensory decussation when the secondary neuron synapses with the tertiary neuron in the thalamus during the thalamo-cortical interplay.

All these stimuli from the five senses must be rapidly, that is, in milliseconds, received by the brain as impulses, involving not just millions of neurons for the incoming impulses, which are the results of the decomposed stimuli, but also the combination and/or the re-combination of these inchoate masses of impulses for interpretations as percepts (i.e., images). Such combination and re-combination of the inchoate masses of impulses may be termed the perceptual organization or the perceptual re-organization of impulses in the brain. These reconstructed images, as a result of the perceptual organization or the perceptual re-organization, are 'potential resources' of background noises in the brain, unless they are 'erased' (i.e., forgotten).

The question here is how the decomposed components of a stimulus (visual, auditory, olfactory, tactile, or the like) come together in the brain to become a single whole, so that the individual can perceive the stimulus as it exists in the real world. Put differently, if binding and coherence of impulses can put together a blue square in the brain so that the individual can perceive that as BLUE SQUARE, I believe binding and coherence also apply to auditory stimuli, olfactory stimuli, tactile stimuli, and the like. The process of decomposition simply allows the brain to increase its capacity for memory.

The process of decomposition can also be verified in the reception and the production of sounds, especially linguistic sounds, like vowels and consonants. Linguists have touched on this process when they talk about prosodies, components, or features without knowing the neural mechanisms involved. For instance, in articulatory phonetics, linguists are familiar with high, mid and low pitches or rising and falling pitch contours in tonal languages when they train students to hear such sounds or when they transcribe a foreign language into phonetics by differentiating aspirated vs. unaspirated, or voiced vs. voiceless stops. In production, linguists are also familiar with articulators, points of articulation, and manners of articulation for consonants, and front or back, high or low, and rounded or unrounded for vowels, and voiced vs. voiceless for both consonants and vowels. But they do not know how the brain, the brainstem, and the cranial nerves function in relation to these components.

In neuroanatomy and neurophysiology, however, these sounds are differentiated in the brainstem by undergoing the process of decomposition to become phonetic features or components or prosodies which can then be received and combined by the cerebral cortex for perception as consonants or vowels. These consonants and vowels, however, become acoustic images in the brain and are mapped onto their corresponding meanings (or concepts) to become coherent sound-images when they come out in accordance with the features or components of decomposition by way of the appropriate cranial nerves working in coordination to become physical sounds; otherwise, they remain decomposed. For instance, articulators in the images of consonants are motoric, involving the trigeminal nerve (Vth), the facial nerve (VIIth), the glossopharyngeal nerve (IXth), and the hypoglossal nerve (XIIth), coupled with the vagus (Xth) for the muscles of the pharynx and the larynx, which also controls the movements of the vocal cords (manipulated by the recurrent laryngeal nerve in the vagus).

It is, I believe, because of decomposition that a native speaker of a language can detect foreign accents when hearing the sounds of a non-native speaker or of lisping from another native speaker. Linguists, unaware of the neural mechanism of decomposition, think that the foreign accents are a result of allophonic displacement (or maladjustment) on the part of the non-native speaker. For instance, if in English the initial aspirated sound [th] for the word *time* is pronounced as an unaspirated [t], the component of aspiration [h] is missing, and therefore the native speaker, when hearing the word *time* pronounced as [taym], instead of [thaym], will decompose the initial alveolar stop [t] as unaspirated (i.e., without the component of [h]), thereby detecting the foreign accent. He/she will then have to re-organize the decomposed features of [t] as equivalent to his/her percept of [th] in the images of *time* in his/her brain, so that he/she can adjust the accented [taym] as [thaym] in order to realize it as *time*, because there is no word in the native speaker's brain as images that correspond to [taym]. The same is true of lisps.

5.2 Forgetting

If images keep piling up in the brain, they will soon overflow. Thus, Mother Nature has built in a process in each individual's brain called forgetting. Because of this, no human adult can remember what he/she did as a child, say, at three years of age. There may be exceptions. For instance, Mozart was a genius who could compose music, at the age of two; for example, the tune of 'Twinkle, Twinkle, Little Star', if the story is true, which he expanded into a beautiful piano sonata when he became an adult.

However, a genius may not forget as easily what is experienced or learned or invented as a non-genius (i.e., an ordinary person). But resistance to forgetting may not be a bliss, as will be shown shortly. What I want to stress here is that an important trait of genius is the extraordinary speed of maturation (which will be explicated further below as an important process of the brain functions of memory as capacity), a speed that is faster than that of an average person's maturation. But if the speed is too fast, say, one year in real time speeding to seven to eight even ten years, the consequence will not be a bliss but a detriment, called progeria (the syndrome of premature aging), which is pathological. It is a rare disease and the incidence is one in eight million infants; there are only 40 or so known cases in the world, and the child's life expectancy is 13 years.

Forgetting, of course, does not have to go all the way back to childhood. Just imagine what happened yesterday or two days ago. Few people, if any, can remember every event or details of such events other than breakfast, lunch or dinner, or some important appointments. Even so, only a summary of each such event is remembered, not its entirety. For instance, when dinner was served yesterday, the food may be remembered the next day but how the dinner was served is usually forgotten.

However, if a person cannot recall what he/she ate yesterday for breakfast, when confronted with such a question one day, and fails to name what he/she ate for breakfast or lunch or dinner, three days in a row, something serious may be happening to his/her brain functions of memory. This is pathological, and is not what I mean here by forgetting which may be called 'normal forgetting'. What is 'normal' and what is 'abnormal' forgetting is, of course, a clinical issue which is difficult to judge with pinpoint accuracy. Fortunately, the issue I am raising here is not clinical but ontological in nature; that is, forgetting is an important process for the brain functions of memory as capacity, because it makes room for selective new experiences to be retained in the form of impulses as background noises in the brain.

5.3 Replication (or Copying)

If an individual keeps losing or forgetting what he/she has already learned or experienced, or cannot remember or repeat what he/she said two minutes or so ago, that person is on his/her way to dementia which is pathological. In other words, memory as capacity is not like bookshelves in a library where, once a book is borrowed, the bookshelves no longer have that book. There must be a built-in process, which I believe is biochemical in nature closely associated with neurotransmitters, whereby the brain can replicate or copy repeatedly the same or similar action potentials on demand each time after one has already been transduced to manifest as a behaviour (verbal or otherwise); or else, the brain would have to accommodate millions of the same acoustic images and visual images in order to last through the individual's lifetime. After all, there is a similar, though not identical, process called hyperplasia, accompanied by mitosis, whereby cells multiply in number; mitosis refers to the duplication process of chromosomes whereas hyperplasia refers to the multiplication process of cells. And there is a complementary process called hypertrophy by means of which cells grow in size. All organisms must have these two processes for growth. I am willing to speculate that CREB (cAMP-Responsive-Element-Binding) protein plays an important role in this regard. This protein is known to sustain the chemical substances called neurotransmitters when they make synaptic changes across the synaptic cleft, resulting in the post-synaptic transduction of impulses as signals. Unless these neurotransmitters, more than 100 are now known, remain active pre-synaptically and post-synaptically, there will be no impulses as signals for neuronal communications, hence, no memory.

Nobody knows exactly how this process of replication works *vis-à-vis* CREB proteins and the brain functions of memory. I would suggest that it seems to counter 'normal forgetting' and helps the mechanism of rehearsal in the brain functions of memory as mechanism. For instance, when a word or a sentence cannot come to mind right away in the midst of a conversation, we all have the experience of saying, 'I was going to tell you something but I can't remember what it was', but after a search for it in the brain, for a few seconds, all of a sudden it 'pops' up. On the other hand, if and when this process of replication is disordered, because of the dysfunction of CREB proteins, the disorder will lead to abnormal forgetting which becomes pathological as in dementia.

However, I must add that without the contiguous neuronal supply of the same or similar impulses, no individual can repeat the same word or sentence twice; nor can he/she transduce any signal in the neuronal network for either production or reception, a behavioural act that requires the repetitious depolarization for the 'same' or similar impulses, without which once an impulse as a signal from a neuron becomes a manifestation in behaviour that impulse is gone for good.

In any case, this is a lifetime work for me and I shall stick to it for a very, very long time, because the brain functions of memory in relation to language in the brain are the greatest enigma in neuroscience. Linguistics and semiotics can no longer afford to overlook the importance of memory in relation to language behaviour, if they are to survive without getting philosophical, which can skip the brain functions of memory and cognition.

5.4 Dreaming

Every human (even a non-human mammal or a lower vertebrate, say, a chicken) dreams. Some dreams can be remembered the next day, or later, but most dreams cannot be remembered the following morning. In the Bible, the Book of Genesis, there are descriptions of dreams by several people, which were remembered: Chapter 37, Joseph's dreams: Chapter 40, the Cupbearer's and the Baker's dreams; Chapter 41, Pharaoh's dreams.

The point I am making is not so much about the contents or interpretations of these dreams as about the neurophysiology of dreaming and of sleep as well as the relationships of these dreams (in content plane) and language behaviour (as manifestation through expression plane in the sleepers).

Most dreams occur during sleep. But what is sleep? And what is the mechanism of sleep that causes the sleeper to dream? These are enigmatic questions which still await a clear definition and plausible answers. For instance, will the observation that the sleeper ordinarily exhibits relative inattention to the environment and is usually immobile suffice?

But some people sleep-walk at night and others may day-dream. Not only that, dolphins and other marine mammals swim while sleeping, and some birds may sleep through long migrations (Siegal, 2003: 72). Fortunately, a few clues have become available regarding the relationships of dreaming and sleeping. So, I will now explore such relationships a little in respect to the brain functions of memory as capacity.

In the neurophysiology of sleep, there are two stages, called REM (Rapid Eye Movement) sleep, or paradoxical sleep, and non-REM sleep, or orthodox sleep. Periods of REM sleep alternate with periods of non-REM sleep, of which four stages of increasing depth are recognized. Thus, in layman's term, the former may be called 'shallow or light sleep' while the latter may be called 'deep or heavy sleep'.

Dreams occur in both REM and non-REM sleep, but in the former, dreams occur more frequently and yet are seldom remembered, because they do not reach normal consciousness in the reticular formation, although a human adult usually spends about a total of two hours each night in REM sleep, which spreads over several periods; in REM sleep, however, if the sleeper awakes while dreaming, the dream is remembered, albeit usually very transiently and fading quickly, unless an effort is made to 'rehearse' the dream, for instance, by telling someone about the dream. The latter, in contrast, for most people, has few dreams which tend to be remembered (Crick and Mitchison, 1983). The authors, then, suggest that unlike normal forgetting, REM sleep has a mechanism which they call 'reverse learning' or 'unlearning'.

Their theory may be substantiated by a recent revelation (Siegal, 2003) that the brain behaves completely differently in the two states of sleep. Three points are worthy of mention here: regional activities in the brain during each state; the consumption of energy in relation to electrical activity in each state; and the overall pattern of activity.

5.4.1 Regional Activities

During waking, neurons are behaving individually, each doing more or less its own business. For instance, most neurons in the forebrain and the brainstem regions are quite active, because the individual must be kept conscious, subserved by all the nuclei including the reticular formation in the brainstem and alert at all times, subserved by the cerebrum including the basal ganglia, the thalamus, the limbic system and the cerebellum.

During non-REM sleep, however, neurons in different brain regions do very different things. Most neurons in the brainstem, immediately above the spinal cord, reduce or stop firing, whereas most neurons in the cerebral cortex and adjacent forebrain regions reduce their activity by only a small amount. In contrast, during REM sleep, brain activity resembles that during waking; that is, neurons are behaving individually. As a result, most neurons in the forebrain and the brainstem region are quite active, signalling other nerve cells at rates as high as rates seen in the waking state (Siegal, 2003: 73).

5.4.2 Consumption of Energy

During non-REM sleep, because most neurons in the cerebral cortex reduce their activity slightly, they fire synchronously, with a relatively low frequency rhythm. But this synchronous electrical activity in non-REM sleep generates higher-voltage brain waves than waking does. As a result, breathing and heartbeat tend to be quite regular during non-REM sleep (ibid.: 73); perhaps, for this reason, the individual dreams much less frequently and, even when he/she does, vivid dreams are rare.

In contrast, however, during REM sleep, because its brain activity resembles that during waking, brain waves remain at low voltage, and the consumption of energy during REM sleep is also as high as during waking. Such neuronal activity accompanies the familiar twitches and eye movement that gave REM sleep its name (ibid.: 73); perhaps, for this reason, the individual dreams more frequently but, when he/she does, the dreams are seldom remembered.

5.4.3 Overall Pattern of Activity

Although in non-REM sleep synchronous electrical activity occurs, a very small group of brain cells, around 100,000 in humans, at the base of the forebrain is maximally active during non-REM sleep. They are called sleep-on neurons whose function it is to induce sleep, although the precise signals that activate the sleep-on neurons are not clear (ibid.: 73).

On the other hand, even though there are also brain cells called REM sleep-on neurons located in the brainstem, they become especially active during REM sleep and appear to be responsible for generating this state of sleep. In addition, however, because dreaming is accompanied by frequent activation of the brain's motor systems (ibid.: 73), not to mention sleep-walking by some individuals, these motor systems must not be left unchecked. Siegal reasons that most movements during REM sleep are inhibited by two complementary biochemical actions involving neurotransmitters: the brain stops releasing neurotransmitters that would otherwise activate motoneurons (the brain cells that control muscles); and the brain also dispatches other neurotransmitters that actively shut down those motoneurons. However, such mechanisms do not affect the cranial nerves which control the muscles that move the eyeballs.

In view of the revelation by Siegal, I will now return to the theory of unlearning (or reverse learning) proposed by Crick and Mitchison (1983) with some comments. The basis of their theory is this:

1. They assume that in viviparous mammals the cortical system (the cerebral cortex and some of its associated subcortical structures) can be regarded as a network of interconnected cells which can support a variety of modes of mutual excitation.
2. Such a system is likely to be subject to unwanted or 'parasitic' modes of behaviour, which arise as it is disturbed by either the growth of complexity in the brain or the modifications produced by experience (e.g., background noses – FCCP).
3. Such modes of behaviour are detected and suppressed by a mechanism of what they call reverse learning or unlearning which operates during REM sleep and has the character of an active process which is, loosely speaking, the opposite of learning.

Since it is during REM sleep periods that the sleeper dreams, but occasionally during non-REM sleep periods as well, the question that can be raised is, 'How can reverse learning occur during dreaming?' The answer, I believe, lies in the undoing of what has been done to become the brain functions of memory as content through the brain's motor systems.

Recall that I have said in connection with phantom limbs that the body schemata are built up in the brain by way of both sensory and motoric experiences, perhaps more so by motoric than by sensory experiences. Such being the case, the brain's motor system plays an important role in both learning and unlearning. This role, however, hinges on two inhibitory mechanisms: the brain stops releasing certain excitatory neurotransmitters –

presumably with glutamatergic functions – which would otherwise activate motoneurons in wake; at one and the same time, the brain also releases certain inhibitory neurotransmitters – presumably with GABAergic functions – to actively inhibit motoneurons which would otherwise be activated by dopaminergic neurotransmitters in wake.

If this is true, and I should add that there is no reason why it is not, each time an individual dreams in REM sleep periods as well as in non-REM sleep periods, the dream makes more room in his/her brain to accommodate new experiences that will be forthcoming. In other words, dreaming is an important process for the brain functions of memory as capacity, because it is preceded by REM sleep-on neurons in the brainstem and sleep-on neurons at the base of the forebrain during non-REM sleep, thereby triggering reverse learning arising from the inhibition of excitatory motoneurons.

5.5 Maturation

This concept seems to be associated with the notion of aging, which implies the weakening of body functions. I have, therefore, avoided the use of 'aging' as the cover term, reserving it only for the process of weakening in body functions which will become apparent shortly. The reason is that life from one zygote onward is a continuous process, the most significant portion of which is the changes of brain functions in neural complexity over time for each individual. For instance, 'the average weight of the brain at autopsy falls from 1,375 grams (3.03 pounds) to 1,232 grams (2.73 pounds) between 30 and 90' (Shock, 1962: 100). This constitutes a 10.4 per cent loss over a span of 60 years. Hence, I have chosen the term 'maturation' to take into account the total continuous neural process of life itself.

Since the change in neural complexity has to do with the individual's maturation, I have divided it into Growth and Aging. There is evidence which indicates that in humans the age of 18 is the cutting point (Peng, 1995, 1981). I have, therefore, referred to the change of brain functions in neural complexity prior to age 18 as growth and the change of brain functions in neural complexity after age 18 as aging. I am, of course, aware that the total process involving time is a continuum.

However, maturation has to follow the development of neural complexity smoothly as each individual's brain changes, not only from birth to death but also from one zygote to a newborn baby. If there is a disruption or alteration in the continuous development, the consequences become a birth defect or hypermaturation; both abnormalities are detrimental to the individual in all behaviours, including language behaviour.

I have mentioned progeria (also known as Hutchinson-Gilford Syndrome) as a case in point arising from a detrimental pathology, because of the disruption or alteration, in the process of maturation, in which case the individual starts aging during childhood, long before the age of 18, at the rate of eight to ten biological years for one calendar (or chronological) year. The case I have introduced was a boy of no more than ten years of age but he looked like an 80-year-old man, because his brain cells aged ten times faster than his real-time physical aging by calendar years.

The pathology must have started during the mother's pregnancy, because she became pregnant as a 17-year-old and had been smoking pot, taking drugs and drinking every day since the age of 15; thus, the pathology was congenital, a birth defect, when she gave birth to the boy.

The son was named 'Ashuri' and appeared 'normal' at birth and age one. But soon after that his premature aging showed through. The child would never exceed the size of a normal five-year-old, because of dwarfism affecting the master gland, even though he was ten years old and looked like an 80-year-old. The median age of death is around 13. As a result, the mother was converted to Christianity and wrote a biography in Japanese entitled '*Mijikai Inochi wo Dakishimete*' (Embracing Tightly A Short Life), which is published by Fuji TV. Her story was televised by Fuji TV as a documentary, entitled 'Science Mystery II: The Human Truth and Love Explicated by DNA' (DNA *ga tokiakasu ningen no shinjitsu to ai*).

The point I am trying to make is that the boy did learn to speak Japanese to some extent, which is rudimentary, but that he has serious language disorders. That is, a man of 80 years of age normally has had plenty of experiences and developed a sufficiently large vocabulary and, therefore, his content plane and expression plane have all the needed background noises for the brain functions of memory as content. In the case of Ashuri, however, his life will be short, because his brain cells have already prematurely aged close to the end point, and therefore his brain functions of memory as content are insufficient to be comparable to his peers at the age of 10. The reason is that the sped up maturation has altered the normal development of the brain functions of memory as capacity for the enrichment of experiences to become the needed background noises in his brain functions of memory as content without the sophisticated brain functions of memory as mechanism which a normal 80-year-old man is expected to have developed.

Now, when the development of neural complexity is normal, there is no denying that ten-year-old children do not have many experiences compared to adults. Thus, it can be said for sure that children's brain functions of memory as capacity are not up to the level of those of adults, because adults' brain functions are much more complex. A genius as a child may be an exception, because such a child at the age of nine may have already graduated from college with a BA or BS in mathematics. In that case, the child's development of neural complexity has been greatly expedited because of genetic factors.

But when an adult in his/her thirties is compared to another adult in his/her seventies, because of brain weight losses, there is no question that the younger adult's brain functions of memory as capacity are greater than those of the older adult, even though the latter may have had more experiences than the former. Put differently, I am not talking about a comparison of the amount of experiences each adult has had; rather, my crucial concern is the changes in complexity of the neural circuitry, which decline steadily after the age of 18. The reason is that the neuron population at birth is already determined, which can only decrease when aging starts, that is, after the age of 18, thereby leading to the decline of changes in the complexity of brain functions. Such changes are what I mean by maturation as an important process that determines the brain functions of memory as capacity which is time-sensitive.

6. Brain Functions of Memory as Mechanism

The brain functions of memory as mechanism include what have traditionally been thought of as the brain functions of cognition, and more. They handle the goings-on of the here-and-now by relying on the brain functions of memory as content through synaptic changes of impulses (or action potentials) in neuronal communication by means of excitation, inhibition and disinhibition which are the only forms of neuronal signals the brain recognizes; hence, they are based on the time factor mentioned earlier.

Typically, the brain functions of memory as mechanism include the following:

1. retrieval of memory as content from the past to the present;
2. rehearsal of memory as content in the present on the basis of the past;
3 repetition of events (or behaviour, verbal or non-verbal) for memory as content in the present;
4. problem-solving regarding memory as content in the past (including mathematical problem-solving, arithmetic calculation, etc.);
5. the decision-making of memory as content in the present (including what to say and what not to say);
6. judgement of conflicting memories as content in the past and the present;
7. ability to orient oneself in time and space;
8. (most important of all) ability to think in order to utter and understand sentences and words for human interaction.

6.1 Retrieval of Memory as Content

The term 'retrieval' is often used by psychologists in most theories of memory. The term implies that something that has been 'stored' as memory is taken out of the 'storage' for whatever purpose, as if memory is a thing and retrieval is a 'tool' like a fork or a pair of forcepts which can pick up the 'thing' from storage. In the present context, however, the term employed is not in keeping with this usage. Rather, retrieval implies on-going neural activities that change the status of impulses on demand from the background noises (which include memory as content in the content plane) to a certain region of the brain to accomplish an objective; that objective may or may not come out through the corresponding expression plane. For instance, if a man is about to leave the door to the garage but suddenly, as he puts his hand in his pocket, he realizes that he left the car key in the kitchen, so he goes back inside to pick up the car key. Here, the neural activities in his brain involve his brain functions of retrieval of memory as content from the past to the present. Specifically, the involvement may be depicted as follows:

1. His background noises include the following:
   (i) a car to be driven needs a car key;
   (ii) he has the key but has left it in the kitchen, which is a background noise in the past;
   (iii) the only way to get it is to go back to the kitchen, which is a background noise in the present.
2. His retrieval includes the following neural activities to bring the past to the present, if he wants to achieve the intended objective which is to drive the car:
   (i) he did not realize that he had left the key in the kitchen until he put his hand in his pocket, which was his habitual behaviour in the background noises;
   (ii) the motoric and the sensory functions of his hand trigger or reactivate the background noises from the past mentioned above;
   (iii) at one and the same time those motoric and sensory functions enable him to make a here-and-now decision, that is, to handle the goings-on, in order to properly adjust to the external environment, that is, to either give up the idea of driving the car (i.e., to leave the house by calling a taxi) or to re-enter the house to get the car key.

There are many instances of such retrieval of memory as content in our daily life, which we encounter routinely without paying much attention to what is going on in the brain or how we handle the situations. When they are analysed systematically, as I did above, all fall into place and the mechanism of retrieval of memory as content begins to make sense. I should add, however, that the brain functions of memory as mechanism seldom operate independently. For instance, the mechanism of retrieval nine times out of ten leads to the mechanism of decision-making which, in the example above, is euphemistically depicted as 'making a proper adjustment to the external environment'.

6.2 Rehearsal of Memory as Content

In layman's terminology, rehearsal requires going over the same things (i.e., behaviour) at least more than once, as in orchestra rehearsal or ballet rehearsal. However, I have reserved this sense of behaviour for the repetition of memory as content. Thus, rehearsal of memory as content in the present context suggests the utilization of new impulses in combination with old impulses which have become memory as content in the background noises, either instantaneously or over time, in a mental 'exercise', without any overt manifestation of behaviour in the present, so as not to forget (i.e., lose) them or to improve what has been done in the past in anticipation of what may happen in the future.

A good example of rehearsal in this sense is 'day-dreaming' a recent experience, such as an erotic encounter, or 'practising' mentally in the present the new moves of chess recently acquired in the past from one chess game in order to improve the skills for the next game. Maybe psychologists would want to humorously call this 'the hypnagogic as fullest reservoire for creativity', a line suggested by Professor Roger Matthews (personal communication).

It should be noted that unlike dreaming which occurs in sleep, be it REM or non-REM sleep, day-dreaming occurs in wake, albeit the day-dreamer is relatively inattentive to the surroundings. Therefore, reverse learning does not take place, because his/her brain cells are active in the forebrain and the brainstem and, therefore, are functioning independently rather than synchronously. Thus, day-dreaming does not make room for the brain functions of memory as capacity, for it is an example of the mechanism of rehearsal in the brain functions of memory.

6.3 Repetition of Events for Memory as Content

Repetition of events is in line with the layman's sense of going over the same thing more than once in order to improve the skills or vocabulary of a new language being learned as the goings-on of the here-and-now. However, as the layman's sense of repetition and that of rehearsal overlap, I have made an effort to separate these two terms, because their brain functions are different. In another sense, laymen also have another term, called 'practice' as in practising a musical instruction, for example, violin or piano. All these brain functions (repetition and practice) suggest the manifestation of overt behaviour, indicating the involvement of both motoric and sensory functions of the body, by going through the same motoneurons and sensory receptors. The results are the same, that is, the retention of memory as content in memory as capacity for a longer period of time. Thus, in the present context, repetition may be regarded as synonymous with 'practice'. Traditionally, however, repetition is used to explain the transfer of recent or short-term memory to long-term memory, an idea that is partially adopted here.

6.4 Problem-solving Regarding Memory as Content

When an event occurs, which cannot be handled or solved here and now as a going-on, it becomes a problem; if it can be taken care of on the spot, it does not become a problem. For instance, taking a train to go to New York from Chicago is an event that can be handled here and now, if you catch it in time. However, if you miss the train, the event becomes a problem in your memory as content, because you have to attend a meeting the next day. Problem-solving regarding memory as content is to remove the problem from your memory as content, for instance, finding an alternative way of getting to New York, such as taking an airplane from O'Hare Airport.

I have extended such brain functions to problem-solving in mathematics, which presuppose memorization as a part of the background noises in the past of certain formulaic calculations. If those formulae cannot be remembered by the individual, implying that they do not exist as part of his/her background noises, the mathematical problems cannot be solved. However, I should add that the brain functions for solving mathematical problems are much more complex and may be of a different kind, because they do not involve human interactions. Thus, there are people who are very good at solving mathematical problems but are usually quite poor at solving contextual or administrative problems involving human interactions, such as some professors at university, and vice versa.

6.5 Decision-making of Memory as Content

The brain functions of decision-making overlap to some extent those of problem-solving. But there is a distinction. In decision-making, the brain functions are engaged in choosing one of at least two or more events, for instance, what to say and what not to say, whereas the brain functions of problem-solving are technically limited to one problem at a time. If your family has planned to go to New York from Chicago for quite some time, that plan has become memory as content in the background noises of your brain for your family. However, your brain functions of decision-making are engaged in the choice in the present of going by train, car or airplane. If the choice is taking an airplane, and you and your family catch the airplane in time, there is no problem to be solved.

On the other hand, if you and your family miss the flight, your brain functions of problem-solving will have to take over to remove (i.e., solve) the problem. The overlap of decision-making and problem-solving can be seen or will happen when no decision can be made by you and your family regarding the transportation, because one member wants to fly, and another member wants to take the train but you want to drive. In that case, decision-making becomes a problem in the present, which will have to be solved first. However, decision-making may overrule problem-solving by postponing the trip to New York, in which case, the problem is tabled for the time being, which will become the past in the present when it is taken off the table in a week or so by you or your family for another round of decision-making.

6.6 Judgement of Conflicting Memories as Content

Unlike the above-mentioned mechanisms which do not create conflicts in the individual's brain, the brain functions of judgement of conflicting memories as content are solely concerned with the individual's own conflicts within his/her memory as content; those conflicts may be cumulative from the past but may happen in the present and are quite prevalent in every society among individuals in many sectors. Examples are: accepting or rejecting bribes by a government official or fraud by the CEO of a company; a woman having two or more suitors of whom she has to choose one; embezzlement of money by a manager or a clerk in a company or a bank, respectively, and the like.

In the case of bribery, the government official has to judge the pros and cons of the consequences, if and when caught or exposed; that is, the pros of the next election which will need campaign money and how tight the family's purse strings are must be weighed against the cons of the consequences of being put behind bars when exposed or caught. An example of the pros and cons of fraud by the CEO can be illustrated in the case of Enron, whose executive, Mr Lay, finally decided to give himself up to the legal authorities resulting from his own judgement of conflicting memories as content, although he pleaded not guilty.

In the case of flirtation with two or more suitors, the judgement of conflicting memories as content must be made when marriage becomes an issue or when each one of the suitors becomes aware that rivalry exists and that he is not the only one. This conflict also exists when a married man is seeing another woman behind his wife's back or a married woman is seeing another man behind her husband's back. In a community of polyandry, the woman can marry both or all suitors without having any conflict; likewise, in a community of polygyny, as in an Islamic country, the man can marry up to four wives, and therefore there is no conflict.

Embezzlement is an interesting example, because I witnessed a case in 2002 by the assistant manager of a well-known prestigious boutique shop in Honolulu through an internal exposé. It is interesting because it involved not just the judgement of conflicting memories on the part of the culprit, who is usually an employee, but also problem-solving and decision-making on the part of the employer.

The assistant manager, who is a Korean woman, embezzled more than US$100,000 over a period of three years by means of manipulating the receipts from customers on certain days through the computer for the bookkeeping and falsifying the inventory. When her wrong-doings were exposed, of course, she was dismissed. During that period of three years, she must have had a series of judgements of conflicting memories in her brain each time she stole money from the company. It can be summarized as follows.

When she first nullified a receipt by not registering the sale on the computer, in order to steal the money, I believe she was somewhat nervous and had to weigh the pros and cons to see if her behaviour would be detected by her colleagues. She succeeded the first time. As a result, she was emboldened subsequently. By then, for each subsequent stealing, she had less and less of a guilty feeling because her judgement of the conflicting memories became 'numb'. I was informed that prior to the exposé she even boasted that the employer in the headquarters could not care less how the boutique shop was run, even though it was in the red, because the manager, her immediate superior, left everything to her, so much so that she felt that she could fool everybody in the store. But the exposé happened because someone notified the headquarters of her wrong-doings with just one piece of evidence. That cracked open the whole scenario and the employer in the headquarters sent a team to investigate the bookkeeping and the inventory.

Now, the employer had a problem when her wrong-doings were exposed.

Prior to the exposé, the store had been running in the red for quite some time, especially during the three-year period, and the employer was contemplating solving the problem by making a decision as to whether or not to close the shop. The exposé took care of the employer's problem of losing money, because the cause of the 'leak' was found and the 'leak' was plugged up by dismissing the assistant manager. However, the employer at the same time faces the decision-making of whether to litigate the former assistant manager or not, knowing that she probably had spent all the $100,000 plus and that the company could not get the money back. Not only that, litigating her would cost money and probably inflict commercial damage on the prestige of the well-known boutique shop.

What I am trying to emphasize through this vivid example is that more often than not the judgement of conflicting memories on the part of one individual may trigger problem-solving and decision-making on the part of another individual. The reason is that these brain functions of memory as mechanism seldom take place independently of one another, because of interdependencies, in just one person in a vacuum, as they will most likely involve human interactions of more than one person in varying contexts of situation.

6.7 Ability to Orient Oneself in Time and Space

This ability is too often taken for granted, but actually affects every individual's life and death because it must constantly monitor the past against the present and vice versa for the individual to be aware of where he/she is and the time line he/she is in. For instance, having made several appointments, the individual must keep the appointments in the order in which they were made, but if he/she goes to the second or third appointment before the first one, by mistake, the time line is mixed up.

The ability to orient oneself in time and space may be tied to proprioception facilitated by the spinal cord. Imagine how to figure out the directions on the ground surface which has several paths without any signs when you are underground. On the ground surface, there are different buildings and other landmarks, beside road signs, to aid your sense of direction, East or West, North or South, and left or right, which comes primarily from the visual channel, although other channels may also be of help. When you are underground, however, all these landmarks are not available to facilitate your brain functions for the ability to orient yourself in time and space.

In this sense, then, a deaf person may have a better sense of direction than a blind person, because in the blind person's brain, the ability to orient him/herself in time and space is greatly compromised. To supplement this deficit, either a cane to switch the sense of direction from the visual to the tactile channel or a guide dog is used, which also employs the blind person's tactile functions. Thus, when a person begins to lose this ability, as in dementia, that person lives in constant danger with a time bomb, because the deterioration is neurodegenerative.

In AD, FD or Pick's disease, the patient's first symptom is the loss of recent memory, thereby repeating the same thing, as in cooking or shopping or asking a question, over and over again. For instance, when cooking, the patient may forget that she has already put salt in the food and therefore will add more salt; when shopping, he/she may forget that a loaf of bread has already been put in the cart and therefore will go back for another loaf; and the most obvious behaviour as the first symptom of dementia is that the patient will ask his/her spouse 'what day is today?' every twenty minutes or so or 'where are we?' when they go out together. However, the patient is likely still able to describe certain events which happened during childhood.

The symptom of the second stage in dementia is getting lost in a familiar territory and not knowing how to come home. When the condition becomes worse, the symptom of the third stage is that the patient does not remember familiar faces, including his/her children, and cannot recall their names. Of course, the patient's content plane is now severely impaired and may gradually lose the ability to change clothes by putting trousers on his/her head and lose motoric function to become bedridden in the final stage before expiration.

6.8 Ability to Think

I have mentioned above the traditional view of the relationships of memory and cognition, in which cognition is said to consist of learning, thinking and memory. Having delineated to some extent the issues surrounding memory and cognition in my framework, I have already made it clear that there is a time factor involved in the relationships of memory and cognition; namely, memory deals with the past and the past in the present (never with the future which can only be talked about, that is, speculated) but cognition handles the goings-on of the here-and-now. It is an important factor that is missing in all other theories of memory.

At the same time, I have also made it clear that learning need not always precede memory, which is regarded by some as the recollection of that which was once experienced or learned. Or else, if there is no learning by an individual, what that individual possesses in his/her brain is not memory but something else. Put differently, to most psychologists, learning is the prerequisite to the existence of memory in the brain. I have taken exception to this traditional view, because memory is also regarded as the recollection of that which was experienced. I have shown that there are some other ways, besides learning, in which the brain functions of memory can be observed, especially when learning is but one kind of experience in the brain functions. Such observable experiences which contribute to the brain functions of memory cannot be experimented by means of a simplistic testing design which ignores the highly complex neuronal interconnections within the cranium; nor can the brain functions of memory be localized as a result of any such simplistic experiment because neurons communicate with one another in milliseconds.

In this section, I should now address the relationships directly by raising one relevant question: is thinking possible as an important brain function without the brain functions of memory? From my point of view, the answer is negative, especially when the ability to think is an important mechanism of the brain functions of memory, because it involves the construction and the reconstruction of meaning. The following is my reasoning in neurophysiological and neuroanatomical terms.

The ability to think is a mechanism of the brain functions of memory that is closely tied to the ability to orient oneself in time and space, but is not limited to patients with dementia, when it is impaired, because the impairment of this ability in the early stage affects mostly the handling of the goings-on of the here-and-now, as in patients with schizophrenia or other psychoses. This ability is, therefore, interrelated to all the other brain functions of memory as mechanism. After all, inside the cranium all neurons are interconnected directly or indirectly with high-speed communication among themselves, even though the individual may be asleep; when the individual is awake, they function independently rather than synchronously. Thus, it would be absurd to contemplate the ability to think as a separate faculty controlled or manipulated by a specific brain structure.

In this vein, I have mentioned the importance of the extrapyramidal tract, the looping of which is where thinking takes place, because any impulse from the expression plane that is destined to come out as active behaviour goes through the loop at least twice; if it does not come out as active behaviour, the looping of all impulses from the expression plane continues in the brain as passive behaviour, which may be what is known as inner speech or intrapersonal communication in communication theory (i.e., the individual 'talks' to him/herself, as it were). However, I would like to call this state of neural activities language potentiation.

But in order to think properly the cerebello-cerebral circuit and the Papez circuit must also take part in both active and passive behaviour. Recall that the extrapyramidal tract and the two circuits all go through the thalamus, which is not just a relay station; rather, it is an important brain structure that integrates all brain functions, even during REM and non-REM sleep. I am willing to speculate that when an individual loses the ability to think properly to the extent that he/she fails frequently to make proper verbal or non-verbal adjustments to his/her dyadic partner in the family, so much so that his/her family members begin to worry, notice or complain about his/her behaviour as irritations, he/she has lost the normal functions of the extrapyramidal looping and the two circuits, all of which contribute to the brain functions of memory as mechanism in particular and to the brain functions of memory as content and as capacity in general.

The reason is that the symptoms of the impairment of this ability to think is most obvious in ideation with respect to the mechanism of integration (to be explained shortly). That is, the individual is likely to misinterpret speaker's well-intended utterances (i.e., reconstructed erroneously the meanings on the basis of the utterance produced by speaker) not once but frequently.

There are many instances in our daily life, be it at home, in politics, or playing poker, or gambling in a casino, to illustrate the ability to think. For the present purpose, let me cite one real example, from World War II taken from *Hawaii Chinese News* (16–31 July 2004, p. 4).

It reports a story of intelligence/espionage, showing the contest of the brain functions of the ability to think on the part of the people concerned. The contest involved USA and Japan, with the supporting roles of Great Britain and Nazi Germany after the attack on Pearl Harbor. It is now known that the US Navy cracked the secret code used by the Japanese Imperial Navy but the story gives a background description of how the US Navy was able to crack the code to turn the tide so as to win the war.

After Pearl Harbor, the United States government mobilized a large amount of manpower to concentrate on the gathering of intelligence about the Japanese Imperial Navy. Such mobilized efforts required a great deal of the brain functions on the part of the planners, brain functions of the ability to think in particular. Their brain functions included seeking the cooperation of the British Intelligence. As a result, they found out that the Japanese Imperial Navy was quite worried about the mounting efforts on the part of the US Navy; that is, the Japanese became concerned that their intelligence might be leaking to the US.

To safeguard their intelligence system, the Japanese Imperial Navy got in touch with Nazi Germany, Japan's ally, and acquired a new spy ship equipped with the 'latest' and most advanced secret code operation system and was assured by Nazi Germany that nobody would be able to crack the new system. But the British Intelligence had already gathered the information about the transaction of the spy ship from Nazi Germany to Japan and passed it on to the United States. The US Navy was delighted to learn that the Germans made such an offer to the Japanese.

Upon receiving the new equipment, the Japanese Imperial Navy started to operate a new secret code by sending telegrams in that code. One of the telegrams was intercepted by the US Navy; the telegram contained a secrete code 'AF' as the next target of attack. The US Navy was not sure what it was, guessing that it may be The Aleutian Islands, the Hawaiian Islands, or the Midway Islands.

The Commander of the Pacific Fleet, Admiral Nimitz, guessed by using his ability to think that it could mean the Midway Islands. To test the accuracy of his own brain functions to think, he ordered the commander stationed in the Midway Islands to cable the headquarters in Honolulu, openly reporting that the islands had a severe shortage of drinking water and was in desparate need of supply, so as to test the Japanese reaction.

Sure enough, the Japanese Imperial Navy responded by notifying its Pacific Fleet that 'AF' was in need of drinking water, thereby verifying unequivocally the accuracy of Admiral Nimitz's brain functions of the ability to think. As a result of the verification, unwittingly offered by the Japanese Imperial Navy, the US Navy was ready and prepared when the Japanese fleet attacked Midway Islands, a battle that eventually led to Japan's defeat and turned the tide against her to lose the war.

7. More Brain Functions of Memory as Mechanism

It is clear from the above-mentioned that the brain functions of memory as mechanism are interrelated; there is no such thing as a single mechanism that operates alone independent of the others. For instance, in the case of Admiral Nimitz, he had to make daily decisions, including the cooperation from the British Intelligence, of how to counter the Japanese Imperial Navy's intelligence in order to avoid another attack, which was a constant problem in his mind; his brain functions, however, enabled him to think in order to solve the puzzle of 'AF'.

There are more brain functions of memory as mechanism of which most neuroscientists are not aware; namely, rapid inhibition mechanism (i.e., RIM), function enhancement mechanism (Peng, 1994), reinforcment mechanism, recall mechanism, and consolidation mechanism (Stevens, 1994) or integration mechanism (Peng, 1994).

Some elaborations of these mechanisms are in order to avoid confusion, because several of them appear redundant, when they are not, and a few of them are quite new: that is, retrieval vs. recall; repetition vs. rehearsal; RIM; function enhancement; reinforcement; and consolidation or integration.

7.1 Differences between Retrieval and Recall

The mechanisms of retrieval and recall both involve or make use of the brain functions of memory as content; however, they differ in the 'depth' of memory as content or the extent to which memory as content is involved or made use of. In other words, retrieval involves memory as content to the extent that what is retrieved, in the form of impulses, interacts with other motoric or sensory impulses or incoming sensory stimuli for the purpose of realizing certain meanings required of the individual; but recall involves memory as content only to the extent that what is recalled, also in the form of impulses, is a mere response to what was called for, to manifest as behaviour on demand or voluntarily, without any interactions of the recalled impulses with other motoric or sensory impulses or incoming sensory stimuli. For instance, any kung fu behaviour depends entirely on the mechanism of retrieval, coupled at least with the mechanisms of Orient Oneself in Time and Space and of the Ability to Think; without such mechanisms, the kung fu expert simply cannot fight. On the other hand, when a person is asked his/her name, the oral response involves only the mechanism of recall. However, if that person is required to write down his/her name or fill out an application form, the mechanisms of retrieval must take over.

7.2 Differences between Repetition and Rehearsal

The mechanisms of repetition and rehearsal may sound redundant but they differ in whether or not the receptors in the sensory organs, for instance, the ears, the eyes, etc., are involved. When an individual uses one of those organs to receive the same stimuli, as in listening to a tape from a tape recorder or viewing slides from a projector, he/she is activating his/her mechanism of repetition in the brain functions of memory. On the other hand, if he/she utilizes only his/her memory as content, by relying on recall, without making use of any receptor in one of the sensory organs, as in mentally practising the multiplication table, without verbalizing it, only the mechanism of rehearsal is involved. On the other hand, if the individual verbalizes or writes down what is being rehearsed, the mechanism of repetition takes over. An alternative way of looking at those differences is this: repetition relies on retrieval in the way in which rehearsal relies on recall. In other words, repetition is multiple retrievals and rehearsal is multiple recalls.

7.3 The Characteristics of the RIM

The RIM is absolutely necessary if a person wants to speak or write smoothly without stuttering or perseveration in the manifestation of his/her verbal or written behaviour. That is, when a series of impulses goes through the extra-pyramidal looping to come to the pyramidal tract, the impulse that goes first must be instantaneously erased to allow the one that comes next to go through, and so on, or else that person will stutter or perseverate. This characteristic is efferent.

Likewise, it should not be misunderstood that the RIM is needed only in production. Quite the contrary, it is also needed in reception. Or else, those impulses that have already entered the brain will interfere with what come later. However, those which come first will have to be retained to some extent long enough for the hearer to bind those impulses with the impulses that follow to undergo perceptual organization or re-organization in order to have a coherent reconstruction of meanings in his/her brain regarding speaker's utterances. If those impulses which have already entered the hearer's brain cannot be retained long enough, or are erased too quickly, the hearer cannot bind them with those that follow, for perceptual organization or re-organization, resulting in the failure to reconstruct his/her own meanings of what speaker said. Typically, such a consequence is often referred to as a confusion or misunderstanding.

But how quickly or slowly the afferent impulses in reception should be erased successively by the RIM is an empirical question that will require more investigation. However, examples of interference, if erasure is not appropriate, can be found in cases of heated quarrels between members of a dyad. Such examples will illustrate the fact that the excitations of neurons in both parties cannot be inhibited fast enough to calm down each party; the consequence, in the worst possible scenario, may lead to a fist fight. On the other hand, examples of a confusion or a misunderstanding can be found in listening to a high-brow lecture above the audience's head because each listener in the audience simply cannot retain each impulse or series of impulses long enough for coupling in order to bind with those that come successively afterward, for perceptual organization or re-organization, to make any coherent sense. To some extent, confusion or misunderstanding has its source in the lack of function enhancement which is elaborated below.

7.4 The Mechanism of Function Enhancement

As I have speculated, the mechanism of function enhancement makes extensive use of the aborization of neural activities in the cerebral cortex, especially when impulses go through at least twice the extrapyramidal looping in milliseconds to return to the cerebral cortex for understanding in reception with respect to meaning, as in puns, jokes, irony, or sarcasm. In one sense, the mechanism in the brain of function enhancement may be said to include at least the collective effect of two neural mechanisms; namely, the RIM mentioned above and the Status Upgrading Mechanism (SUM), which can be commonly observed in the utilization of the vocal cords for singing and/or speaking, or of the tongue for the same purpose.

The basic brain functions of the vocal cords, controlled by the recurrent laryngeal of the Xth cranial nerve, is to stop the ventilation for the increase of physical strength, for instance, in weight-lifting. In the brain functions of language, the SUM pertains more to reception, which upgrades the concept of a sign – for example, *that* or *this* – from its linguistic meaning (i.e., dictionary meaning) to an enhanced meaning to cover what has been said, heard, seen, written, or touched previously, when hearer/qua speaker reconstructs his/her meaning. In production, however, function enhancement also plays a significant role when a man wants to pun, joke, or perhaps sweet-talk a lady, or soft-pedal his superior or when he summarizes what has been said or written. This mechanism in both production and reception will be illustrated with more examples later.

7.5 The Mechanism of Reinforcement

This mechanism involves the recruitment of additional impulses, either motoric, sensory, or both, when those impulses which are already recalled or retrieved are insufficient to enable the individual to accomplish what he/she intends to say, do, write, or know. For instance, if a person in the midst of writing an article cannot think of the right words to finish a sentence or the right sentence to finish a paragraph, or is not sure of the spelling of a word, he/she may consult a dictionary, a thesaurus, or rest to let it sit for a while in order to wait for some kind of inspiration to 'pop-up' (from the background noises); when the right words are found or when an inspiration 'pops up', he/she has activated the mechanism of reinforcement.

7.6 Consolidation or Integration

The term consolidation is used by Stevens (1994) to refer to the interplay of the CREB protein and memory. In my terminology, however, I have employed the term integration to refer to a broader mechanism which, in tandem with the ability to think and function enhancement described above, includes the collective effect of three series of specific brain functions:

1. Summarizing (i.e., the ability to summarize what has been seen, read, heard, or told into a logically coherent whole, most certainly on the basis of perceptual organization or re-organization, because nobody can reproduce what has been seen, read, heard, or told *in toto*).
2. Paraphrasing (i.e., the ability to reproduce, coupled with perceptual organization or re-organization, what has been read, heard, or told in a form sufficiently different from the original as distinguishable from copying and quoting verbatim).
3. Inferencing, *not* inferring (i.e., changing deliberately or under duress the original meaning or proto-meaning, that is, intent, when circumstances change, into some other meanings which are different from or even contradict the original meaning). Note that the difference between inferencing and inferring is on a par with that between servicing and serving or that between referencing and referring.

A good example of the mechanism of integration can be found in Admiral Nimitz's brain functions when he integrated the Japanese Imperial Navy's secret code 'AF' with the 'shortage of drinking water', by way of his ability to think, on the basis of perceptual organization or re-organization, in order to inference, as a result of function enhancement, the meaning of 'AF' through reconstruction that 'Midway Islands would be the next target of attack by the Japanese Imperial Navy'.

The integration mechanism, if and when combined with non-language behaviour by activating the SUM in relation to memory as content and memory as capacity, will lead to Acting (or Histrionics, suggested by Professor Roger Matthews, which is probably a better term) as in opera or theatrical acting, the discussion of which, however, falls outside the purview of this monograph. It will be introduced and elaborated on a separate occasion, for instance, in respect to Chinese opera, which differs considerably from Western opera.

13 Language in the Brain is Meaning-Centred

As was shown above in the various definitions of language given by linguists after Saussure, and by a nine-year-old, language teachers, or neuroscientists, only the Hallidayan definition is concerned with meaning. The erroneous definitions of language from the medical point of view, therefore, will not be taken up again here. However, as is purported by Thibault and repeatedly demonstrated by Saussure himself, the Saussurean framework is concerned more with the speaker than with the hearer in terms of meaning. Thibault's own phrasing of Halliday's 'meaning-making', although occasionally 'construal' is used as well, tends to also emphasize the speaker.

A typical example is Saussure's well-known speech circuit (1959: 134). Although in this example Saussure uses A (speaker) and B (hearer) to illustrate the speech circuit, and the diagram of phonation and audition seems to balance the two, unknowingly he favours the speaker; that is, the hearer is depicted to take what is given by the speaker for granted as if the concept in A's brain before the phonation is the same as the concept in B's brain after the audition.

This assumption of Saussure's has become the model or precursor of all post-Saussurean frameworks in modern linguistics. When the individual aspect of language (i.e., *langue* and *parole*) is carefully examined, however, the conclusion has to be quite different from Saussure's assumption. That is, the speaker's concept before the phonation and the hearer's concept after the audition may or may not be the same; more often than not they are different. The reason is that speaker constructs meaning, as part of his/her active behaviour in the brain, but hearer reconstructs meaning, as part of his/her passive behaviour in the brain. That is why people quarrel between husband and wife or between the plaintiff and the defendant in court through their lawyers.

In this section of the monograph, I emphasize in some detail what goes on in the speaker's brain, for his/her active and passive behaviour, because he/she is at the same time a hearer as well when producing utterances, and what goes on in the hearer's brain, for his/her passive behaviour. The speaker's production and the hearer's reception will then be demonstrated in Part V.

The two meanings differ, moreover, because of several very important but often overlooked neuroanatomical and neurophysiological facts.

First, when the speaker utters words or sentences through phonation, via the cortico-bulbar pathways (including the cortico-striato-pallido-thalamo-cortical looping), only the sounds come out of his/her mouth, and the meanings are left behind in the speaker's brain. In other words, the meanings and the sounds in the speaker's brain must be separated again to allow the sounds to come out through the cortico-bulbar pathways. Therefore, the sounds have no meaning in and by themselves; during the looping, because that is when thinking takes place irrespective of whether words are uttered (i.e., come out as sounds) or not, the speaker monitors and/or adjusts his/her wording. The same fact applies to sign language, except that the signer utilizes the brachial apparatus, rather than the vocal apparatus.

Second, when the hearer receives the sounds through audition, which have no meaning, he/she must reconstruct his/her meanings on the basis of the sounds heard irrespective of whether or not he/she decides to respond, this time as speaker; either way, the reconstruction of meanings on the basis of the sounds heard is influenced by his/her memory of the past which is reactivated, that is, brought back, by way of the brain functions of memory as mechanism (e.g., retrieval of memory as content from the past to the present), in hearer's brain to participate in the reconstruction of meanings. The same fact applies to sign language, except that viewer now utilizes the retino-thalamo-cortical pathways, rather than the bulbo-thalamo-cortical pathways.

Imagine how President Bush as hearer reconstructs his meanings when he receives briefings from his staff and the military: on Afghanistan or Osama bin Laden; on the reconstruction of Iraq and Saddam Hussein and his henchmen all of whom either were killed or have been captured; and on the 9/11 Commission's Report, more than 500 pages made public on 23 July 2004, which cites FBI and CIA failures. He has to respond or react to each report he has just heard from the staff and the military. The dyadic interactions, back and forth, between the President and his staff during a Cabinet meeting can be quite involved or even heated. In particular, the impact of the Commission's Report, which was destined to become a best seller, on the Presidential Election in 2004, regarding the worthiness of the Iraq War waged by President Bush in relation to the weapons of mass destruction (WMD), will remain an important issue for many years to come in American history.

Now that Saddam Hussein's two sons were killed, and Mr Hussein is in the legal custody of the Iraqi interim government for the 'Trial of the Century', President Bush's reconstruction of meanings on Iraq would be quite different when receiving further briefings from the intelligence in Iraq. For instance, the sons' deaths gave President Bush the confidence to declare emphatically at the White House on 22 July 2003 that Saddam Hussein's return to power is nil: 'He will not be coming back'. It was a declaration that assured not only the allies but also the Iraqi people of a positive future and alleviated their minds of any remaining fear.

Third, the reconstruction of meanings is also influenced by other expressions, such as facial expressions and gestures which hearer is likely to pick up (or which is 'stolen' by the hearer without the speaker's awareness).

And, fourth, even other events occurring simultaneously with the dyadic interactions of A and B in each context of situation are likely to enter the hearer's brain in order to help him/her reconstruct his/her own concept.

It is in the sense given above that I have advocated that language in the brain is meaning-centred. The differences between the speaker's construction and the hearer's reconstruction of meanings, in terms of the neuroanatomy briefly described above, are one of the main foci in this monograph. These differences will be further elaborated in a later book, *Language Disorders: A Critical Perspective.*

Before I go on to the next section, I will add that two or more receivers in an audience (hearers or viewers) may also differ in their respectively reconstructed meanings, even more so between speaker (or signer) qua hearer (or viewer) and hearer (or viewer). A good example is the different reactions to the American and coalition forces in Iraq from the different groups – for example, the Islamic Shias, the Islamic Sunnis to whom Saddam Hussein belonged, and the Kurds – even though there was only one war, Operation Iraqi Freedom. Such differences were further verified in the general election on 30 January 2005 for the Iraqi parliament.

The differences in the construction of meanings (or intended meaning by the speaker or the signer) and the reconstruction of meanings (or perceived meaning by the hearer or the viewer) are always 'translated' into or 'transferred' to actions, each of which is a sequence of mixed behaviours, language behaviours and/or otherwise, for human interactions. Nothing can show such human interactions more clearly than election campaigns in which different political parties are engaged in 'dog-eat-dog' battles (or negative campaign strategies).

President Bush and Mr Gore were engaged in such battles until the very last minute (shortly before the inauguration in 2001), each side refusing to acknowledge defeat. The 2002 mayoral elections of Taipei and Kaohsiung in Taiwan, set on 7 December illustrated even more clearly the differences of constructed and reconstructed meanings between the candidates of the ruling party and the opposition party, each accusing the other for fraud, smear, and/or fabrication of facts; the mass media, such as TV and newspapers, were not exempted from the 'mud-slinging' language behaviours either.

In Taiwan, there was an election set on 1 December 2001 for which not only parliament members were up for re-election but also all 23 city mayors and county governors. The campaigns waged by all candidates were becoming more and more fierce each day, as I observed on TV and in the newspapers, until the last minute on 30 November. In each campaign speech, a political figure attacked the opponent(s) by reconstructing a meaning that was *not* intended by the opponent in order to smear him/her.

When the election was over and the results came out on 2 December those who won made speeches in jubilation because their limbic systems were stimulated and transduced impulses to their cortices to select words for the appropriate occasions; however, those who lost were in no mood for jubilation, and therefore their limbic systems were also stimulated and yet transduced different sorts of impulses to their cortices to select words, accompanied by tears, for the appropriate but emotionally opposite contexts of situation.

In 2004, the presidential election in Taiwan on 20 March almost got out of hand, because an assassin on 19 March fired two bullets in an attempt to kill the incumbent president and vice-president. The candidates of the opposition parties, moreover, having twice lost their ambitions, became the sore losers by orchestrating a nasty violent social unrest that lasted more than two months in an attempt to nullify the process of the election and even to deny the constitutional legitimacy of the duly re-elected president and vice-president so as to force a revote.

There was even an attempt on the part of the sore losers to ask China to send the Red Chinese troops to Taiwan to take over in the event of a riot in Taipei incited by the sore losers and their supporters. President Chen called that attempt, 'A Soft Coup *d'etat*' because it did not succeed as had been plotted even though emails from the opposition camp and a couple of retired generals, including a former minister of defence, called upon the military to attack the headquarters of the ruling party and to kill the president and the vice-president.

I have, therefore, postulated that there are different shades of meaning for each utterance of the speaker, which the hearer can reconstruct. But the hearer qua speaker tends to or can only reconstruct one of them and translates it into something that can only be reconstructed by the opponent qua hearer as just the opposite of the original meaning. I have called the 'real' or original meaning intended by the speaker's 'proto-meaning'. Nine times out of ten the hearer's reconstructed meaning is not the same as the speaker's intended proto-meaning. Hence, the negative campaign battles go on and on between the candidates, each blaming the other(s) for not telling the truth.

The following is an illustration, via the visual facet, to demonstrate such differences. Bear in mind that in non-visual facets, the differences may be more acute or pronounced and varied but are difficult to illustrate visually here. When the same sounds are perceived differently by two hearers, there is no technology available that can illustrate such differences on a piece of paper in black and white other than describing them verbally or in writing.

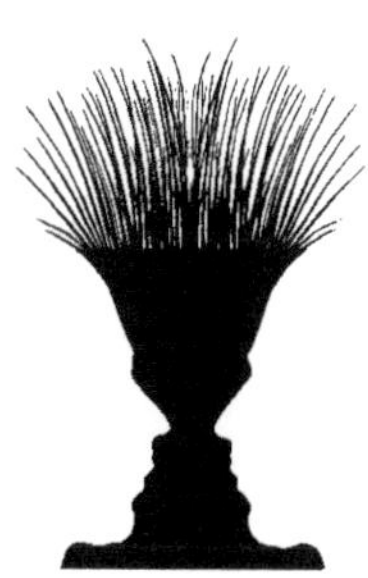

Figure 13.1 *Reconstructions of meaning through the visual facet* (From *The Brain: A User's Manual*, copyright © The Diagram Visual Information Group Ltd. Used by permission.)

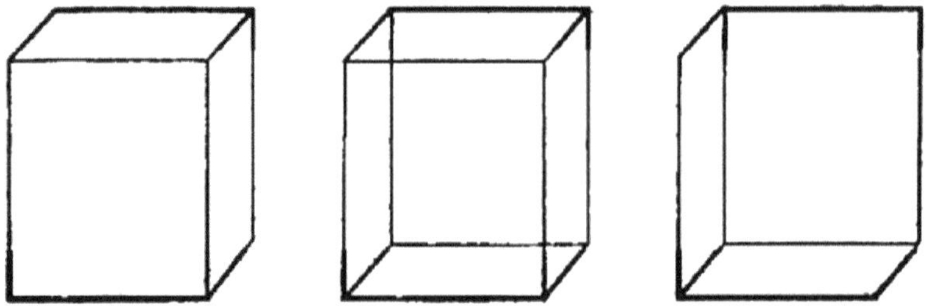

Figure 13.2 Reconstruction of meaning illustrated by Hockett (1958) (From *A Course in Modern Linguistics*, by Charles F. Hockett, New York: Macmillan Company, 1958. Courtesy by permission of Pearson Education.)

Notice that there are two views (or meanings) which can be reconstructed from Figure 13.1 one at a time: a vase or two faces looking at each other. Nobody can have the two views simultaneously. Neuropsychologists use such a picture, along with many others, to illustrate the 'distortions' in the visual mode. For semioticians, this picture is a good illustration that the interpretation of any signs lies in the viewer's brain functions. That is to say, the proverb of 'beauty lies in the eyes of the beholder' must be reckoned with seriously.

Hockett, however, uses Figure 13.2 in his book as an analogy to illustrate the differences in the 'depth' of meaning of spoken Chinese or English, saying that 'The depth that we perceive lies in us, not in the figure' (1958: 149). He adds that 'the experiences by virtue of which we read "depth" into utterances are specific to the particular language' (ibid.: 150). Again, anybody can see the left and the right boxes simultaneously but nobody can see two boxes simultaneously in the middle one without shifting the focus. Likewise, nobody can reconstruct two meanings simultaneously without shifting the focus in the perceptual organization.

I should caution that the two illustrations are not examples about semantic ambiguity; rather, they depict the different shades of meaning that can be reconstructed in the brain from the same utterance (or stimulus, visual or otherwise); one of the different shades of meaning is the constructed meaning which is the 'real' meaning (i.e., meaning intended by the speaker or signer or producer) and the other, the 'inference', thereby illustrating that all behaviours, language in the brain as behaviour in particular, are meaning-centred.

From my point of view, however, these illustrations are but a tip of the iceberg for the whole inchoate mass of impulses called Thought in language behaviour. That is to say, different opinions between the speaker and the hearer or between two and more hearers exist when looking at or hearing presumably the same thing. When such reconstructed meanings from the same thing differ, naturally the differences lead to quarrelling if expressed. The different opinions (or meanings) held by France, Germany, Russia, Great Britain and the USA regarding the role of the UN in rebuilding post-war Iraq constitute a pivotal manifestation of what I have described above.

14 Language in the Brain is Multifaceted

Recall the structuralist definition of language. It was confined to one facet, that is, oral language, as a rebellion against the long tradition of language being written words and texts. Recall also Saussure's dismissal of Whitney's suggestion to include sign language, although linguists after Saussure have acknowledged the importance of written language; however, written language to many structuralists was only a surrogate. Why should I then propose that language in the brain is multifaceted? Here the relevance of the neuroanatomy briefly described in Chapter 11 will come into being readily and vividly; the relevance also hinges on the significance of memory and meaning described in Chapters 12 and 13.

There have now appeared several important questions of which most linguists and semioticians are not even aware. One is: What are the differences between oral language and sign language? Another, for semioticians, is: What are the differences between auditory signs and visual signs? I shall answer these questions below.

1. What are the Differences between Oral Language and Sign Language?

Ostensibly, most linguists would probably say that they differ in modality: oral versus manual. But such a difference is superficial, to say the least. There are important differences that go deeper than this superficial difference.

First, from the point of view of production, oral language and sign language differ in the pathways utilized: oral language takes the cortico-bulbar pathways whereas sign language takes the cortico-spinal *and* cortico-bulbar pathways. In the central nervous system, the cortico-bulbar pathways stop at the brainstem but the cortico-spinal pathways go all the way to the spinal cord.

The cortico-bulbar pathways in the brainstem take the medial routes and make synaptic connections with five important cranial nerves:

1. the VIIth (facial) cranial nerve (which controls the facial movements, the lip movements in particular);
2. the IXth (glossopharyngeal) cranial nerve (which controls the posterior

tongue movements and the pharyngeal, the uvular, and the epiglottal movements);
3. the Xth (vagal) cranial nerve (which controls the glottis and vibration of the vocal cords, that is, the recurrent laryngeal nerve, and the pulmonary ventilation from the lungs);
4. the XIth (accessory) cranial nerve (which monitors the largyngeal movements and the neck movements);
5. XIIth (hypoglossal) cranial nerve (which controls the anterior tongue movements, the most movable body part).

The number of fibres in the cortico-bulbar tracts, including those distributed to sensory relay nuclei and parts of the reticular formation, are estimated to be around five million (cf. Nauta and Feirtag, 1979: 88–111).

The cortico-spinal pathways take the lateral routes and the anterior routes (at the pyramid where motoric decussation takes place), making synapses with thoracic and lumbar nerves for limb (including hands, fingers, feet and toes) movements and torso movements. And the number of fibres in each tract of the cortico spinal pathways are estimated to be over one million of which some 700,000 are highly myelinated (cf. Carpenter, 1976: 255). In sign language, however, both the cortico-bulbar pathways and the cortico-spinal pathways are utilized, the former being for rich facial expressions, which are part of sign language, and tongue display, which is also a part of sign language.

Second, in the cortico-spinal pathways, since the active behaviour entails the impulses to cause the limbs to move, it has been known in neurology that the impulses do not come directly from the cerebral cortex, via the pyramidal tract, to the spinal cord; rather, they pass through a loop, called the extra-pyramidal tract, in each of two subcortical structures, the basal ganglia, and go back to the cerebral (motor) cortex via the thalamus. Then and only then do such impulses come down to the spinal cord on the contralateral side via the ipsilateral posterior limb of the internal capsule as the pyramidal tract because of decussation in the medulla oblongata. The use of Braille also employs the same cortico-spinal pathways for punching. So does writing for written language and painting (excluding mouth-painting which utilizes the cortico-bulbar pathways, although foot-painting also utilizes the same cortico-spinal pathways, albeit not the same spino-cortical pathways). In both cases (punching and writing), however, the spino-cortical pathways must also be actively involved for sensory feedback to guide production through the motor system. But, for such sensory feedback in hand-painting, the fasciculus cuneatus in the spino-cortical pathways is involved, whereas the sensory feedback in foot-painting must come not from the fasciculus cuneatus but from the fasciculus gracilis in the spino-cortical pathways.

Third, such being the case, I have repeatedly suggested that if phonation is considered to be a kind of movement, as it should, to result in language behaviour, the impulses that cause phonation must also go through the extrapyramidal subcortical looping (i.e., the cortico-striato-pallido-thalamo-cortical loop) before the individual can utter any sound. Even if sounds are not to be made, the looping must take place for thinking (or abstract thinking) in a state which I have called language potentiation.

Fourth, in facial expressions for sign language, the impulses take the cortico-bulbar pathways which include the said looping; that is why sign language utilizes both the cortico-spinal and the cortico-bulbar pathways, even though people may think of sign language as using only the two hands.

Fifth, from the point of view of reception, however, oral language utilizes the bulbo-cortical pathways while sign language utilizes the retino-thalamo-cortical pathways. Recall that I have said that the two retinae are part of the brain. The spinal cord is not involved. But if Braille is used for 'reading with fingers', or writing is employed, then and only then will the spino-cortical pathways be utilized for sensory input involving the fasciculus cuneatus for sensory feedback.

2. What are the Differences between Auditory Signs and Visual Signs?

Since oral language and sign language are relevant to auditory signs and visual signs, respectively, what I have said about the differences between oral language and sign language also apply here. However, there should be more differences which go beyond oral language and sign language; that is, non-language differences must be included, which of course incorporate or are applicable to language differences. Four major differences come to mind.

First, in the case of oral language it makes no difference where the sounds of a speaker come from – left, right, front or back; the hearer can still hear them without too much difficulty. On the other hand, in the case of sign language, signing must be conducted within the viewer's visual fields of both eyes. A signer cannot sign to a viewer from the viewer's back and expect the viewer to see the signing. Moreover, the visual fields must be right side up; if the viewer is lying down or 'standing on his/her head with the visual fields upside down', the signer's signing or any visual object cannot be properly understood. All this is because visual stimuli from the outside world to the two retinae are registered upside down (because of the lenses) on the retinae, decomposed, as I have already described, and the impulses thereby going through the IInd (optic) cranial nerve must be corrected, after the optic chiasm, in the brainstem (superior colliculi) and the two thalami (lateral geniculate bodies), through interplay with the cerebral cortex for perceptual organization or re-organization in the process of coupling.

Second, but, in the case of oral language or auditory signs, there is no right side up or upside down for sounds, although they must also be adjusted: first, they are adjusted after they enter the VIIIth (vestibulo-cochlear) cranial nerve from the ear; second, they are adjusted when they ascend to the two inferior colliculi in the brainstem and the two medial geniculate bodies in the thalami; third, some of them decussate in the brainstem, by going to the contralateral side, and others do not decussate, thereby remaining in the ipsilateral side; and finally they reach the respective auditory cortex in each temporal lobe of the two hemispheres for perceptual organization or re-organization in the process of coupling in order to reach a reconstruction of meaning. Both perceptual organization and perceptual re-organization differ in that the former handles someone else's voice or sounds while the latter handles the speaker's own voice.

If written language is added, the production and reception in the brain as active and passive behaviour, respectively, will be all the more complicated. Linguists in the 1950s and 1960s, however, did not even recognize the existence of written language, just like they refused to recognize sign language as language until 1962. Be that as it may, there is no denying now that oral language, sign language and written language (including the use of Braille) are different facets which all belong to language. But, in the individual aspect, such multifaceted language can only be accounted for properly if and when neuroanatomy is taken into consideration.

My research has been to explore or ascertain such differences of the various facets in terms of the first two components of language in the brain just mentioned; that is, language in the brain is memory-governed and meaning-centred in each facet and may vary from one facet to another. However, it may have common grounds in all facets because there is only one brain in each person even though that person may be a polyglot. Some localizationists, who think they are familiar with neuroanatomy, have claimed one brain two languages in bilinguals by assigning the second language to the left parietal lobe; it is a fallacy that cannot be taken seriously.

When one of the facets is impaired, the individual will have language disorders of one form or another in that facet. Thus, a congenital blind person may learn to speak and can hear sounds without any difficulty, but his/her content plane is not the same as a seeing person's. For example, the blind person may have learned to talk about 'colours' such as 'red' and 'blue', but the 'red light' at a crossroads will have a different reconstructed meaning, when the sounds are heard, or a different constructed meaning, when he/she utters the sounds of 'red light'.

Third, mention must be made that because of the differences in neuroanatomy and neurophysiology, coupled with the fact that each person has only one tongue but two upper limbs for production, sign language has the characteristics of simultaneity, reversibility and directionality which no oral language can have.

For instance, in 'John and Mary are brother and sister' brother and sister cannot be uttered simultaneously in any oral language but in Japanese sign language (JSL), they are signed together with two hand-configurations and movements, one representing 'brother', and the other, 'sister'. For reversibility, no oral language uses reversed articulation to indicate that two words refer to opposite meanings: if *dog* is played backward on a tape recorder, it may come out as 'god'; but if *good* is played backward, it may come out as 'doog' which is nonsensical. In JSL, however, *dark* and *bright* are signed with the same hand configuration but opposite movements, that is, 'opening movement of the two hands' for *bright* but 'closing movement of the two hands' for *dark.*

Likewise, no oral language utilizes directionality of the tongue for articulation, but in JSL 'a woman getting married to a man' is signed with one little finger moving to the other thumb, while 'a man getting married to a woman' is signed with one thumb moving to the other little finger.

Fourth, the differences between auditory signs and visual signs are not limited to oral language and sign language for both production and reception; they exist in sounds other than linguistic sounds and anything that is written or drawn. In the latter sense (non-linguistic signs) the differences are not so great for production, because the same (if not identical) body parts are employed for the production of linguistic sounds and other sounds and the same (if not identical) body parts are also employed for the production of linguistic signs (as in writing) and other signs (as in painting pictures). However, the differences are greater for reception, not only between auditory signs and visual signs but also between varying auditory signs and between varying visual signs. These differences are the main domain of interest in semiotics.

15 Language in the Brain is also Stratified

Stratification is an important component in the Saussurean framework of language; namely, Content Plane and Expression Plane. However, these terms were not his, because he was not precise. That is, he talked about thought and sound (Thibault, 1999: 166–7) with the characteristic role of the language system to serve as the intermediary between thought and sound, on the one hand, and he also discussed in some detail the notion of *le signe* consisting of concept (or *signifié*) and acoustic image (or *signifiant*), on the other.

Since Saussure's time, however, the notion of stratification has been expanded by structuralists, generativists, systemicists and, of course, stratificationists for their methodological purposes. The European schools of thought, such as the Firthian school (which influenced the Hallidayan theory of systemics) and the Hjelmslevian school (which influenced the stratificational theory in North America), also took part in the process of expansion for their methodologies. In fact, it was Hjelmslev who proposed to replace concept and acoustic image (or sound-image) with content plane and expression plane, respectively.

Be that as it may, the Saussurean dichotomy of content plane and expression plane (*à la* Hjelmslev) still holds because it works best for the individual aspect of language (i.e., *langue* and *parole*) which has been depicted into four strata, except that the two planes are no longer intimately related as were originally proposed; hence, they have been modified by me (1992b, 1994) and the modification has become such that the two planes subsume concept and acoustic image, respectively. As a result, the four strata of language in the brain (or the individual aspect of language) may be schematically depicted as shown in Figure 15.1.

1. Stratification: Is there an Intermediary between Thought and Sound?

Earlier, mention was made about Saussure's dichotomy of content plane and expression plane (via Hjelmslev) which have been modified by me. The two planes are generic terms of his stratification within the sign. But a closer examination of *CLG*, which is thoroughly re-examined by Thibault, reveals that he has another stratification with the language system (*langue*) between

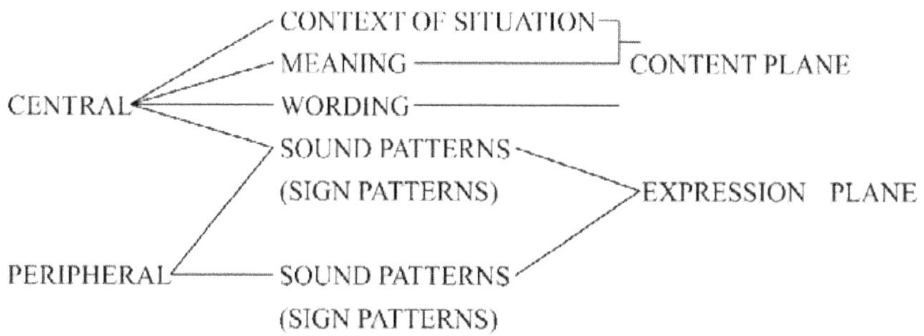

Figure 15.1 *Corresponding relationships between the nervous systems, the four strata of the individual aspect of language, and the two modified Saussurean planes*

thought and sound (Thibault, 1997: 166), 'the characteristic role of which *vis-à-vis* thought is not to create a material phonic means for the expression of ideas, but to serve as the intermediary between thought and sound (...), so that their union necessarily brings about reciprocal delimitations of units' (Thibault, 1997: 167; Saussure, 1959: 112). I will quote some more directly from *CLG* (1959).

> Thought, chaotic by nature, has to become ordered in the process of its decomposition. Neither are thoughts given material form nor are sounds transformed into mental entities; the somewhat mysterious fact is rather that 'thought-sound' implies division, and that language works out its units while taking shape between two shapeless masses. (p. 112)
>
> Language can also be compared with a sheet of paper: thought is the front and sound the back; one cannot cut the front without cutting the back at the same time; likewise in language, one can neither divide sound from thought nor thought from sound; the division could be accomplished only abstractedly, and the result would be either pure psychology or pure phonology. (p. 113)

It is this very characteristic role of the language system purported by Saussure as the intermediary (or social-semiological system, in the Hallidayan terminology) between thought and sound that has influenced and dominated the contemporary theories of linguistics, including of course Halliday's theory of systemics; the stratification in the sign or of the content plane and the expression plane as modified by me has simply been brushed aside until my modification of them as the pivotal notions in my theorizing of the individual aspect of language for the brain functions of language.

However, the language system has become syntax in the early form of generative transformational theory and is equated with lexicogrammar in the Hallidayan theory; in neuropsychology, and lately in the cognitive approach (or cognitive linguistics), syntax (or grammar) is the interface between semantics, on the one hand, and phonology, on the other; each of them is said to represent a 'module' of brain functions. Since generativists want to claim that language (or the language system) is rule-governed and innate, not learned, many of them have sought the long-lost course of 'representation of rules in the brain' but they will never be able to find such a representation; the human brain does not work that way, although some have brought in language template to replace the ideal speaker/hearer as being innate, a claim that is just as nonsensical.

Here, a word of alarm is needed. In addition to 'Thought and Sound', Saussure has used two more pairs of terms, that is, Concept and Acoustic (or Sound-) image and *signifié* (signified) and *signifiant* (signifier); these two pairs of terms are used more or less interchangeably.

From the neurolinguistic perspective as advocated by me, however, content plane and expression plane are no longer the substitutes of concept (or signified) and acoustic image (or signifier), respectively. There are two main reasons for the change in usage:

1. Throughout *CLG* Saussure never goes beyond the domain of *le signe*, which is merely exemplified by the French word *arbre*, into lexicogrammar (or, more specifically, syntax), although the language system is mentioned in relation to thought and sound.
2. The two sides of *le signe* are intimately linked and the one calls up the other, that is, they are inseparable. Even Hjelmslev, in his substitution, has also upheld the inseparability of the two functives, expression and content, an opinion which is no longer in line with my usage of the two terms. It is this departure from the Saussurean tradition (*à la* Hjelmslev) that will give me the freedom to posit my own framework of the relationships between thought and sound, a new framework that will probably irk many traditionally minded linguists and semioticians.

In fairness to Saussure, however, it must be added that the language system as the intermediary between thought and sound does go beyond *le signe* for reciprocal delimitations of units of the union between thought (*à la* concept) and sound (*à la* acoustic image). Such being the case, two interesting questions immediately arise:

1. What is the distinction, if any, between 'thought' and 'concept', other things being equal?
2. Is the sign function of the two functives the same as the intermediary between thought and sound?

Asking these questions is tantamount to saying that I have cast serious doubt about the existence of the intermediary in the brain from the ontological point of view.

2. Modification of Saussure's Notions of Stratification

Having sensed the problems involved, when I raised these questions, I decided to modify Saussure's notion of *le signe* and its function on the basis of neurolinguistic findings as follows:

1. Saussure's notion of *le signe* must be expanded to become *text* in the Hallidayan sense;
2. *signifié* (or concept) and *signifiant* (or acoustic image) are separable, because in the brain (or brain functions of memory as content) they do not stay together; they are separated in the first place;
3. as I have already proposed, the terms acoustic image and sound-image must now be differentiated, with 'acoustic image' referring to the impulses collectively in the expression plane, in relation to the impulses in the content plane (or proto-meanings), and 'sound-image' referring to each impulse in the linguistic sign bound to its corresponding concept prior to language potentiation.

On the basis of the modification, thought and sound are not the front and the back of a sheet of paper, which is what Saussure regards as language; rather, they are two separate masses of impulses capable of coming together selectively for mapping and of separation again when acoustic images via sound-images are ready to come out as physical sounds. However, Saussure has a different metaphor which is closer to what I am proposing here but contradicts what he has said about language being compared with a sheet of paper:

> Visualize the air in contact with a sheet of water; if the atmospheric pressure changes, the surface of the water will be broken up into a series of divisions, waves; the waves resemble the union or coupling of thought with phonic substance. (1959: 112)

Put differently, thought from which the signified is derived and sound from which the signifier is derived are two separate masses of impulses, as background noises, roaming around in the brain; a proto-meaning as a part of thought and an acoustic image as a part of sound are brought together temporarily as a concept (or linguistic meaning) and a sound-image prior to language potentiation. The union is temporary because a concept is catalytically mapped onto a sound-image only to be separated again from the sound-image in production when they are no longer in a state of language potentiation, as the sound-image must now enter the extrapyramidal loop by leaving the concept behind in the cerebral cortex. Likewise, the union of acoustic (or other sensory) stimuli in the process of coupling with their corresponding linguistic meanings is also temporary in reception, because of the process of decomposition in the brain functions of memory as capacity, in order to undergo the perceptual organization and re-organization to become percepts for comprehension. Consider the visual binding of the impulse of 'blue' and the impulse of 'square' for BLUE SQUARE in reception explained on page 174.

Given Saussure's second metaphor, unlike that of a sheet of paper, there is no intermediary between thought and sound to be called language. Even so, this metaphor of atmosphere and water in contact depicts only the catalytic mapping, and not the separation, of proto-meanings and acoustic images in production of language; the reception side of language cannot be depicted by this metaphor.

The reason is that thought belongs to the strata of Context of Situation and Meaning, while sound belongs to the Stratum of Sound Patterns. Hence, the signified and the signifier are separate impulses (or series of impulses) in the first place but are brought together only to be separated again to allow the concept (i.e., meaning or *signifié*) to remain in the brain of the speaker while he/she transmits the sound-image (as an impulse or a series of impulses) to the vocal apparatus via the extrapyramidal loop to come out as a physical sound in production. Conversely, a physical sound has no meaning in the first place before it becomes an impulse, when it is heard, because it has to be first recognized and then identified with an existing acoustic image in the expression plane where the acoustic image has a potentially corresponding meaning. Therefore, when a physical sound is recognized through the sensory receptor to become an impulse (or series of impulses), it cannot be put together with any meaning until it is properly processed in reception through identification and coupling, so that a meaning after coupling (appropriate or not) can be reconstructed by the hearer as a result of his/her perceptual organization or re-organization.

Now, what does the stratum of Wording do in my framework? Is it the same as or another version of the intermediary proposed by Saussure? The answer is 'no', because it is not the interface between meaning and sound patterns, nor is it a module. Rather, it is the phenomenon (or the consequence of neural activities of two masses of impulses) when these impulses are brought together in either production or reception. Therefore, there is no corresponding plane.

Saussure uses the air in contact with a sheet of water to explain that 'thought-sound' implies division and that language works out its units while taking shape between two shapeless masses (1959: 112). He also compares language with a sheet of paper: thought is the front and sound is the back; one cannot cut the front without cutting the back at the same time; likewise, in language, one can neither divide sound from thought nor thought from sound; 'the division could be accomplished only abstractedly, and the result would be either pure psychology or pure phonology' (1959: 113). I depart from his analogies for two reasons: first, thought and sound are *not* two shapeless masses; rather, they are two inchoate masses of impulses which are ontologically real in the brain; second, I do not equate wording with language, like a sheet of paper, nor is it synonymous with lexicogrammar, serving as an intermediary, because thought without wording is *not* pure psychology; *nor* is sound without wording pure phonology.

So, I will use a metaphor, too, to explain a similar phenomenon, which is limited to the analogy of wording, nothing more, because no metaphor no matter how elegant can sufficiently or adequately explain the entire production or reception of the complex brain functions of language involving wording.

Simply put, when threads of silk or cotton are woven into a decorative band or when three or more strands of hair are interlaced into a length of hair, the result is called a braid. The threads of silk or cotton or the strands of hair are separated to begin with; they are not inseparable in a band or a braid. Thus, when they are put together into a decorative band or an interlaced braid of hair, the decorative band or the interlaced braid is constructed. The analogy is clear. While the threads of silk or cotton or the strands of hair are ontologically real and visible, when they come together, the phenomenon of weaving or braiding is invisible without the moving activities of the threads or strands; when the threads of silk or the strands of hair are constructed into a decorative band or an interlaced braid of hair, the constructed result is equally ontologically real and visible.

In the same vein, wording is included as a stratum in my framework, not because it is a set of rules or a module comparable to an inchoate mass of impulses, like thought (which comes from the strata of Context of Situation and Meaning in the brain) or sound (which comes from the neural activities of the cerebral cortex and the brainstem). Rather, it is a stratum of language in the brain, because it is a phenomenon that takes place when two inchoate masses of impulses, which are ontologically real, roaming around in the brain, come together to look for each other in order to construct a meaning, in production, or to reconstruct a meaning, in reception.

It follows that (proto-) meanings and acoustic images must undergo two processes in production – catalytic mapping and separation – and two processes in reception – recognition and coupling; recognition, however, has two steps, namely, initial contact with stimuli from either the external or the internal environment, and identification. The initial contact is needed because some stimuli cause the individual to respond with reflexes while some other stimuli allow the individual to take more time to respond in order to identify the incoming stimulus or stimuli from the external or the internal environment.

The process of separation is contrary to Saussure's idea of inseparability of thought and sound, because he thinks that the separation leads to 'pure psychology' (for thought) or 'pure phonology' (for sound). His misgivings are unwarranted, neurophysiologically (i.e., ontologically) speaking, because thought (or meaning) and sound are mapped onto each other catalytically, as they are separate masses of impulses to begin with, and must be separated again because of the looping when acoustic images have become sound-images which are produced as physical sounds via the vocal apparatus.

In light of the modifications, the answers to the two questions become quite apparent: thought and concept (i.e., *signifié*) are *not* the same thing, because thought subsumes *signifié*; the sign function of the two functives now refers to the two processes in production, on the one hand, and to the three processes in reception, on the other, and therefore it cannot serve as the intermediary between thought and sound (nor does the interface as a module between semantics and phonology exist in the brain). Wording as a stratum, however, is *not* a module between meaning and sound patterns; rather, it refers to the contact (or binding and coherence, in the terminology of clinical neurophysiology) of the impulses of meaning and those of sound (or sign) images, for both production and reception.

In spite of the above modifications, there remains the question of whether sound and sound- (or acoustic) image are the same or not. Here, Saussure is ambiguous. Judging from his statement, 'a series of contiguous subdivisions simultaneously patterned on the undefined plane of inchoate ideas (in his A) and on the no less indeterminate plane of sounds (in his B)' (1959: 167), they are not the same; that is, the no less indeterminate plane of sounds refers to the unlimited number of vocal sounds the human vocal apparatus is capable of producing, including yawning, hiccoughing, sneezing, or the like; an acoustic image, in contrast, is learned by each individual and the number of such acoustic images are cumulatively maintained through decomposition in each individual's brain functions of memory as capacity, long term or short term, but are subject to forgetting; therefore, they are limited (no more than the vocabulary a person can acquire or accumulate during his/her lifetime); the vocabulary changes in size during a person's lifetime. Hence, I have said that 'infinity' (in the sense of 'a set' or 'length') as asserted by TG-ers is nonsense, because no human individual in any language can or will ever combine those limited vocabulary items into an infinite set of sentences or a sentence that is infinitely long during his/her lifetime. Such being the case, what is the scientific value of infinity when it is nonsense and out of touch with reality?

Earlier, mention was also made in Chapter 12 that language in the brain is memory-governed (not rule-governed, because there are no such things as 'rules' in the brain) and meaning-centred. What, then, is Saussure's 'thought' now that it is said to subsume *signifié* (concept)? Saussure, once again, leans to psychology for a 'solution' by saying 'Psychologically, (...), our thought is no more than an amorphous and indistinct mass' (Thibault, 1997: 166) or it is 'the undefined plane of inchoate ideas (ibid.: 167): 'Amorphous and indistinct', yes, but 'psychologically', no. The reasons are as follows.

2.1 Thought as the Undefined Plane of Inchoate Meanings

Thought is built up and maintained in the brain functions of memory as content on account of memory as capacity through decomposition and of memory as mechanism through perceptual organization by way of experiences in varying contexts of situation to result in the brain as background noises. It consists of hundreds of thousands of impulses, lurking (or roaming around) in the cerebral cortex waiting to be 'picked up' (i.e., 'unlocked', to use Saussure's terminology). Neurophysiologists use the terms 'binding' and 'coherence' for similar neural activities in the brain, when two or more impulses come together in the brain for comprehension, as in the sensory processing of BLUE SQUARE, via the retino-thalamo-cortical pathways.

The impulse of the colour, BLUE, and the impulse of the shape, SQUARE, must come together in the brain to allow the individual to form the proper meaning of a 'blue square', which constitutes a part of his/her content plane; it becomes a part of the background noises in his/her brain if retained (i.e., not forgotten). I have called the coming together of different impulses to form a single, coherent whole in the brain perceptual organization.

The meaning, if it is to be catalytically mapped onto a series of acoustic images [blùw skwèr], in production, must look for (or unlock) the acoustic images first for the catalytic mapping, so as to form a linguistic sign consisting of the concept (or linguistic meaning) of 'blue square' and its corresponding sound-images; and, then, they separate again, that is, the linguistic sign splits, to allow the sound images to go through the extrapyramidal looping in order to reach the exit (i.e., the motor cortex) so as to come down inside the pyramidal tract of the internal capsule to the vocal apparatus for emission as physical sounds.

If the meaning fails to 'unlock' (or find) the needed corresponding acoustic images to form a coherent linguistic unit, for lack of experience in his/her vocabulary (i.e., expression plane), because he/she is not a native speaker of English, then there is no catalytic mapping nor is there separation; consequently, there is no emission of physical sounds, although the individual can still perceive the object as BLUE SQUARE in his/her brain. The electro-neurophysiological concept of binding, which is confined to reception, is herewith extended to production in the process of catalytic mapping.

On the other hand, a person may have a false start, when attempting to speak or sign to another person. When and if that happens, the speaker or signer may or may not be aware that he/she made a mistake.

In the case of awareness, which usually occurs in a split second, the speaker or signer will have to correct the mistake, with an apology to the hearer or viewer (e.g., 'I beg your pardon') or without it, because he/she has the instant feedback as speaker qua hearer or signer qua viewer of the mistake. At that point, when he/she reiterates or resigns what was originally intended, his/her brain functions have the perceptual re-organization which is to rely on the brain functions of memory as mechanism (e.g., the mechanism of repetition) to find the right (or correct) corresponding acoustic image (or visual image) for the process of catalytic mapping again.

In the case of unawareness, however, the speaker/signer's erroneous language behaviour would be the same as in the case of no mistake made, until the hearer/viewer qua speaker/signer points out the mistake. When the mistake is pointed out – for example, 'Did you say A? I thought it was B' – the speaker/signer then simply starts the utterance or signing again, with perhaps an apology like 'Sorry, I meant to say B.'

Linguists who are innatists have proclaimed the irrelevancy of experience to language because they have denied the importance or the essential ontological nature of human memory to language in the brain. The truth of the matter is that the brain functions of memory as content are experience-based and time-sensitive. Without experience of any kind, internal or external, the brain functions of memory as content in the individual would be 'empty', primarily as a result of the dysfunction of memory as capacity, long term or short term.

The brain functions of memory are also time-sensitive, primarily as a result of forgetting as a normal function of memory as capacity. The fact that a person can talk smoothly (without stuttering) in a linear fashion, an important function of the vocal apparatus, in contradistinction to simultaneity which is an important function of the brachial apparatus for sign language, is because the impulse that goes (or comes out) first must be erased instantaneously in the pathways to allow the impulse that comes next to go through the pathways. This instantaneous erasure of successive impulses in the cortico-bulbar pathways or the cortico-spinal pathways I have called Rapid Inhibition Mechanism (RIM for short). The instantaneous erasure of successive impulses is a form of normal forgetting that belongs to the brain functions of memory as capacity. Stuttering is a form of impairment of this process arising from inhibitory disorder, so is perseveration that is often observed in patients with brain damage; for example, aphasic patients.

Stuttering, it should be emphasized, is a wording problem arising from disorders of the RIM. But it can be temporarily 'loosened' up by stimulating the 'hand area' in the cortex to disinhibit the on-and-off inhibition of impulses, in the cortico-bulbar pathways, from the 'mouth area' of the cortex (cf. Figure 15.2). These areas were mapped out by Penfield and Rasmussen in 1950, thereby 'repairing' temporarily the wording problem as long as the stimulation lasts. Put differently, the RIM is important to wording, in production (i.e., efferent), and since stuttering is a disorder of the RIM, it hampers wording, although the stutterer's content plane and expression plane are intact. However, I should add that stuttering does not happen to reception (i.e., afferent), although the RIM is relevant to both efferent and afferent impulses.

Clinically, it has been observed that a pianist/entertainer, who is also a stutterer, can play the piano to entertain the audience while talking to them without any sign of stuttering, but the moment he/she stops playing the piano,

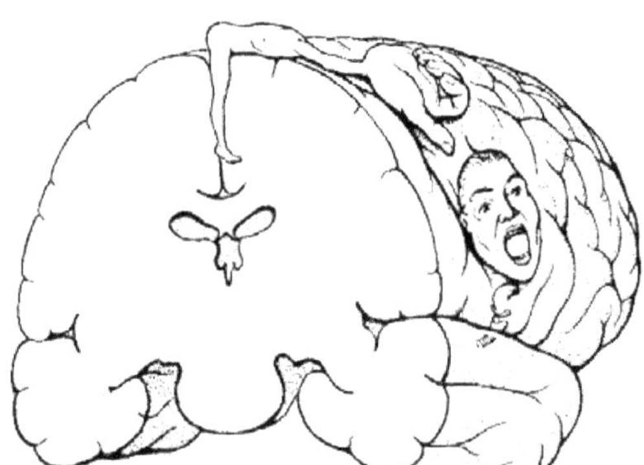

Figure 15.2 *Somatotopic localization of parts of the body in the motor cortex. Parts of the body are drawn in proportion to the extent of their cortical representation (after Penfield and Rasmussen, 1950)* (From *The Cerebral Cortex of Man: A Clinical Study in Localization of Function*, by W. Penfield and T. Rasmussen, New York: Macmillan Company, 1950. Used by permission of Thomson Gale.)

his/her stuttering returns immediately. Professor Roger Matthews has suggested that 'the reading aloud of verse (i.e., rhythmic patterns) may have the same therapeutic effect'.

If his idea is proven clinically effective, then the stutterer may have the acoustic feedback working to help enhance the perceptual re-organization in order to improve the impaired RIM, albeit temporarily. However, there is a catch. English verse relies heavily on its various metres (based on the stress system in the English language) and rhyming scheme for rhythmic patterns, such as an iambic pentameter; the Japanese or Chinese verse, on the other hand, does not use metre for expression; instead, it relies heavily on the arrangement of the number of syllables and/or rhymes and tonal patterns (in the case of Chinese). It would be nice if the recitation (or reading aloud) of poems in any language, written or unwritten (e.g., Ainu Yukar) could prove useful in the treatment of stuttering.

2.2 Experiences as the Source of Thought

The experiences so maintained in the brain functions of memory as content, via memory as mechanism in memory as capacity, become the individual's background noises which are, therefore, quite personal. For instance, those astronauts who have been to the moon have the kind of experiences which most of us do not have. The same goes for families whose members have suffered from AD, FD, HD or PD, for instance, Mrs Reagan, the former First Lady; her experience is unknown to most of us with regard to caring for the former president who passed way in July 2004 and was diagnosed to have had AD, although there was no autopsied proof; more likely, he had dementia which had been neurodegenerative caused by neurofibrillary tangles (i.e., AD) or senile plaques (i.e., FD); both diseases have been mixed up in the literature as Alzheimer's disease when the latter should have been designated as Fischer's disease (FD). But other families whose householders have the same disease, or I should say, dementia, most certainly share similar, if not identical, experiences with Mrs Reagan.

Likewise, most of us who watched TV for the repeated reports of the terrorists' attacks on September 11 2001 shared the same experiences but those family members of the 3,000 or so victims, killed in the attacks or aftermath, have traumatically permanent experiences which most of us cannot share; thus, we cannot in any way express words that can correspond to the deep-felt meanings they can construct. When the Commission's Final Report came out on 22 July 2004, it is difficult to imagine (i.e., to reconstruct the meanings of) how family members of the victims felt as they reviewed the report which concludes that 'failure of imagination', not government neglect, allowed 19 hijackers to carry out the deadliest terrorist attacks in US history.

When on July 7 2005 four terrorists attacked the underground and a bus in London, killing more than 50 people, the Londoners' experiences were reminiscent of the New Yorkers' on September 11, 2001 as the source of thought in their brain functions of memory for proto-meaning.

2.3 Proto-Meaning

Since such experiences have entered the individual's brain via the five senses for safe keeping in the brain functions of memory as capacity, subject to modification on account of time-sensitive forgetting, I have called them proto-meaning, too, as part of the individual's background noises in his/her brain functions of memory as content. They are amorphous and/or indistinct in the sense that they are not in a state of language potentiation; once they are in such a state or ready to be expressed to the hearer via catalytic mapping, they are not shapeless.

However, within each individual different experiences do exist, as he/she can recall as part of his/her thought, without verbalizing them, in respect to the origins of certain experiences; for example, a woman's beautiful necklace bought during a visit to Japan by her husband for their twentieth wedding anniversary. Even without an anniversary, most people can remember where and when a photo was taken or where and when they bought certain dresses; they can reminisce on occasions with their close friends by retrieving these experiences as proto-meaning into verbalization (via catalytic mappings) for a lively conversation.

Likewise, those family members of the victims on September 11 2001 will never forget the pains and sorrows for the losses of their loved ones; when they reminisced on occasions, for instance, after they had reviewed the Commission's Final Report, and then shared with their relatives or close friends their anguished experiences in their background noises as proto-meanings into verbalization (again, via catalytic mappings), their language behaviours, it can be absolutely certain, were not lively conversations; rather, they were sad, resentful and weeping conversations.

2.4 Meanings in Memory as Content

When these experiences are maintained in the brain functions of memory as content, they are not 'pictures' or icons of the original shapes and/or configurations or movements; nor are they packed into book forms placed on bookshelves. Rather, they are decomposed into impulses of different sorts, after the initial contact, not 'tucked away' in the two hippocampi, as most specialists working on memory would like us to believe.

These decomposed impulses are registered or encoded for shape, colour, order, and the like, as proto-meanings, in neurons of different parts of the brain, depending on the types/kinds of experience encountered, for example, visual, olfactory, auditory or the like. But they must combine through binding and coherence to also undergo perceptual organization or re-organization for perception as whole percepts. They can also be recalled, or retrieved, as needed, from maintenance on the basis of the brain functions of memory as mechanism to reach the state of language potentiation so as to become linguistic meanings. If a person cannot retrieve (i.e., remember) a certain experience (or proto-meaning) on demand or on free will, to the extent of more than 50 per cent failure, or repeats the same thing over and over again in his/her daily life or gets lost in a familiar territory, while driving home, it is likely that dementia has already set in.

Those reasons, and there may be more, all point to the fact that thought is not a psychologically amorphous and indistinct mass; it consists of neurophysiological entities called impulses (which are action potentials caused by biochemical substances known as neurotransmitters and travel rapidly in milliseconds as brain waves for neuron-to-neuron communication or thinking).

In other words, thought is ontological in nature and made up of neural activities which, in the form of brain waves, combine with or bind other brain waves coming from different regions of the brain. These other brain waves are the signals or impulses of neurons which have been referred to above as acoustic (or sound-) images (not at all sounds which are the physical phenomena coming out of the mouth). There is quite a distance, because of the cortico-striato-pallido-thalamo-cortical looping, before an acoustic image (in the brain) as an impulse can be transduced to become the sound-image in a linguistic sign (also in the brain) in order to come out as a (physical) sound in the air via the vocal apparatus.

2.5 Language Potentiation

I have postulated that when impulses from proto-meaning (i.e., from the content plane or thought) are catalytically mapped onto their corresponding acoustic images, which are also impulses (i.e., from the expression plane), resulting in a linguistic sign (consisting of a concept and a sound-image) or a series of such linguistic signs, there is a mental state of preparation which follows before allowing the sound-images to enter the loop; I have called that mental state of 'preparation', language potentiation. Once the sound-images in the linguistic signs are separated from their corresponding concepts to enter the loop, the sound-images must go through the looping where thinking takes place before words can come out of the mouth as physical sounds via the pyramidal tract (from the motor cortex where large pyramidal cells of Betz are activated); thinking takes place because the sound-images through the looping go back to the cerebral (motor) cortex for 'confirmation', 'reconfirmation' or 'fine-tuning' of meaning the speaker has constructed or intended. For this reason, thought (i.e., content plane) and Sound (i.e., expression plane) are not at all shapeless.

Such being the case, there is no intermediary between a meaning as an impulse or a series of impulses (from thought, i.e., content plane) and a sound-image or sign image as an impulse or a series of impulses (from sound or expression plane). However, as thought consists of hundreds of thousands of impulses in the cerebral cortex, it can be regarded as a mass of impulses which are neurophysiologically amorphous and indistinct before any catalytic mapping takes place. Be that as it may, the mass varies in size from one individual to another depending on each individual's age and, proportionately, his/her experiences. In like manner, there are also hundreds of thousands of acoustic images in sound (or expression plane), each of which is either an impulse or a series of impulses. But these acoustic images remain indeterminate unless they are catalytically mapped onto their corresponding meanings to become the sound-images in a linguistic sign or a series of linguistic signs, in which case, the sound-images are not at all indeterminate even though they belong to the expression plane just the same; rather, they are quite specific and their number may be large, but varies from individual to individual, and therefore it can never be larger than each individual's vocabulary size at any given time, that is, during childhood or when he/she has become an adult.

2.6 Linguistic Meaning

Once an impulse from thought (or content plane) is catalytically mapped onto, that is, bound to, an acoustic image from sound (or expression plane), in production, the impulse can no longer be amorphous either; it becomes quite specific, so much so that it is this specificity that has led me to call the bound impulse linguistic meaning, as it now refers to what Saussure calls concept (i.e., signified). It is posited in contradistinction to proto-meaning.

2.6.1 Different Shades of Meaning

Between linguistic meaning and proto-meaning, there are different shades (or degrees) of meaning, which may be called, technically, enhanced meaning as the result of what I have called function enhancement in the brain. The different shades of meaning for any particular utterance in a dyadic interaction vary in number; they come and go, depending on the circumstances under which the speaker constructs his/her meaning (which may be proto-meaning or linguistic meaning) and the hearer reconstructs his/her meaning (which may be the speaker's proto-meaning qua linguistic meaning but is more likely the hearer's own 'presumptuous' proto-meaning for the speaker). A good example is what President Truman said during his re-election, 'If you can't stand the heat, get out of the kitchen.' The 'real meaning' (or proto-meaning) underlying this expression is what laymen would call inference; a person with a different linguistic and cultural background is likely to miss it, even if he/she speaks good English, thereby getting only the linguistic meaning, although sociolinguists might want to call the expression as a whole a perlocutionary act. The same goes for puns, jokes, satires and a host of other examples.

However, a linguistic meaning from the content plane and an acoustic image (or a visual image) from the expression plane do not come out together to reach the vocal (or brachial) apparatus; they must be separated, again, to allow the linguistic meaning to remain in the brain while permitting the sound-image (or the visual image) to come down, as in the example of BLUE SQUARE, via the loop, to the vocal (or brachial) apparatus for the actual phonation (or signing). The result is a sound or a series of sounds (or a hand configuration and/or movement) which has no meaning in and by itself, because the corresponding meaning (linguistic meaning or proto-meaning) is left behind in the speaker's (or signer's) brain. The hearer or viewer must reconstruct his/her own meaning (which may be linguistic meaning, speaker/signer's proto-meaning, or enhanced meaning) in the brain on the basis of the sound heard or sign seen in the course of reception.

2.6.2 Further Modification

If this specific binding of a linguistic meaning and a sound-image (or a visual image) in production (for catalytical mapping) or in reception (for coupling) is what Saussure calls Signification, then another modification must be made, which pertains to what linguists call lexicogrammar (or grammar for short). I have used the term Wording for the purpose of modification, even though systemic linguists make no distinction between lexicogrammar and wording.

In my modification, however, wording is *not* the same as lexicogrammar, because there is no lexicogrammar (as a module) in the brain. It is the creation of linguists (or an artifact of data processing) for their purposes of referring to what they want to discuss in the social aspect of language; it is neither an ontological entity in the brain nor a module of any brain function. It is an entity of epistemology created by linguists from the data-processing of texts, and not an ontological given. That is why there are so many different grammars for English or any other language in the linguistic literature.

On the other hand, wording refers to what is happening in the brain, when impulses from the content plane come into contact for binding with impulses from the expression plane, in either production or reception; it is when (catalytic) mapping or coupling of thought and sound takes place, respectively, that wording can happen, which is to say that wording is *not* a built-in mechanism but a phenomenon in the presence of catalytic mapping or coupling.

Lexicogrammar, of course, does not exist in the brains of other animals; nor does it exist in the human brain. But wording as a stratum of brain functions exists as a phenomenon in the brains of all animals, vertebrates and mammals, because they all have content plane and expression plane in their brains. However, I should add that wording varies in complexity from one species to another, because of the differences in the complexity of neuronal organization in each species.

Creating a lexicogrammar for any human language is a perfectly legitimate enterprise, because it is the result of data-processing from texts (transcribed phonetically or written); with computer-aided data-processing, the result may become even more minute and complicated. Chomsky's *Syntactic Structure* was created that way in 1957, patterned after computation for machine translation. But to turn around and assert that other animals do not or cannot have that creation in their brains, and therefore they do not have language, is self-deceiving. Worse still, to claim that the 'rules' as grammar in the creation are innate and universal becomes a farce.

2.6.3 Catalytic Mapping and Separation

In catalytic mapping for wording, on the other hand, thought (in the form of various concepts from the content plane governed by the brain functions of memory) and sound or sign (in the form of sound-images or sign-images from the expression plane also governed by the brain functions of memory) look for each other, so that each concept can 'unlock' or find its corresponding sound-image or sign-image. The nervous system of any other mammal, or even vertebrate, is equipped with this kind of capability, obviously not to the same level of sophistication for the volume of thought and variety of sound. The result is a coherent linguistic sign which is modified from Saussure's idea of *le signe.* However, this linguistic sign consisting of a concept and a sound-image must be split, so that the concept and the sound-image are separated again to allow the sound-image to go through the looping in the extrapyramidal tract.

2.6.4 Recognition, Identification and Coupling

In coupling, likewise, for wording, each incoming stimulus must have the initial contact with the receptors (auditory, visual, olfactory, gustatory or tactile) to become an impulse as a part of the process of recognition. Such an impulse must look for a corresponding acoustic, visual, olfactory, gustatory or tactile image in the expression plane first, which is a process involving identification, and then locate each corresponding meaning (or concept) in the content plane for coupling. If a needed image in the expression plane cannot be located, then the individual's brain is likely to look for a close-enough but similar image. In other animals, such brain functions exist to enable them to make proper adjustments to the internal and the external environments. Or else, they cannot survive. The fact that they have survived is evidence that they are well equipped with the needed brain functions.

From the initial contact to the coupling of the incoming sensory impulses with their corresponding meanings I have said that there are two processes in between, which are worthy of some elaboration; namely, the recognition of each decomposed stimulus, and the identification of the components of each such decomposed stimulus, now as a perceptually organized or re-organized whole, with an existing acoustic image in the brain functions of memory as content (i.e., expression plane). In the case of oral language, I have already mentioned the roles played by the inferior and superior colliculi and the two medial geniculate bodies. I am willing to speculate that the second process is conducted in the interplay of these subcortical structures with the cerebral cortex, and that the first process is handled by the auditory receptor organ, consisting of one row of inner hair cells and three rows of outer hair cells, and the auditory nucleus of the VIIIth cranial (i.e., vestibulo-cochlear) nerve. I will give an example here from oral language.

When a person makes an utterance in English, it is not made up of just what linguists call consonants and vowels; it also contains intonation, stress, tone of voice, timbre, voice quality (of a man, a woman, a child or an elderly person) and the like. The hearer must recognize all these components in the speaker's utterance, consciously or subconsciously. I believe these components are first detected in the hearer's auditory nucleus, after they pass the receptors – for example the hair cells – and are then identified as such in the midbrain and the thalamus when adjustments are required therein, because the medial geniculate bodies (i.e., the thalamus) are the places where the incoming impulses are matched, through the interplay with the cerebral cortex, with the existing acoustic images. From the thalamus onward, the process of coupling takes place for perceptual organization or re-organization in which wording must take part; the corresponding meanings (which are also impulses) can be found for coupling with the incoming auditory impulses, thereby resulting in the hearer's reconstruction of his/her meanings for the speaker's utterance, including not only the linguistic meanings but also the nuances, the age and sex of speaker, or to some extent even the speaker's socio-economic and/or educational background and the like.

Thus, wording in production and wording in reception differ in terms of the brain functions for each species, whereas in linguistics no distinction is made between lexicogrammar for production and that for reception, although attempts have been made by some linguists, such as Hockett (1986), to characterize the hearer's grammar; such attempts were unfortunately overlooked.

Some researchers in Florida have tried to 'decipher' the sounds made by dolphins. It has also been known that marine mammals, such as dolphins and whales, make different sounds in their vocalizations to communicate among themselves. Perhaps, these researchers can 'write' a grammar of dolphin's code, even though we can never know exactly what goes on in a dolphin's brain. However, it was learned during Operation Iraqi Freedom that dolphins were used in the war for military purposes; they had been trained to search or find mines in the Persian Gulf or elsewhere, and seemed to have done a good job. Sea lion's code has also been studied. The result shows that sea lions produce and receive their own sounds for different behavioural purposes. It would be interesting to find out how a sea lion's brain works in comparision with that of a dolphin's.

2.7 Summary: Departure from the Tradition

I have in the previous chapters taken the stance which drastically departs from two traditions: the tradition in linguistics, and the tradition in neuroscience. In the former, I depart from the tradition about wording and lexicogrammar or language in general, by making a mild proposal from the point of view of brain functions; in the latter, I depart from the tradition of memory and cognition, by regarding them as two sides (i.e., heads and tails) of the same coin which governs language in the brain, or any other behaviour, thereby abandoning the cherished notions of cerebral dominance and cerebral laterality.

Since these departures are rather new, I shall spend most of my remaining time dealing with or elaborating those ideas expressed especially in connection with the brain functions of memory as content, memory as capacity, and memory as mechanism. The result will be the reconsideration of regional specializations because brain structures are interdependent in regards to their functions which are not exclusively specialized for any particular region.

Most contemporary researchers dealing with memory seem to be preoccupied with the classification of memory as content, for example, Squire (1987). There is one exception, namely, Working Memory, which advocates one central executive and two slaves which are the articulatory (or phonological) loop and the visuo-spatial scratch-pad (Baddeley, 1986). I have already briefly commented on this model. However, as it is fundamentally flawed from the neurolinguistic point of view, with conflicting results, because of its simplistic view of what language in the brain is, I shall elaborate below my objections further in terms of language in the brain and other related behaviours.

First, I should mention that brain impulses travel in milliseconds and yet all experiments in working memory were conducted in reaction time (from half a second or so to a couple of seconds for each subject's reaction) or even performance time, without realizing that by the time a subject reacts to any stimulus, the brain impulses activated have already travelled in all directions several times over in his/her brain. (See Goldman-Rakic (1992) in comparison with Gitelman (2003) for the claim of involvement in the prefrontal cortex and the conflicting results between these studies.)

Second, it also completely neglects the role of subcortical structures in the brain functions of memory, such as the basal ganglia, the cerebellum, and the Papez circuit, presumably because working memory is thought to be concerned only with very brief short-term memory, however brief it may be, and therefore the two hippocampi, the thalamus, the basal ganglia and the cerebellum are not the major 'players' in working memory. For these reasons, it does not and cannot account for the brain functions of memory as purported in this monograph in the sense of memory as content, memory as capacity, and memory as mechanism.

16 Evolution of Language: What Evolved?

It should be clear from the preceding chapters that the brain functions of memory play a crucial role in language behaviour, which is to say that any discussion dealing with language in the brain in particular or other behaviours in general for humans must take the brain functions of memory into consideration. This requirement is tantamount to the fact that language is memory-governed; so are all other behaviours. Therefore, it is not an exaggeration to say that any study of language origin must be based squarely on the ontogenesis and phylogenesis of the brain functions of memory in all animals, human or non-human, because they have their brain functions of memory which govern their behaviours.

Such being the case, any attempt to consider the evolution of language cannot avoid the question of whether or not non-human behaviours include such behaviours that can be called their language behaviours which are also governed by their brain functions of memory. But, unfortunately, none of the works on the evolution of language or language origin so far have faced up to such a question.

On the other hand, the question of when language started and how it has evolved to the present has intrigued many investigators over the past two millennia or so in various fields which I have described briefly in the preceding chapters, especially Part I. However, because such a question depends on the answer to another more fundamental question of 'what is language?', the question of the evolution of language cannot be properly answered unless or until the fundamental question is dealt with squarely. For this reason, more than ten thousand 'theories' of language evolution and language origin had been documented in the past by one count (Hews, 1974), but some of them were reworked in the twentieth century. Since the issue of evolution of language now reappears as a new trend in the twenty-first century (*Science*, 2004), bringing in medical gadgets, like PET and fMRI as tools to support the proponents' assertions, I shall devote this chapter to express my views in response to 'Evolution of Language' in *Science* (2004).

1. The Notion of Evolution of Language

The evolution of language has always been tied to human evolution in the belief that only humans possess language and other animals do not, and therefore the belief becomes a fascinating issue which inevitably triggers the search of what differentiates humans from non-human animals. The search has had its ups and downs in the past but a special edition of *Scientific American* (2004) appeared recently, entitled 'Human Evolution' containing 12 articles which took a fresh look at the old issue in order to challenge and intrigue the readership. Despite the new look, regrettably the old issue remains; that is, the search for the criterion that can separate humans from non-human animals continues with no definitive conclusion in sight. This old issue is discussed in one of the articles, entitled 'Where did people come from?' and is touched on in another, entitled 'Why we walk on two legs'. I will forefront the old issue here as it is related to the notion of the evolution of language.

Anthropologists thought at first that the criterion was the use of tools, which involved the evolution of intelligence. The idea failed, because they found that other animals, like a certain kind of birds, not to mention non-human primates, can use a twig to stick into a hole of a tree to force the worm inside to come out, after listening carefully to the movement of the worm inside the tree. They then changed the criterion to the making of tools, which also turned out to be false, because non-human primates were found to be able to make suitable tools for crossing a river or getting food beyond the reach of their forelimbs.

Having failed twice, anthropologists now joined by linguists, psychologists and neuroscientists turned to language as the sole criterion and asserted that only humans possess language and this separates them from non-human animals. As will be shown in Chapter 17, this criterion is intimately linked to the cherished notions of cerebral dominance and cerebral laterality in neuroscience, which do not apply to non-human animals, because these animals are also said to have cerebral asymmetries, a notion that should be distinguished from the cherished notions.

The new trend in the twenty-first century, although it is now equiped with new medical tools not available in the past, invariably steps into the old 'shoe'; that is, no attempt is made to clarify what language is, as if everybody knows what it is. Therefore, language is implicitly taken for granted as either a thing or an organ that can evolve by itself, rather than as behaviour which depends on the characteristics of neuroanatomy and neurophysiology in the varying individual organisms of each species for production and reception. Thus, the idea of 'mirror neurons' – whatever they may be – was proposed by some investigators in the evolution of language.

They then claimed that these 'mirror neurons' were for imitation as the origin of language or clicks believed by some to be the first language in humans, without recourse to those characteristics; that is, they do not realize or are not aware that non-human primates can also make clicks; if an attempt is made to refer to such characteristics in order to uphold their claim, the attempt is erroneous. I will now state my response from the point of view of what has evolved phylogenetically and what can evolve ontogentically by recapitulating some of what I have already described earlier.

2. What has Evolved Phylogenetically?

I should point out first that language as behaviour does not evolve by itself nor on its own; what can and does evolve are the characteristics of neuroanatomy and neurophysiology of the varying individual organisms of each species. The neurophysiological properties, such as the exchange of positively charged and negatively charged ions (i.e., cations and anions) within a single neuron do not change from non-human animals, such as a squid, to humans. Thus, the electric activity called impulse running through the giant axon of a squid cannot be distinguished from the impulse running through an axon in a human nervous system. However, when the complexity of neuronal circuitry (resulting from gross anatomical alterations) changes through evolution, the patternings (i.e., the functions) of impulses, as may be shown in the complex summation of impulses, greatly change to the extent that the change gradually alters the manifestations of behaviour in varying contexts of situation.

As is pointed out in the special edition of *Scientific American*, there are many anatomical changes resulting from evolution, chief among them being the following: from quadrupedal to bipedal locomotion; the change of facial features (or the shape of the skull); and the change of skin colours. Since the first two changes are closely related to the change of language as behaviour, I shall confine my discussion to these two changes which are interrelated.

2.1 The Change from Quadrupedal to Bipedal Locomotion

As may be seen in a circus or animal show, a four-legged animal such as a poodle, a monkey, or a chimpanzee can be trained to walk on its hindlegs, resembling bipedal locomotion. Such a locomotion, of course, cannot alter the head shape or the neuronal circuitry inside the cranium within a short period of time, that is, the animal's lifetime. However, anthropologists now believe that the bipedal locomotion of some primates started millions of years ago, not at once but gradually building up the new habit through many generations, to adapt to the new locomotive style: walking upright. There are two prerequisites for the needed phylogenetic changes to take place:

1. The change to locomotive style started millions of years ago, which was initiated not by all primates but by some whose motivation for the change varied.
2. The newly adapted locomotive style had to continue for many generations, through hundreds if not thousands of years, in order to allow mutations to occur in the gene pool.

Many people claiming the origin and evolution of language are either unaware of the long time frame the mutant genes had to take in order to start working or simply naively take some mutant gene, such as FOXp2, for granted as if it existed millions of years ago. Worse still, unlike the gene in Huntington's disease which took geneticists ten years to unfold or the many genes now discovered in SCA (Spino-Cerebellar Ataxia), all of which have the trinucleotide repeat expansion as the genetic marker of each disease, FOXp2 is tied only to a few individuals in a single pedigree, who were said to display certain grammatical errors, involving the past tense marker, in their language behaviour which is English. The curious question I will raise is: what are the trinucleotide repeat expansions in the affected members of the pedigree? Without specifying such expansions, the proponents then jumped to an unfounded and, I should say, naive generalization to claim that the gene is a language gene for all humans in their languages, only to retract it later.

Using an error in the behaviour of a grammatical feature within a few English speakers and linking it to the mutant gene of those individuals as the origin of the normal language behaviour of many peoples in the world, whose languages do not have the tense inflection, is barking at the moon. I should reiterate that there is no grammar in the brain, because it is an epistemological creation of linguists for data-processing and not an ontological given in the brain. Therefore, there is no language gene, because a gene is a functional concept and not a structural one, which will be explained in greater detail further below.

2.2 The Change of Facial Features

This change includes the alteration of the shape of the cranium (or skull) and of the vocal apparatus as a result; it is a direct consequence of the locomotive change just described. Upright locomotion, after thousands of years, gradually changed the shape of the cranium, first among some individuals in the offspring of the primates who had adapted to it and subsequently the appropriate genes mutated in one chromosomal locus or even in more than one chromosomal loci. The facial and cervical musculature also had to change accordingly in order to accommodate the facial body movements that affected the lips, tongue and jaw.

A slight alteration of the shape of the cranium can be observed in a human individual who has the congenital torticollis (*tortus* 'twisted' + *collum* 'neck') because the cervical muscle (sternocleidomastoid) on one side was injured at birth. There is no mutation of the individual's genes, however. Therefore, his/her offspring will not inherit the trait, if born without the same injury.

Facial features and stature may also be altered genetically. For instance, people with Down's Syndrome, with 47 chromosomes rather than 46, look more like each other than they do their own siblings; the stature is usually short and the facial features are peculiarly similar among them, so much so that they can be recognized on the spot.

2.2.1 Alteration of the Shape of the Cranium

When the genes that direct the shape of the cranium after birth started to mutate millions of years ago, the neuronal circuitry inside the cranium had to change as well. I have already mentioned the differences between humans and non-human animals in their nervous systems, namely:

1. more bending of telencephalon to accommodate the gradually increased number of neurons;
2. the increased formation of gyri to accommodate the connections of the increased number of neurons;
3. delayed myelination to adjust to the ontogenetic development of the vocal apparatus and the increased intelligence;
4. the increased complexity of aborization to accommodate and facilitate the connections of the increased number of neurons for the elevation of function enhancement in behaviour.

2.2.2 Alteration of the Vocal Tract Shape

The vocal tract shape refers to the function of the vocal apparatus for the production of speech. The vocal apparatus consists of a set of body parts which include not just the larynx but also the whole system of respiration (the lungs, the trachea, the mouth and the nose) and the articulatory system (the vocal folds, the thyroid cartilage and the muscles attached to it, the cricoid and the muscles attached to it to control various movements of the vocal folds innervated by the recurrent laryngeal nerve of the vagus, the buccal cavity, the teeth, the tongue, the upper and lower mandibles, the uvula, the pharynx, and the epiglottis).

The intricate coordination of expiration and inspiration in conjunction with the following body parts is very important for speech production:

1. the articulators;
2. the points of articulation;
3. the manners of articulation, for consonants;
4. the tongue heights and movements;
5. the lip shapes and movements, for vowels;
6. the movements and control of the vocal folds for voicing, voicelessness and glottalization, or even pharyngealization.

Instructions to do all these come from the cerebral cortex, which not only induce the appropriate cranial nerves but also act on the lower respiratory centre (in the floor of the fourth ventricle) in the medulla oblongata to change spontaneously the normal respiratory pattern to a pattern concerted to the actions of articulation and combine them for breathing (not abandoning it, as some would have us so believe) at the same time. In other words, when a person speaks his/her speaking is a part of his/her breathing as well, or else that person will die of not breathing (or of suffocation). Put differently, the system of respiration is innate and exists in all mammals and vertebrates; but utilizing the system for speaking in combination with breathing depends to a large extent on the phylogenetically evolved and highly complex cerebral networking and the sophisticated vocal apparatus in humans.

I have already mentioned that all body parts have their body schemata in the brain; thus, the functions of such body parts to make speech had to increase in the brain because of the alteration of the shape of the cranium just described, because it depends on the close coordination of such body parts which are controlled by a few cranial nerves under instruction from the cerebral cortex. In other words, one single body part alone from the set cannot make speech sounds; alternatively, the loss of just one such body part, as in laryngectomy to remove the larynx because of cancer caused by smoking or because of cleft palate, will disable or distort speech production.

It seems confusing, then, that one of the proponents of language evolution, Pinker, should note that 'both breathing and articulation are directed by brain areas quite separate from those associated with human speech' (*Science*, 2004: 1317). Another perplexing remark has been made by MacNeilage about phonetics, phonology and syntax in the following way: 'The next stage ... was to give voice to these behaviors by bringing the larynx into play. This theory fits well with the fact that the unique sounds of click languages, which some speculate may have been the original mother tongue, do not use the larynx. Once the larynx was involved, a phonology – a set of sounds that could be combined in endless ways to form a large vocabulary – developed, and this in turn paved the way for the emergence of syntax' (*Science*, 2004: 1319). Three points are open for criticism.

First, clicks do involve the larynx. One can find this out by pressing one finger on the Adam's apple and clicking a sound (bilabial, dental, or retroflex click). The larynx has to move to pull down the mouth air in order to make the click. In *Manual of Articulatory Phonetics* (Smalley, 1983) clicks are described in great detail, including voiceless clicks (aspirated and unaspirated), nasalized clicks and voiced clicks. Such clicks are used in Zulu, which are the results of motor functions. But for non-linguistic purposes, similar click activities appear in kissing (voiceless bilabial click), expressing mild reproval: 'tsk tsk' (voiceless dental click), 'giddeap' (voiceless lateral affricated click) and the like (ibid.: 428). Such clicks are the results of motor activities. Is kissing the origin of language, then?

Second, phonology is another technique created by linguists in the late 1930s for analysing each language on the basis of phonetics; there is no such thing as a universal phonology.

Anyway, the technique employed in phonology does not combine sounds in endless ways, because each language has its own sound sequences, which linguists have called phonotactics; they are limited and finite. Phonetics, however, may allow an individual to make as many different sounds as he/she wishes in his/her lifetime, none of which is identical with the rest. Put differently, phoneticians believe that a person cannot make the same sound twice in his/her lifetime.

Third, syntax, which is also a cherished creation of linguists, albeit not without merit for data-processing when linguists talk to one another for the sake of referencing, does not emerge in the brain, which recognizes only impulses. There are no such impulses in the brain which can be identified as nouns, verbs, adjectives and the like, or Subject and Predicate, or Topic and Comment. Impulses are electric activities which roam around in the brain and are transduced from one neuron to many other neurons more or less simultaneously via neuronal interconnections in a linear fashion or from many neurons to converge on a single neuron. However, if two presynaptic impulses are transmitted along the same axon, separated by a very short interval, they will result in a summation postsynaptically. Thus, it is totally nonsensical to formulate $S \rightarrow NP + VP$ as a rule, or any other rules Chomsky or programmers designed for the computer, pretending that it exists in the brain, when it does not, because impulses in the brain do not work that way. To claim otherwise is a farce.

3. What has Evolved Ontogenetically?

In Chapter 10, I described the appearance of the cranial nerves and the formation of the vocal apparatus and pointed out the species-specific function of the human vocal apparatus. Although non-human primates also have their cranial nerves and vocal apparatus, the functions of their cranial nerves and vocal apparatus differ considerably from those of human cranial nerves and vocal apparatus. It is true that the existence of these nerves and the organ is as a result of phylogenetic evolution over millions of years. However, the human vocal apparatus has its own ontogenic evolution (i.e., timetable) which is phylogenetically predetermined. Two points deserve recapitulation here.

First, a newborn human infant's vocal apparatus is shaped like a chimpanzee's. It starts to change its shape and size ontogenetically through two important processes which are necessary for growth in all animals: hyperplasia (increase in the number of cells) and hypertrophy (increase in the size of each cell). The change starts at the age of six months, with the exception of the tongue, which remains more or less the same size; the larynx to which the epiglottis is attached starts to descend in order to reach its adult shape at two years of age. Nonetheless, the manoeuvre (or exercise) of the vocal apparatus, especially the tongue, or the articulatory sucking of a thumb by some foetuses, starts before birth inside the uterus.

Second, it has been frequently demonstrated by psychologists that a two-year-old human child's intelligence is lower than that of a two-year-old chimpanzee, because of the slower myelination and aborization on the part of the human child. However, after that, the speed of myelination and aborization, on the strength of the phylogenetically determined formation of more gyri, substantially increases in momentum on the part of the human child and, therefore, its intelligence (or brain function) quickly surpasses the chimpanzee's. As a result, the human child will probably go to college while the chimpanzee may end up in a zoo.

17 Cerebral Dominance and Cerebral Laterality: Fact or Fiction?

In Chapter 16, I repeatedly pointed out the erroneous pursuit of the evolution of language because it is based on a wrong definition of what language really is. Worse still, language is taken for granted as if everybody knows what it is, and therefore it is tacitly assumed to be 'a thing' or 'an organ' or even 'an organism' or a set of rules or similar by scholars in different disciplines or lay people for the claim of evolution of language. This chapter will assess the consequence of such views about language which have led to the notions of cerebral dominance and cerebral laterality in neuroscience.

The origin of the notion of cerebral dominance or laterality goes back to Broca (1861), if not earlier to phrenology. The notion was pretty much established in 1874 when Wernicke showed a different area in the superior gyrus of the left temporal lobe of another patient with a different kind of language disorder. On the basis of his own findings and those of Broca's, he classified aphasias into three types:

1. Inability to understand language despite fluent speech because of lesions in the auditory area of the left superior temporal gyrus; he then called this receptive aphasia.
2. Inability to speak despite the ability to understand utterances by others because of a lesion in Broca's area; this was then called expressive aphasia.
3. Inability to repeat utterances by others, select appropriate words, read or write despite adequate understanding of utterances by others, because of destruction of the arcuatus fasiculus; this became known as conduction aphasia.

In the context of such a development, and on the basis of its results, there can be no denying that Broca and Wernicke made two heuristic assumptions for their findings.

First, the abnormal behaviours of their patients arose from the loss of proper functions of the lesioned sites, an assumption that was only partially right. It was this assumption that subsequently led to the notion of cerebral dominance. However, I should add that it was partially right because it is based on the one-to-one 'discrete' association between a causative lesioned site and a resultant abnormal behaviour without taking into consideration the effect of the lesion upon the functions of its neighbouring cortical and subcortical structures.

Second, the original functions of the lesioned sites must have been solely responsible for the total normal behaviours lost as specializations, had the tissues involved been kept intact. This second assumption was implicit as a corollary but erroneous because of the erroneous discrete association. It is erroneous because it led Broca and Wernicke to draw their conclusion leading to their notions of language in the brain; their conclusions have unfortunately been inherited by all subsequent investigators, that is, expressive language (for Broca's area) and receptive language (for Wernicke's area), as if language is a thing that could be divided into two pieces. Quite the contrary, language is what the brain does through its neurophysiological properties, called impulses, as behaviour, and not at all a thing that can be sectioned into smaller pieces and stored in or controlled by so-called language centres in one hemisphere alone.

Because of this historical perspective, in the discussions below I shall start with the first consequence of the two heuristic assumptions, a consequence that has given rise to varying impacts upon subsequent investigators who then carried out the 'mission' of proving the notion of cerebral dominance in their own ways. The consequence I have in mind is known as the Lichtheim–Wernicke's model which was mentioned earlier but will be reviewed in brevity with criticial assessments. However, I shall limit my descriptions of the impacts to four realms with critical assessments as well; namely, split-brain research in relation to language in the brain, dichotic listening test, the brain functions of music, and the brain functions of painting.

1. Lichtheim–Wernicke's Model (1885): Built-in Flaws

Lichtheim was a student of Wernicke's and, therefore, was greatly influenced by Wernicke regarding how Wernicke thought the brain worked at that time *vis-à-vis* language disorders, especially aphasia, rather than language in general, because the idea of localization of expressive language and receptive language had already been firmed up. Thus, what I shall discuss below is not so much in respect to the various aphasias proposed in the model as in respect to the theoretical construct proposed in connection with the model underlying the language disorders. For this reason, only the main thrust of the model has been introduced.

There are two fundamental flaws in this model: first, the place where concepts are formulated, which has been assumed by later investigators to be Wernicke's area; second, exclusive lateralization of all centres to one (left) hemisphere. One of the centres, that of auditory images, is often confused with Wernicke's area when in fact, as the model shows, it is a separate centre, now known as the gyri of Heschl. I shall now go over these flaws with criticisms supported by others in the literature.

1.1 The Place Where Concepts are Formulated

Wernicke thought that the posterior third of the left superior temporal gyrus, that is, Wernicke's area, was a particular area giving meaning to words or sentences (Honjo, 1999: 41). In fact, this area was considered to be the site of the dictionary in the brain, where meanings were said to be attached to words (ibid.: 40). However, Howard *et al.* (1992) and Honjo and his colleagues tried to confirm Wernicke's idea but have had great difficulty in locating Wernicke's area. Thus, whether or not such a place where concepts are formulated (or elaborated) exists in a particular cortical area is now seriously questioned, because its presumptive existence has become one of the criteria for the notion of cerebral dominance. But if that place is not lateralized exclusively to one hemisphere and is diffusely distributed throughout the whole brain, the criterion for the notion of dominance evaporates.

As I have already advocated with evidence the diffuse distribution of the brain functions in the preceding chapters, which formulate concepts as the background noises, cerebral dominance will have to disappear. Here are evidence in the literature which are taken to support my idea that the alternative view to Lichtheim–Wernicke's claim is to consider the cerebral cortices of both hemispheres as a whole to be the place where concepts are formulated by abandoning the attempt to localize and prove such a lateralized cortical area as proposed by the model. For instance, in an attempt to do so, Howard *et al.* (1992) found that it varied from the anterior to the middle part of the auditory association area or angular gyrus, and to an area posterior to the angular gyrus (Honjo, 1999: 41). Likewise, three from 12 normal subjects in Honjo's study were found to have no particular area in the brain which could be identified as a candidate for Wernicke's area.

1.2 Lateralization of the Centres of Expressive and Receptive Language

Since Wernicke thought that Wernicke's area was the place where concepts were formulated and was lateralized to the left hemisphere, the difficulty in locating it by various subsequent investigators proves only one point: Wernicke's area is *not* the place where concepts are formulated. However, two residual problems remain: first, the claim of Wernicke's area (wherever it may be, if it exists at all) as the site of receptive language which is thought to be lateralized to the left hemisphere; and second, the confusion of the centre of auditory images with Wernicke's area, thereby mistakenly equating receptive language with the centre of auditory images.

Because of these two residual problems, another term has appeared as a result, called cerebral laterality. The two terms, dominance and laterality, have subsequently been used interchangeably by many investigators, although some of them have indicated the differences in usage:

1. The differences hinge on the notion of lateralization of language in the brain, as both views accept functional dissimilarity of the two hemispheres in humans and non-human animals.
2. If language is thought to be lateralized to the left or right hemisphere, the differences lie in the introduction of two new terms, namely, dominant hemisphere, which exclusively controls or manipulates language (left or right), and non-dominant hemisphere, which is also called the silent hemisphere because it is believed to have no language; thus, cerebral laterality applies only to dominant hemisphere.
3. Only humans have language, and therefore the term cerebral dominance does not apply to non-human animals, even though they are thought to have cerebral laterality without language in either hemisphere.

At this point, it is important to distinguish receptive language which was claimed to reside in Wernicke's area from the centre of auditory images. Although the place where concepts are formulated is certainly not Wernicke's area, because the equation is suspect, the centre of auditory images is not, because the centre of auditory images is represented bilaterally in Heschl's convolutions of each hemisphere. In Chapter 19 I provide greater detail on the issue of where concepts are formulated in relation to the role of the centre of auditory images (or impulses).

The separation of receptive language from the centre of auditory images implies two things: the whole brain is responsible for the formulation of concepts which I have called thought or meaning; and receptive language pertains to both auditory and visual stimuli bilaterally. The resulting impulses must formulate acoustic (and sound-) images or visual (and sign-) images in relation to the brain functions of memory; one hemisphere may be superior to the other in respect to a particular behaviour, but the two hemispheres are interdependent. However, in the processing of the stimuli when they are received as impulses, because of hemispheric functional asymmetries, such impulses are not lateralized exclusively to one side for either the processes or the perceptual organization of the impulses.

I must add that my criticism that receptive language (as claimed to be represented in Wernicke's area) is suspect is not tantamount to saying that concepts are not formulated in the brain. Rather, language as behaviour, receptive or expressive, is memory-governed as an integral part of language in the brain, not a separate or independent entity, because language in the brain is also meaning-centred on account of the hemispheric interdepencies. It is through the brain functions of memory and cognition, which are two sides of the same coin, that concepts are formulated and elaborated in the brain. Thus, by analogy and in addition to the bilateral existence of the centre of auditory images, the occipital lobe (especially the striate cortex) is the centre of visual images, which is also bilaterally represented.

On account of such evidence, there is no specific centre of receptive language (i.e., the place where concepts are formulated), because the whole brain is responsible for it, nor is the centre of auditory images lateralized exclusively to the left (or one) hemisphere, albeit the bilateral representations are asymmetrical. From the point of view of this corrected historical perspective on receptive language, the notion of cerebral dominance is herewith abandoned and the rejection will be reinforced later when split-brain research and dichotic listening test are brought up for discussion. However, the notion of cerebral laterality in relation to the centre of auditory (or visual) images remain viable for the time being, if the centre in either sense is bilaterally represented, but will have to be changed to cerebral asymmetry.

1.3 Expressive Language and the Centre of Motor Images

In like manner, Broca's area, historically regarded as the site of expressive language, has also been regarded as the centre for language production (i.e., motor images) which, along with the centre of auditory images, are lateralized to one (i.e., the left) hemisphere. But there are problems, too.

First, as the model shows, Broca's area receives input from B (the place where concepts are formulated) and A (centre of auditory images). Such being the historical perspective, expressive language should include B, A, and M in the model. However, for some peculiar reason, Broca had not thought of the inclusion which was actually proposed not by him but by Lichtheim in consultation with Wernicke; he simply regarded the area as the centre of expressive language, a notion that was rejected by Pierre-Marie in 1906.

Since I have already pointed out that the place where concepts are formulated is not the same as, nor does it reside in, Wernicke's area, I should reiterate that the formulation is the responsibility of the whole brain. One piece of evidence comes from Wise *et al.* (1991) who show that Broca's area is not just a centre for language production; in the verb generation task, which is to think of a verb associated with a presented noun without pronouncing it, activations of the area posterior to the left auditory association area, Broca's area, and the supplementary motor area were noted.

Such being the case, the notion of cerebral dominance in connection with the centre of motor images (i.e., Broca's area) as the site of expressive language also becomes suspect; at the same time, the true nature of cerebral laterality must be seriously reconsidered.

The above-mentioned critical assessments give room for argument against the species-specific capacity of language that is lateralized exclusively to one side of the brain while the other side does nothing to contribute. The reason, as is supported by the above evidence, is that it is the wrong view of language that has led to the assertion of language being lateralized exclusively to the dominant hemisphere and being a unique human capacity. Put differently, when language in the brain is *not* lateralized to one hemisphere (left or right), the notion of cerebral dominance will collapse. But before I move on to the impacts of this classic model upon split-brain research, dichotic listening test, music and painting, I will comment briefly on cerebral and/or regional specializations which are relevant to such impacts.

1.4 The Claims of Cerebral and/or Regional Specializations

Because of the two heuristic assumptions made by Broca and Wernicke, I have pointed out the weaknesses of the claims of receptive and expressive language in Wernicke's area and Broca's area, respectively. Such claims subsequently led to the notions of cerebral dominance and cerebral laterality, which have also been critically assessed by me. However, as a result of these notions, more claims are made of cerebral and/or regional specializations which are different brain functions assigned to discrete brain regions and then dubbed higher brain (or cortical) functions – for example, language, music, painting, facial recognition, calculation, verbal vs. non-verbal activities, logical analysis – as if other brain functions, such as memory, play no role in these so-called exclusive specializations. I should mention that these are based on the view that each is regarded as one behavioural unit as if it were a thing or a single whole which could be manipulated exclusively by a designated brain structure purported to be responsible for it as a discrete specialization.

An example follows: 'Production of language is a so-called "recall" process of previously stored language' (Honjo, 1999: 139). In this view, then, where language is stored in the brain has largely been mystified and becomes an enigma. Since I disagree with such a view, because all behaviours are memory-governed and those so-called 'specializations' are no exceptions, I regard language in the brain as what the brain does as behaviour, including production and reception. Thus, I shall with my disagreement in mind move on to my critical assessments of split-brain research, dichotic listening test, music and painting, in that order.

2. Split-Brain Research

Split-brain research actually started out with non-human animals. The initial idea was to test the possibility that when the midline commissures were sliced by the surgeon's knife, the result would produce two separate, but equal, cognitive systems each with its own abilities to learn, think and act (Gazzaniga, 1970: 1–2). This initial idea was put to test by Myers and Sperry (1953) in their now classic experiment in which they 'demonstrate that midline sectioning of the optic chiasm and the corpus callosum and anterior commissure in the cat produced an animal who was unable, using the untrained eye, to perform a visual discrimination learned through the opposite eye' (Gazzaniga, 1970: 2).

The idea of doing split-brain research on human subjects was promoted by Akelaitis 'who had examined a series of some 26 patients with the corpus-callosum and anterior commissure completely or partially sectioned in an effort to control the interhemispheric spread of epileptic seizure' (Gazzaniga and LeDoux, 1978: 3). But he concluded that 'sectioning these structures did not result in any significant neurological or psychological sequels' (ibid.: 3).

It should be noted ahead of time that not every epileptic patient is permitted or eligible to undergo split-brain surgery. Such a surgery cannot be performed on temporal lobe epileptic patients with intractable seizure (partial or generalized which involves the reticular formation) whose surgery is limited to anterior temporal lobectomy (or amygdalo-hippocampectomy), but is performed on patients with extra-temporal epilepsy or status epilepticus (which is usually frontal). The success rate of the patient becoming seizure-free post-operatively, nevertheless, is not very good, even though the interhemispheric spread of epileptic seizure may be said to have been 'controlled'. Moreover, these patients usually develop psychosis (or even schizophrenic psychosis), which is common among epileptic patients at large.

In 1960, however, Josphe Bogen, another neurosurgeon, after a careful review of Akelaitis' studies, proposed that 'the brain could be split for the purpose of controlling the interhemispheric spread of seizure' (ibid.: 3). But, again, Bogen never said that the patient would be seizure-free post-operatively. He then teamed up with Sperry for a series of experiments on commissure-sectioned patients. They claimed that a variety of striking and dramatic effects were observed. The question that can be raised is, 'Were the patients seizure-free post-operatively when the striking and dramatic effects were obtained? Or did those patients have psychosis (or even dementia) pre- and post-operatively?'

The reason for raising such serious questions is that a patient with status epilepticus can have a seizure attack every thirty minutes in one day and his/her commissurotomy can never make him/her seizure-free post-operatively. I had a patient who had 45 seizure attacks in one day according to his mother's count; he was a 27-year-old man and had had the onset from age seven. Consequently, his epilepsy surgery was denied. It was impossible to test him pre-operatively and I doubt that post-operatively he could have been tested with any scientific accuracy had he undergone split-brain surgery.

Those studies were followed in early 1970 by another series of experiments on commissure-sectioned patients known as the Wilson Series, the result of which have become so well-known that they added considerable weight to the notion of laterality, for regional differences and hemispheric specializations, by making use of the notion of cerebral dominance already in vogue. In this section, I shall cast doubt on the conclusion reached regarding language in the brain *vis-à-vis* cerebral dominance and cerebral laterality. Three points may be singled out below:

1. What was the overall aim of split-brain research?
2. What kinds of human subjects or non-human animals were used in the experiments?
3. What were the experimental methods employed?

2.1 Overall Aim

The overall aim has four objectives:

1. to prove or test the hypothesis that each hemisphere when the commissures, especially the corpus callosum, are cut has its own

cerebral functions whose independence is obscured because of the connections;
2. to demonstrate what those cerebral functions are like by isolating them structurally from the interference of those in the other hemisphere;
3. to induce the nature of interhemispheric communication in the belief that an infant is born with a split-brain;
4. to show that those cerebral functions cannot be expressed unless they are in the dominant hemisphere where language as a cerebral specialization is taken for granted or made use of, and that when they are in the silent hemisphere the subject is 'mute' or 'confused' without knowing what to say, in order to ascertain the existence of cerebral dominance.

2.1.1 Each Hemisphere has its own Independent Cerebral Functions

This first objective can by and large be accepted so long as the task involved is for a discrete behaviour, which does not require the continuing efforts of the hemisphere concerned. But such was not the case, because there is no discrete behaviour that can be tested or experimented on.

In one experiment, for instance, the touch information from the left hand projects mainly to the right hemisphere (Gazzaniga, 1970: 26), thereby making the afferent connection; the experiment implies that the right hemisphere, despite the connection, has no language, and therefore the experimenter did not consider the subject's subcortical structures in the connection. In such an experiment, however, the touch involves both motoric function and sensory function in hand movements for tactile contact. I assume that the projection of touch information to the right hemisphere is meant to be the sensory function, which suggests that the motoric function (i.e., what causes or motivates the subject to move the hand) is completely overlooked by Gazzaniga.

But I should add that in such an experiment the optic chiasm is not cut, nor are the two extrapyramidal loops and the two pyramidal tracts disconnected, or else the subject would not have been able to make the visual–tactile association or pointing. Put differently, many more brain functions are involved in the course of the tasks of association and pointing than the mere afferent connection purported by Gazzaniga:

1. The striate cortex of the hemisphere to which a stimulus was projected had to be involved via the optic radiation of that hemisphere.
2. The optic radiation starts from the lateral geniculate body (an important nucleus of the thalamus) as a continuation of the retino-thalamo-cortical pathways and forms part of the posterior thalamic peduncle (a subradiation of the internal capsule) which provides reciprocal connections between the thalamus and the cerebral cortex, and therefore the ipsilateral thalamus had to be involved both structurally and

functionally. But these structures and the participation of their functions were completely ignored.

3. The involvement, through the posterior association area of the hemisphere, had to make contact with the anterior association area of the same hemisphere, as the subject attempted to move the contralateral upper limb, in which case, both the ipsilateral and the contralateral basal ganglia of the moving limb had to be involved as well to activate the cortico-spinal pathways; that is, from the frontal lobe the motoric impulses and from the association area other impulses had to make contact with the striatum to enter the cortico-striato-pallido-thalamo-cortical looping in order to return to the ipsilateral motor cortex for the contralateral exit through the pyramidal tract as part of the cortico-spinal pathways. The participation of these subcortical structures in the processing of brain functions was also completely ignored, as if they did not exist and there was a direct pipe (or hose) from the cortex to the limb.
4. Granted that the sensory impulses from the left hand go primarily to the right hemisphere, and it should be noted that before the hand moves the impulses from the retino-thalamo-cortical pathways have already reached the striate cortex, which is to say that the decision to move the hand, under instructions prior to the test, was made not by the striate cortex but by the extrapyramidal looping where thinking takes place in coordination with the frontal association cortex.

2.1.2 *What are those Cerebral Functions Like?*

The split-brain researchers' overall aim would have been completed, with due reservations just presented, had they stopped at the first objective. But Gazzaniga goes on to claim that a weak 'ipsilateral' component of the input goes to the left hemisphere, which is usually not enough to enable the patient to say (using the left hemisphere) what he has picked up. In other words, Gazzaniga is using this kind of experiments to uphold or make use of the notion of cerebral dominance in order to implicitly support or confirm the notion of cerebral laterality. Conversely, those cerebral functions were taken as evidence of cerebral laterality which, by taking language for granted, was purported to prove cerebral dominance without looking into what language in the brain really is. Thus, there are also problems in the claim of such cerebral functions. Three may be pointed out below.

First, all human subjects were epileptic patients with intractable seizure, usually status epilepticus, whose brains had been abnormal prior to the commissurotomy. Even after the surgery there was no mention of the condition of each hemisphere, such as the epileptogenic focus remaining or not. Recall that the split-brain surgery was purported to control the interhemispheric spread of epileptic seizure and not to remove the epileptogenic focus in either hemisphere. Thus, to treat each hemisphere of such patients as normal is misleading, to say the least, because the success rate of becoming seizure-free post-operatively for such patients is very low and the risk of developing psychosis (or even dementia) is high, but their conditions during the testings were never mentioned.

Second, the fact that the subject could not respond when each stimulus was projected to the 'silent' hemisphere was taken as evidence that this hemisphere contributed nothing to the brain functions of language, an assumption that was similar to the second heuristic assumption made by Broca and Wernicke. In other words, it is not true that the 'silent' hemisphere does nothing; rather, it is the investigator who does not understand or know what the 'silent' hemisphere does that leads to the erroneous assumption. An outlet in the 'dominant hemisphere' does not guarantee that it does everything for language production as behaviour; conversely, the lack of an outlet in the 'silent hemisphere' is no proof that it does nothing to contribute to the production of language.

Third, the role of the subcortical structures, such as the basal ganglia, and the roles of the cerebellum and the brainstem were completely ignored. When these subcortical structures are taken into consideration, I should anticipate that the notion of cerebral dominance will disappear. I have already described in some detail the role of the cortico-striato-pallido-thalamo-cortical loop on pages 145–6 and elsewhere (Peng, 2000) in any production, which contributes to thinking in the brain functions of memory. The cerebello-cerebral circuit also plays an important role in the brain functions of memory, not just passively modulating voluntary movements. The Papez circuit is highly significant for epileptic patients in both production and reception of not only language in the brain as behaviour but also other behaviours, such as music and painting, for example, especially if they have developed psychosis.

All these subcortical structures pertain directly and indirectly to the brain functions of memory, which consist of a tripartite system. However, none of these have ever been mentioned, let alone dealt with, in any split-brain research. Perhaps, they were considered irrelevant to the brain functions of each hemisphere when the corpus callosum was cut.

2.1.3 The Nature of Interhemispheric Communication

It is of some significance to note that many human body parts or organs are paired, for instance, two eyes, two ears, two nostrils, two arms, two breasts, two lungs (two lobes in the left lung and three lobes in the right lungs), two vocal cords, two testicles (for men), two kidneys, two legs, two fallopian tubes (for women) and so on. Within the cranium, there are two cerebral hemispheres, two sets of the basal ganglia, two thalami, two fornices, two mammillary bodies, two lateral and two medial geniculate bodies, two superior and two inferior colliculi, two cerebellar hemispheres, three paired cerebellar peduncles and 12 pairs of cranial nerves, not to mention the paired nuclei in the brainstem. The questions that can be raised are:

1. Why are these body parts, organs or nuclei paired?
2. Can just one of them suffice to take charge of the total functions?
3. Is one of them a spare, just in case the other goes haywire?
4. Must they coordinate (or 'communicate') to make the best of whatever function that needs to be accomplished by their joint efforts?

All these are tough questions that have never been raised before. But some of them can be speculated; for instance, there are two lateral geniculate bodies because they are tied to the existence of two eyes which need to be connected to the striate cortices in the occipital lobes via the optic radiation in each, which starts from each lateral geniculate body; the left eye is partially connected to the right lateral geniculate body, by crossing the chiasm, via the right optic radiation, to reach the right striate cortex, and the right eye is partially connected to the left lateral geniculate body, by crossing the chiasm, via the left optic radiation, to reach the left striate cortex. Is the partial connection (on the nasal side) a joint effort with the opposite eye (on the temporal side) or is it an independent function? Likewise, there are two vocal cords each one of which is innervated by a recurrent laryngeal nerve supplied by one cranial nerve (the Vagus); however, proper voicing requires the joint efforts of both cords; so does the effort of increased strength as in weight-lifting. Such are the reasonings for some of the pairings, beyond which speculations will be difficult.

But why should split-brain researchers take the trouble to show or demonstrate the nature of interhemispheric communication when the joint efforts of the two hemispheres are required to make a normal living for an individual possible? There is only one purpose for their trouble: to ascertain that the two hemispheres are two separate, but equal, cognitive systems each with its own abilities to learn, think and act but that these separate systems also need to communicate with each other for their own specializations one of which is that language is believed to reside in the 'dominant' hemisphere, because of the cerebral laterality effect, or else the 'silent' hemisphere is 'mute'.

Such is the remarkable purpose. However, it has missed many of the functional accomplishments the joint efforts of the two hemispheres can contribute, because it has not proven that language in the brain is the exclusive specialization of one hemisphere (left for most but right for some); rather, it was based on or took advantage of the traditionally purported but erroneous belief that language in the brain was specialized exclusively in one hemisphere. There is another way to uphold the cerebral laterality effect of language, however, without assigning language in the brain exclusively to one hemisphere, which is to say that cerebral laterality effect is not synonymous with cerebral dominance for language and that the whole brain is responsible for language as behaviour in both production and reception in spite of cerebral asymmetries.

I have already argued against the notion of Wernicke's area being the place where concepts are formulated. Thus, the alternative way is to regard the whole brain as the place for forumulating concepts; the cortico-striato-pallido-thalamo-cortical pathways will be involved bilaterally as a result; the looping will, then, involve the centre of motor images (Broca's area) as the exit (in either hemisphere) of the bilateral cortico-bulbar pathways. At the same time, the alternative way also involves the two centres of auditory images (in the case of oral language) as the two entrances of impulses, which are *not* Wernicke's area, leading to the destinations of the bilateral bulbo-cortical pathways in preparation for the formulation of concepts with respect to language in the brain.

In the case of sign language, however, the place where concepts are formulated is the same, that is, the whole brain, but there are many exits and two entrances; the exits are the bilateral motor cortices (involving the cortico-spinal pathways) for the two hands and the bilateral facial areas in the pre-central cortices, involving the cortico-bulbar pathways; and the entrances are the bilateral striate cortices, involving the retino-thalamo-cortical pathways.

2.1.4 Cerebral Functions and the Dominant Hemisphere

Having stated an alternative view as an explanation for the cerebral laterality effects, by denying the notion of cerebral dominance, I should now add that all cerebral functions may have the same cerebral laterality effects which need not depend on the dominant hemisphere for their expressions, because cerebral dominance does not exist. Examples of such cerebral functions, other than language, are music, which will be elaborated in sections 3 and 4, and painting. Of course, music may involve the same exit as oral language as in singing, but shares the same exits as sign language when playing an instrument in more ways than one for the patterning of body movements which must include the extrapyramidal loop. However, music utilizes the same entrances as oral language in listening, because it involves sounds which have the bilateral entrances, encompassing the same bulbo-cortical pathways. As a result, there is no dominant hemisphere to speak of.

2.2 The Subjects Tested

It should be pointed out that all human split-brain subjects tested were adults, which is to say that no children or infants took part in any split-brain experiments, although non-split-brain children were also tested and mentioned. However, those adults were all patients with intractable epilepsy. I have already pointed out that their brains, pre-operatively, were abnormal to begin with. There was no guarantee that post-operatively each subject's two hemispheres would function normally. Of course, no neuroscientist would dare split the two hemispheres of a normal subject in order to find out how each hemisphere works. Likewise, all non-human animals tested were adults. But unlike human subjects they were all healthy animals to begin with.

Since no reference to the subcortical structures of each subject or animal was made and their functions tested – if they could be localized for testing at all – or analysed, it would seem that the results of each testing might not have been as clear-cut as the experimenters claimed. One fundamental flaw is that the epileptic patients' pre- and post-operative memory impairments were not taken into consideration, pretending that such impairments did not exist when in fact every epileptic patient, intractable or non-intractable, has serious memory impairment (Peng, 1995) with a high risk for psychosis (Peng, 2003a). Another fundamental flaw is that all split-brain researches did not use normal human subjects as controls; since, no investigator would dare split the corpus callosum of a healthy human to test the brain functions of the two hemispheres, the lack of such human subjects as controls cannot be said to be the investigators' fault. To compensate, split-brain researchers used healthy animals as substitutes, thereby changing the methods to get the animals to respond manually rather than orally. Thus, to draw a parallelism of human patients and healthy animals on their results from the experiments would seem rather far-fetched.

2.3 The Methods Employed

Since the selection of human subjects in a research involving behaviours is a part of the methods employed, if the research is conducted under a normal situation, other factors, such as age, social status, sex and so on, will usually be taken into account. However, in the case of split-brain research, as it could not use normal subjects, the experimenter had no choice but to take whoever was available, provided that the subject was a candidate for epilepsy surgery. Thus, each subject's condition was predetermined, which is to say that he/she was not a healthy subject irrespective of his/her age, sex and socio-economic background. In other words, the experimenter was testing human subjects even when each one of them may not have been seizure-free and/or may have developed psychosis pre- and post-operatively.

Given this predetermined restriction, the least the experimenter could do was to test each patient pre- and post-operatively for a comparison of results. But as a candidate for commissurotomy, the patient had extra-temporal lobe epilepsy which is intractable (i.e., could not be controlled by medication) and usually had had many years of such epilepsy, most likely from childhood. Thus, another restriction on the methods to be employed was automatically imposed on the experimenter; that is, it is extremely difficult to test such patients pre-operatively, especially when they have status epilepticus. I have already mentioned a 27-year-old patient with status epilepticus whom I attempted to test pre-operatively. I could not even get him to know what I was saying, because he was not only 'uncooperative' but also emotionally 'derailed'. As a result of his condition, he was denied epilepsy surgery, that is, split-brain surgery, because it would not do him any good. The lack of pre- and post-operative materials for comparison is also detrimental to split-brain research.

But, strangely enough, these restrictions on methods were never mentioned in all split-brain researches available in the literature; all that was mentioned was that the surgery aimed to control or stop the interhemispheric spread of seizure, a statement that was more wishful than factual, because of the low post-operative success rate of becoming seizure-free, and the split-brain experiment to be conducted was just a post-operative follow-up. Thus, built-in flaws for the methods employed became inevitable and were unavoidable.

In addition to these restrictions on the selection of human subjects, however, the actual methods employed were based on the traditional techniques of stimulus and response, which required prior instructions, in the case of human subjects, split-brain or not, so that they could follow the testing procedure and prior training, in the case of non-human animals. But, for some peculiar reason, such instructions or trainings were never mentioned to play any role in the analysis of the results of each testing, as if no distortions of such instructions or trainings would happen to, or interfere with, the brain functions, in each hemisphere of a human subject, especially when such a hemisphere might not be seizure-free. Without any ascertainment regarding the pre- and post-operative assessment of the brain damage arising from the epileptogenic focus remaining in either hemisphere, the experimenter of all split-brain researchers jumped from a simple S-R test to a generalization of brain functions, a leap that can only be detrimental to the notions of cerebral dominance and cerebral laterality the experimenter claims to have upheld.

3. Dichotic Listening Test

Unlike split-brain research, the dichotic listening test was originally designed to test normal subjects, although clinical cases were later also reported; the aim was to ascertain whether there existed in the two hemispheres functional asymmetries or not regarding auditory reception. In this test, each ear would receive a series of three digits, such as 1.2.3, which differs from what the other ear would receive, such as 4.5.6. The procedure was that three such pairs were presented in rapid succession, and at the end of the six digits the subject was to respond with (i.e., report) what was heard in each ear in any order he/she liked.

The conclusion was that the right ear (or left hemisphere) was auditorily dominant for perception, and the left ear (or right hemisphere) was non-dominant, thereby seemingly contributing nothing to perception. It was a conclusion that depended entirely on, and took for granted, the notion of cerebral dominance in which speech was equated with language. Such a conclusion immediately presents several theoretical and factual problems:

1. Dichotic listening assumed an all-or-nothing perception, an assumption that is not true.
2. Perception was equated with production when the testing was conducted through reception.
3. It further assumed that the speech centre existed in the left hemisphere, and therefore the left hemisphere was dominant for perception.

4. No consideration was given to the participation of the subcortical structures, such as the basal ganglia, in perception.
5. The brain functions of memory were totally brushed aside when considering the development of dominance.
6. The dichotic listening task was switched from vocal response for digits to stereotactic response for melodies to arrive at a right hemispheric specialization for music, a serious error in the notion of cerebral dominance that has unfortunately prevailed in the literature.

I shall now address these problems below, which are interrelated.

3.1 The All-or-Nothing Assumption

When Kimura (1961) designed the original dichotic listening test, thereby setting the pace for subsequent investigations, it seems strange that she and others had to claim left-hemisphere (or right ear) dominance as if the right hemisphere (or left ear) contributed nothing to the brain functions of perception – and if it did, no mention of its contribution was ever described – even though the results were obtained from both hemispheres. Put differently, the investigators jumped to the conclusion by taking the responses literally without recourse to the process involved from reception to production. This is another error reminiscent of the second heuristic assumption made by Broca and Wernicke. The truth is that the right hemisphere does a great deal in the process to contribute to perception. It is the investigator who was preoccupied with or biased by the overzealous desire to reach or arrive at the notion of cerebral dominance that failed to see or observe the contributions in the process made by the right hemisphere.

3.2 The Equation of Perception with Production

Since the impulses in the so-called non-dominant hemisphere were ignored, each investigator of the dichotic listening test simply took the results from the so-called dominant hemisphere to represent perception, as if the other hemisphere did not perceive anyting. For instance, if left ear had 11.6 and right ear had 21.8 with the *p*-value of .01, the question that can be raised is: 'What did the right hemisphere (i.e., from left ear) do to the impulses of 11.6 when the differences of 10.2 were taken to justify the left hemisphere dominance (i.e., from right ear), thereby representing perception?' Put differently, my misgivings are the underlying but erroneous assumption which is that the 'dominant hemisphere' does everything and the 'silent hemisphere' does nothing to contribute to perception.

Another question that can be raised is: 'If the right hemisphere did something, other than passing the impulses on to the left hemisphere, what were the functions of the right hemisphere in respect to those impulses for the individual's total perception?' In other words, granted that without production there is no way for anybody to know the subject's reception, what the subject produces in response is *not* the totality of what he/she has perceived.

These questions have never been raised or even considered by all investigators of the dichotic listening test; when raised, however, I believe the investigators or even supporters of the dichotic listening test cannot satisfactorily give answers in order to uphold the notion of cerebral dominance.

3.3 Where is the Speech Centre?

If an answer is demanded for this question, presumably the answer would be Broca's area. But, as I have already explained in relation to Lichtheim–Wernicke's model, Broca's area creates so many unanswered problems that the answer cannot be Broca's area, one of such problems being Broca's area as the site of expressive language, thereby equating language with speech.

Recall also that perception in reception activates bilaterally not only the auditory association areas but also Broca's area and the supplementary motor area. The complication is compounded as Broca's area, according to the model to which all investigators of dichotic listening test seem to subscribe, receives impulses from the place (B) where concepts are supposed to be formulated, which have now been corrected to be the responsibility of the whole brain. However, if Broca's area (which is *not* the centre of speech nor is it the site of expressive language) is taken to be the exit for oral language, as I have already proposed above, then the other hemisphere cannot be the 'silent' or non-dominant hemisphere because it takes both hemispheres along with all the subcortical structures mentioned above, including the reticular formation in the brainstem, for each subject to respond in production to any stimulus. These brain structures are interdependent for and in function, because the involvement of the whole brain pertains none other than to the brain functions of memory.

3.4 The Role of the Subcortical Structures

Many subcortical structures, including the brainstem or even the cerebellum, take part in any manifestation of behaviour. For the sake of simplifying the matter, I shall limit the argument to the basal ganglia.

Every impulse in the brain that is destined to come out as behaviour must go through the cortico-striato-pallido-thalamo-cortical loop, so as to go through the pyramidal tract. It is in the looping where thinking takes place. The reporting of digits in all dichotic listening tests required thinking which was not possible without the brain functions of memory, especially when the digits used were from the language the subject knew. This is why I have advocated that the place where concepts are formulated cannot be localized in the brain. Any test designed for the localization of brain functions in behaviour, such as language and music, is sheer suspect, because the formulation of concepts is a dynamic brain function not a static conduit just transmitting the impulses into and out of the brain.

The mistake in the dichotic listening test was the assumption that the so-called speech centre in the dominant hemisphere handled all this formulation, when in fact it is both hemispheres in which the looping takes place that allow the subject to think of what to report in the order he/she liked.

3.5 Development of the Brain Functions of Memory

The brain functions of memory, as presented in Part IV, control or govern all behaviours, including language. But they develop gradually from foetal life and reach the peak post-natally at the age of 18, after which they gradually lose strength until death. I have called the whole process of this development maturation, referring to the period before 18 as Growth and that after 18 as Aging. I may add that Aging is the reversal of the two important processes of Growth, that is, hyperplasia and hypertrophy. Thus, Aging in the form of complex processes may be defined in terms of hypoplasia and hypotrophy. On the other hand, when hyperplasia and hypertrophy are not normal in the brain, the individual gets cortical dysplasia, resulting in double cortex, or megaloencephaly (extra large cortex) or schizoencephaly (one hemisphere larger than the other), each of which causes epilepsy.

There are, of course, individual variations among people of the same sex or even between people of the two sexes, especially when language as behaviour is considered. But such brain functions of memory are completely ignored in all dichotic listening tests.

When the difference between boys and girls was revealed, it was asserted that the data suggested that 'boys may lag behind girls in the development of cerebral dominance'. There are, however, biological foundations for such differences. For instance, boys lag behind girls in the onset of puberty for a couple of years on average. The question that can be raised, then, is this: Why should a slower development of functional asymmetry of the two hemispheres in boys be limited to their slower dichotic development leading to cerebral dominance and not to the other biological factors, including the brain functions of memory that govern language in the brain and, I should add, its development as well, which may be traced back to foetal life? The answer to this question will be difficult to produce.

3.6 The Differences between Digits and Melodies

So far I have limited my discussion of dichotic listening test to digits. But, because of the peculiar impact dichotic listening test has made on cerebral specializations in respect to music, which is claimed to be lateralized to the right hemisphere, I shall devote a little more space to address this issue in the hope that such a specialization can be corrected as a result.

The claim for the lateralization of melodies to the right hemisphere was conducted dichotically in reception but the response was different from that of digits, using instead the multiple-choice method. Kimura justified the switch 'because the melodies were not familiar to most of the subjects, and it was not feasible to have the subjects reproduce them' (1964: 255). The melodies test was conducted as follows (1964: 356):

> The individual melodies were excerpts from solo passages in concertos by Mozart, Telemann, Vivaldi, Bach, and Antonini. Most of the instruments recorded were woodwinds, but there were occasional violin, viola, and cello excerpts. Eighty such passages were tape recorded from commercial records and subsequently classified into 20 sets of four. Within each set of four melodies, the same instrument was used, and an attempt was made to have the pitch range and the tempo very similar, leaving as the main clue the melodic pattern. The original passages were re-recorded to make melodies of 4-sec. duration. For each set, two of the four melodies were first played simultaneously on the two separate channels, so that one melody was heard in one ear at the same time that the other was played in the other ear. There was then a 4-sec. silence and the four melodies were played in succession, in normal binaural fashion, i.e., with the same melody in each ear. There was a 3-sec. gap between melodies. Thus, the two melodies first heard dichotically were repeated separately, and the subject had simply to identify which two they were. He would reply, for example, 'They were the second and third', or 'First and Fourth', whatever he thought was correct. The position of the repeated melodies was varied in a counterbalanced manner from set to set. The score for each ear was the number of correct identifications for that ear. Since the first two were used for practice, there were 18 sets in the test proper, making a total possible score of 18 for each ear.

Given the test procedure with the justification stated, several problems (or flaws) emerged which Kimura did not detect:

1. Unfamiliarity would be the cause of asymmetry in comparison with digits which were familiar to each subject.
2. The length of each stimulus was definitely an important variable that influenced the subject's brain functions of memory in the judgement for responses, four second duration for each melody vs. one digit (at most two syllables).
3. The four second silence after the dichotic listening and the three second gap between melodies were not blanks as they were so assumed by Kimura; rather, the subject's brain functions of memory were actively working, which Kimura did not take into consideration.
4. The adjustment of pitch range and tempo was suspect because even when the same piece of music by one composer is played by two violinists, for example, they have two subtle but detectable differences in both pitch and tempo that are the crucial basis for music rhythms, hence melodic patterns.

First, in the case of unfamiliarity, if digits from a foreign language, say, Japanese or Taiwanese, are played to an English-speaking or French-speaking monolingual Canadian subject with the same multiple-choice method of response, I would not be surprised to see that the results lean towards those of melodies. If so, does this imply that Japanese or Taiwanese is lateralized to the right hemisphere of the subject or any other subject who does not know the language?

Second, even within English or French, if digits were changed to numbers beyond digits – for example, 1,100, 220, and 45 for one ear but 99, 6,200, and 560 for the other ear, each one of which would be longer than two syllables – what would the results be? Left or right dominant? The problem here is that numbers beyond single digits have longer durations which require more brain functions of memory. In other words, continuing efforts of the brain need more brain functions of memory to retain the incoming impulses even when the impulses are familiar to the subject. If unfamiliar, then longer stimuli, say, four or five syllables each, cannot be maintained long enough for response, let alone reproduction.

If, instead of numbers, phrases or sentences were employed as stimuli, each lasting four seconds, even in the subject's native tongue, I wonder whether the subject would be able to reproduce more than one phrase or sentence from either ear as a response; the others would be forgotten. Which hemisphere is the dominant hemisphere, then, if more sentences are reported as a result from the left ear (i.e., right hemisphere), even though reporting is supposed to be done by the left hemisphere in conformity with the tradition?

Third, during the four second silence and the three second gap, since the subject had already heard the melodies presented dichotically and binaurally, respectively, the subject's brain functions of memory in both hemispheres were actively involved to decide which melodies in the binaural listening would match the melodies heard dichotically. The subject's reporting was not equivalent to only one hemisphere's revelation of its activity; rather, the reporting was the result of the concerted and continuous efforts of both hemispheres. It was a serious mistake to equate the reporting (through the oral exit) with the presumed exclusive activity in the contralateral hemisphere.

Worse still, even though Kimura attempted to justify the multiple-choice reporting, the subject's oral reporting of 'They were the second and third', and the process (i.e., the neural activity) of getting the melodies heard to 'They were the second and third' was not a hose transmitting impulses like water unimpeded. Rather, from the auditory impulses received in each ear (the temporal lobe) through the auditory radiation to both frontal lobes (motor cortices) so as to reach the mouth for uttering the words in production there exist plenty of neural activities for the brain functions of memory. These neural activities in the form of impulses must be carried over (or 'translated') as concepts to become linguistic signs in the brain for mapping onto the sound-images of 'They were the second and third' in order to allow the sound-images to enter the extrapyramidal loop for the ultimate production of the actual sounds. All these important neural activities were completely ignored. The mappings of concepts onto sound-images to form linguistic signs are explained further below.

Fourth, when pitch range and tempo were tampered with, the distortion destroyed the original artistic characteristics of both the composer and the player as musicians. As a matter of fact, the distortion of tempo may have also changed the melodic pattern which Kimura said was the only clue to the subject, because the melodic pattern is greatly influenced by its rhythmic pattern; for example, from a tango rhythm to a waltz rhythm.

In music, the player interprets the composer's artistic characteristic through his/her notations, not just the notes but other notations which guide the player to control the pitch range and tempo as close to the composer's intention as possible. What makes a player a good performer depends not only on the accuracy of playing the notes but also on the intepretation of the composer's intention as shown in the other notations which affect the pitch range and tempo. Such interpretations were totally mutilated in the testing.

4. Music in the Brain

In view of the flaws in the dichotic listening test, especially in respect to melodies, it is extremely weird for later researchers to follow suit and conclude that music in the brain is the exclusive specialization of the right hemisphere, all because the notion of lateralization of music to the right hemisphere started with Kimura's dichotic listening test of melodies. The fundamental flaw for the claim of such an exclusive specialization can only be said to be naivety or the wrong idea about music.

Perhaps, she did not mean to infer melodies as music, but the most unfortunate consequence of such a dichotic listening test is that subsequent investigators have changed melodies to music and concluded that music is a specialization of the right hemisphere, an erroneous conclusion that has prevailed to this date, so much so that all textbooks on neuroscience or articles relating to neuropsychology about cerebral dominance have adopted this conclusion. Such a conclusion has now become so established that it is considered 'common sense' to claim that the right hemisphere specializes in music, among other things, and the left hemisphere specializes in language. The 'common sense' has its origin.

It is based on clinical support from Milner's findings (1962) for which Kimura claimed (1964) that 'a clear dissociation of auditory asymmetries existed, depending on the type of stimulus presented, and these asymmetries in turn reflect differences in function between left and right hemisphere'. Asymmetries in function are fine, which require coordination of the two hemispheres to manifest as varying concerted behaviours. In other words, asymmetries are not synonymous with exclusive specializations or monopolies of the functions by one hemisphere. Therefore, it is wrong to jump from asymmetries to exclusive specialization. To follow Milner's findings, Kimura then used melodies, as described above, to assert the cerebral specialization of melodies which later became the cerebral specialization of music.

I should hasten to add that music is not limited to listening. It includes singing, playing a musical instrument, conducting, composing, sight-reading, impromptu (on piano, pipe organ, trumpet, etc.) and the like or even ballet, social dancing and choreography (including tap-dancing with or without singing). When jazz musicians play jazz or blues, with different instruments, three or four rhythms may be used simultaneously, as they improvise the melody for each piece of music. Using a wrong method for the perception of melodies is no ground on which to claim that music is lateralized to the right hemisphere. But the erroneous notion of lateralization of music to the right hemisphere was propagated by subsequent investigators of the dichotic listening test. It is time that this fallacy is corrected because such music behaviours as were mentioned above require the continuing efforts of both hemispheres, which must be integrated in production and/or reception through their interdependencies.

5. Painting in the Brain

Painting, like language and music, requires the brain functions of both production and reception. But, for some peculiar reason, painting has been regarded as a specialization restricted to the right parietal lobe, just like music is regarded as a specialization of the right hemisphere and language as a specialization of the left for most people but right hemisphere for others.

One reason for such peculiarities is that painting was restricted to production, just like music was restricted to melodies in reception; but language was grossly assigned to some unknown cognitive function in the brain, although the notions of receptive language/expressive language have been proposed.

When both production and reception are taken into account, painting cannot be a specialization of the right parietal lobe. There are several reasons for this criticism:

1. the role of reception in artistic work;
2. foot and mouth painting;
3. inability for split-brain patients to paint;
4. possible artistic works by non-human primates.

But I shall limit my discussion to the first two reasons.

5.1 The Role of Reception in Artistic Works

The role of the brain functions of reception should be obvious, because nobody can paint blindfolded. In sculpture, for instance, the sculptor can see a profile (or configuration) of what he/she intends to create in a piece of raw material, say, a rock or a piece of wood. A profound good example is the sculpture of the four American presidents' heads on Mount Rushmore: Washington, Jefferson, Roosevelt and Lincoln. When the sculptor saw the mountain, he could visualize four faces which no other persons could have done. Other examples for the role of reception in artistic works are lettering, calligraphy, designing and architecture. They all require the continuing efforts of coordination and integration of the brain functions of both production and reception.

5.2 Foot and Mouth Painting

If cerebral asymmetry includes handedness and leggedness, it should be clear that when a right-hander paints and writes with the right hand, let us assume for a moment that his/her right parietal lobe is activated. However, in accordance with the principle of coordination and integration of the brain functions of both production and reception, can it be said that his/her painting is accomplished without the activation of the neocortex of the left frontal lobe (i.e., the motor cortex), both occipital lobes and the extra-pyramidal loop as well, not to mention the cerebello-cerebral circuit and the Papez circuit? Of course, not! But somehow the specialization of painting for the right parietal lobe has taken root in the literature, a notion that is inexplicable in any scientific way.

First, if a left-hander now paints and writes with the left hand, can it still be said that his/her right parietal lobe alone is activated without the participation of the neocortex of the right frontal lobe, both occipital lobes and the extrapyramidal loop as well, not to mention the participation of the cerebello-cerebral circuit and the Papez circuit? Second, suppose now that a person has lost both arms or was born without them but has learned to paint and write with the right or left foot. Is his/her painting still a specialization of his/her right parietal lobe without recourse to the medial frontal cortex, both occipital lobes, and the participation of the basal ganglia, not to mention the participation of the cerebello-cerebral circuit and the Papez circuit? I must now add the participation of the spinal cord which is relevant to both sensory and motor functions; for hand-painting, the fasciculus cuneatus is involved in sensory function to guide the motor function, but in foot-painting, the fasciculus gracilis is involved in sensory function to guide the motor function. All these questions cannot be answered scientifically by the notion of the right parietal lobe being specialized in painting.

Now, suppose that an amputee has learned to paint and write with his/her mouth. The brain functions of both production and reception must shift, other things being equal, from the cortico-spinal and spino-cortical to also involve the cortico-bulbar and bulbo-cortical participation. Can it be said in good earnest that the right parietal lobe is the only brain structure exclusively responsible for mouth painting? Put differently, to claim such an exclusive specialization must be none other than a joke.

PART V PRODUCTION AND RECEPTION

General Remarks

In the preceding chapters, I have described in some detail certain insights and clues to the solution of the question of 'What is language?' I shall now demonstrate, on the basis of those chapters, for an overview, how those insights and clues can be put into practice for the description of language in the brain as behaviour. To do so, I shall first briefly demonstrate the construction of meaning from the point of view of production, using examples from English, Japanese and Mandarin Chinese; even with these brief demonstrations, the complexity of the involvement of brain functions can be shown. I shall then turn to demonstrate the reconstruction of meaning from the point of view of reception, using the same and other examples in these languages, so as to illustrate the differences in the involvement of brain functions. Because of the complexities in reception, I withhold the schematic presentations for the time being.

These demonstrations, however, are not intended to be a perfect or complete description of the brain functions of language as behaviour. As I have repeatedly cautioned, since language in the brain is memory-governed, the description of how the brain functions of memory work *vis-à-vis* language in the brain alone will take up thousands of research papers just to show the tip of the iceberg, because it will involve the excitatory, inhibitory and/or disinhibitory activities of some, if not all, of the neurotransmitters in relation to 'normal' and 'abnormal' human behaviour.

Nevertheless, one thing is clear, which can be definitely concluded beforehand; that is, on the basis of the evidence I have presented, there is neither language gene nor grammar in the human brain. The claim of having identified such a gene in humans is sheer fantasy. Therefore, it was the wrong epistemological views of language, as defined by scholars, linguists or otherwise, that prevented other non-human animals from having a language of their own in each species, rather than any phylogenetically determined ontological factor that excluded them. In other words, each species in the animal kingdom has its own language which may not be up to the sophisticated level of human language; we simply do not know what their languages are like, because we have yet to come to terms with our own language. I must hasten to emphasize, however, that 'do not know' is not synonymous with 'does not exist'.

Now that I have proven that the cerebral dominance and cerebral laterality are more fiction than fact, this Part, through the demonstration of the construction of meaning and the reconstruction of meaning for which the whole brain is responsible, is to show what the brain does as behaviour with wording (not lexicogrammar or rules) and how such behaviour comes into being. With these cautious statements in mind, I shall now move on to the two chapters to deal with two major issues, the solutions to which are basic in the answer to the question of 'What is language?' These issues are fundamental in the search for the answer.

18 The Construction of Meaning: Mapping of Content onto Expression

It should be remembered that to Saussure and to linguists after him (in line with Thibault's re-interpretation) the object of study (in linguistics) is constructed and not given, and therefore it is epistemological in nature. This re-interpretation is true if and only if the object of study, which is language, remains in or pertains to the Social Aspect. Hence, a plurality of frameworks can be advocated, each showing a different object of study that emerges according to the particular epistemological framework used to describe it. However, once the object of study falls in line with the Individual Aspect, as in the brand of neurolinguistics advocated by me, it is no longer epistemological but, rather, ontological, so that it can be dealt with squarely on the basis of neuroanatomy and neurophysiology involving the two nervous systems.

In semiotics, however, the object of study is the relationship between signs, the interpretations of signs, and the varying social contexts of situation in which signs exist. In semiotics, therefore, the object of study, in the way it is going at present, is also constructed, but may be given if the black boxes are opened up squarely for scrutiny, in which case, each interpretation, even though it may vary from one individual to another, has its ontological basis in neuroanatomy and neurophysiology. Semioticians should take note of this 'double-edged sword' which their discipline is facing right now.

In the framework being presented in this monograph, on the other hand, the object of study is not constructed but given, consisting of impulses which are the neural activities (or electrical currents as brain waves) emitted from varying structures in the brain in connection with the spinal cord and the peripheral nervous system; without such brain waves, the individual is either in a coma or brain-dead. Thus, the object of study of the individual aspect of language (or language in the brain) is ontological in nature, which manifests itself in behaviour (active or passive), on the basis of the ability to think in the brain functions of memory as mechanism. In other words, such a study is concerned with language in the brain which is what the brain does, not a thing or an organ or a set of rules or networks stored in the brain.

Such is the difference between my neurolinguistic framework and others including Saussure's original suggestion and semiotics. How to put together the ontological framework, which is based solely on the individual aspect of language, and the epistemological framework, which is based on or derived from the social aspect of language, to account for human language as a whole, is the major issue that confronted Saussure to some extent and still confronts many linguists and semioticians today. In other words, the individual aspect of language and the social aspect of language must meet somewhere, but how they meet will probably occupy hundreds or even thousands of like minds throughout this century. Only then can we talk about the origin of human language in connection with languages of other species in the animal kingdom.

1. Wording in Production: Mappings for Constructing Meanings

When a house (or a tree) is ablaze, it is seen by a bird, a monkey, an ape, or a human in exactly the same way, and therefore the proto-meanings are the same. The difference lies in how the proto-meanings as impulses in the content plane are mapped onto impulses in the expression plane to lead to the physical property (which is the manifestation of behaviour). In the case of non-human animals, the mapping results in 'fleeing' (or flying); some of them may chirp or yap, as they flee. We may be able to guess what they are chirping or yapping about, if and when we see them fleeing from a forest fire.

But, in the case of a human being, he/she has a choice: run (or flee) and/or yell 'Fire!' in English, for instance. In the latter case, the proto-meaning of 'a house ablaze' must change into a linguistic meaning first which can unlock [fáyr]. Notice that there is no wording involved. That is to say, the proto-meaning is not cut up and therefore automatically becomes the linguistic meaning which is then mapped onto the sound-image in the shape of [fáyr] that is a series of impulses. Such a mapping may be schematically depicted as shown in Figure 18.1.

Suppose now that the human being is Japanese or Chinese. Of course, what he/she sees is exactly the same, that is, 'a house ablaze'. Put differently, the proto-meanings are exactly identical. However, by virtue of the fact that the proto-meanings are also 'a mass of meanings' (or a mass of impulses), they are

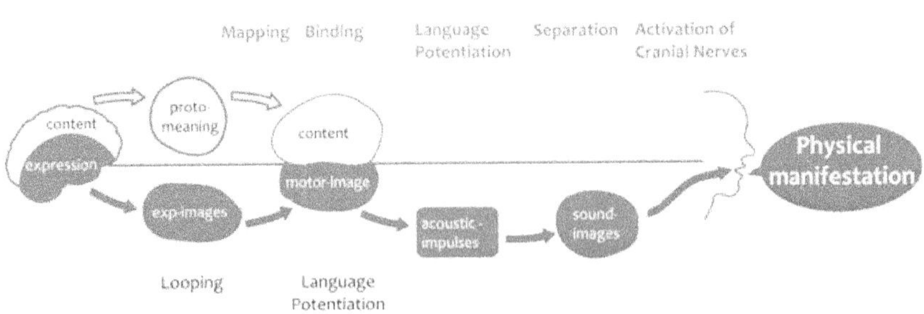

Figure 18.1

mapped onto the acoustic images differently in each speaker's brain – the Japanese, the Chinese, or the English speaker's brain. In other words, the same proto-meanings will have to become different linguistic meanings when they are mapped onto different acoustic images; that is, the proto-meanings are chunked (or parcelled out) differently by the brain functions during the process of mapping. Here are what happens to the Japanese or the Chinese speaker (in Mandarin) in comparison with the English speaker.

A House Ablaze

English	*Fire*
Japanese	*Kajida* 火事だ
Mandarin Chinese	*Shih huo le* 失火了

What has happened to the neurophysiological process of mapping in each brain, then? In terms of the separation of concept (i.e., linguistic meaning) and sound-image (i.e., linguistic sound-image), we can project the three mappings into a prototype as shown in Figure 18.2.

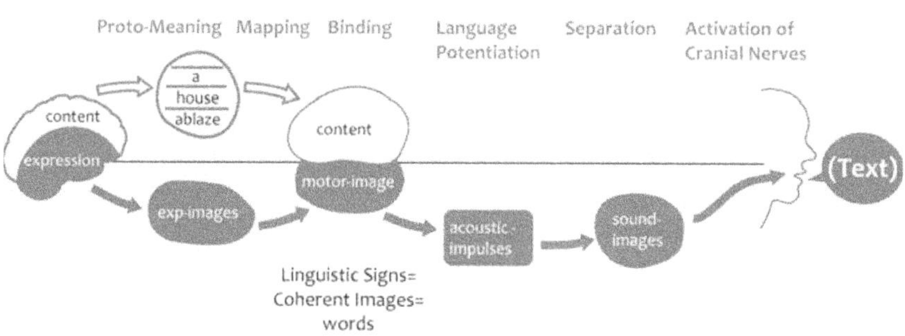

Figure 18.2

This prototype depicts the role of wording in two ways. First, the proto-meaning is chunked (or parcelled out) within the speaker's content plane in as many pieces as are needed by the number of acoustic images (i.e., impulses) onto which the chunked proto-meanings are to be mapped and at one and the same time the cut-up pieces of proto-meanings are lined up, in accordance with the acoustic images, into some kind of a vague time axis. Second, the time axis is set in motion in anticipation of the sequencing of the number of images needed for emission to the extrapyramidal loop; these acoustic images must be selected, by means of the brain functions of memory as mechanism, from a pool of literally thousands of acoustic images in the speaker's expression plane which consists of impulses for the brain functions of memory as content; these impulses are part of the background noises in his/her brain. To select the corresponding acoustic images is what Saussure calls 'unlock'. Wording in neuroanatomy and neurophysiology is defined to depict these two roles and those which will be defined later.

For instance, see Figures 18.3, 18.4 and 18.5.

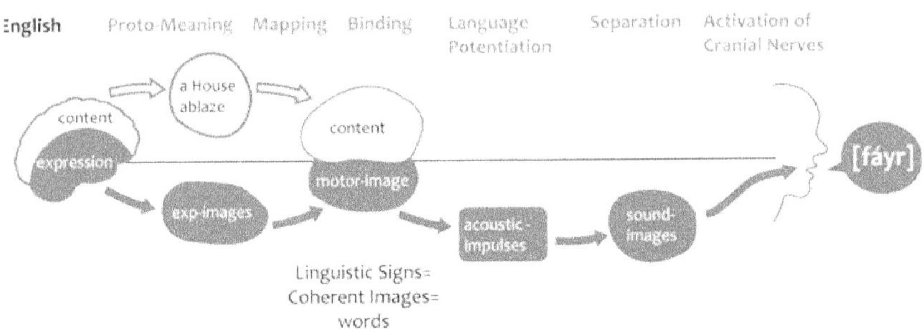

Figure 18.3

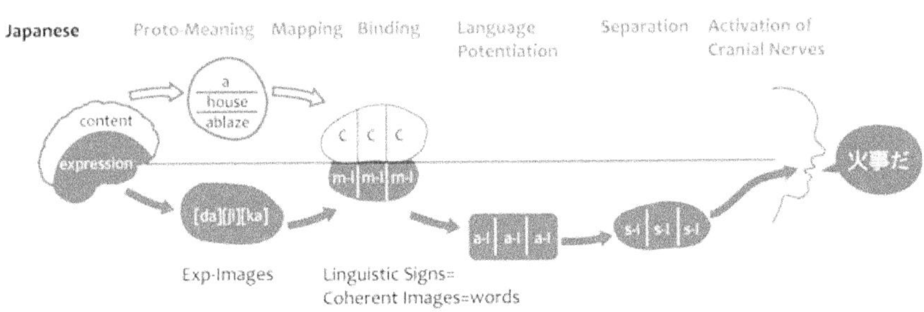

Figure 18.4

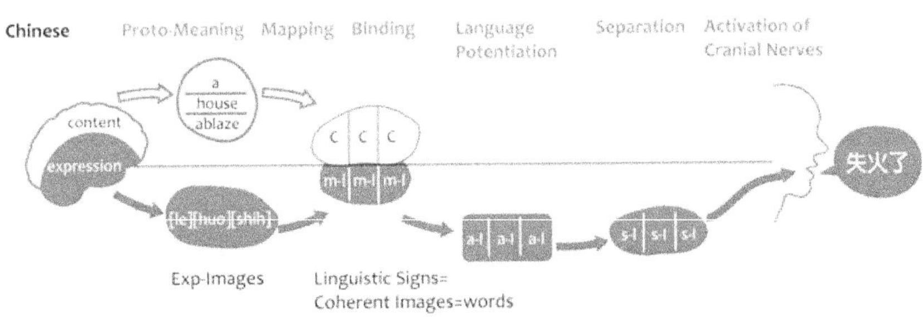

Figure 18.5

In this sense, then, it should be reiterated that wording in neurolinguistics (or behavioural neurology) must not be taken to mean or inferred as grammar which is claimed by some psycholinguists to be 'the interface' between meaning (proto-meaning or linguistic meaning) or semantics and sound patterns or phonology as if they are 'modules'. The brain does not work that way, for it 'understands' or 'knows' only impulses. To me, therefore, meaning (proto-meaning or linguistic meaning) is not semantics and sound pattern is not phonology; rather, meaning in the brain is thought, an inchoate mass of impulses constituting the individual's content plane, and the sound pattern of language in the brain belongs to sound, an equally indeterminate mass of impulses constituting a part of the individual's expression plane.

Neurophysiologically speaking, from speaker's point of view, wording indicates precisely two things: forming the time axis of proto-meanings that are pre-arranged (because they are chunked) in accordance with the corresponding acoustic images; and the phenomenon of unlocking each corresponding acoustic image in the selection of the linguistic meanings into which the cut-up proto-meanings are bound to change subsequently. Wording results in the following neural activities: sequences of linguistic signs (made up of coherent images as words).

Each linguistic sign consists of a linguistic meaning (i.e., concept or the signified) and a sound-image (i.e., the signifier) that are coherently bound, which are in a state of language potentiation, that is, before they are separated again to allow the sound-image to enter the extrapyramidal looping in the brainstem. Once speaker decides to utter the linguistic signs, the concepts (or linguistic meanings) must be separated from the corresponding sound-images; the separation allows the sound-images in the forms of varying impulses to enter the looping in order to reach the vocal organ used in producing the actual sounds, via the pyramidal tract, while leaving the corresponding concepts (or linguistic meanings) 'behind,' as it were, in the brain of the speaker. The over-simplified process (or brain functions) of wording in production are illustrated in Figure 18.6.

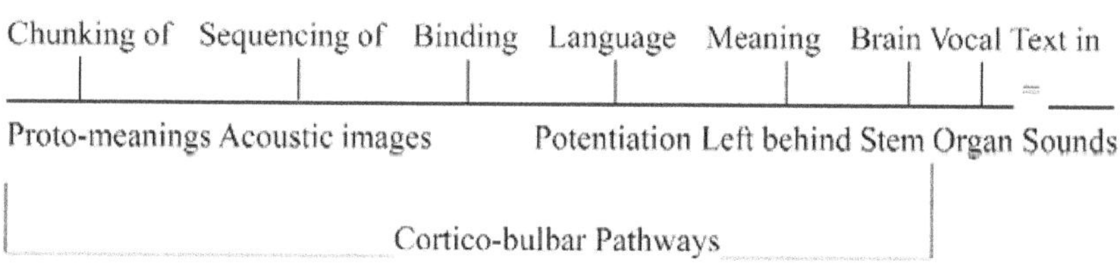

Figure 18.6

However, what happens in the brain, before the text is produced, is much more complex than what I have depicted above, because of the involvement of the time factor in relation to action potentials. In other words, the complexity is caused by the brain functions of wording itself, which is why wording does *not* constitute a plane (or a mass) of impulses of its own in the brain; it involves time for both production and reception. So, let me now conjecture a little about the role of wording, since it is not synonymous with lexicogrammar, in relation to meaning.

2. The Brain Functions of Segmentation

As may be evidenced by the schematization of the roles of wording above, one important role played by wording is the 'sequencing' of concepts. But I should also point out that sound-images themselves must be linearized, too, if words in actual physical sounds are to come out properly. Put differently, nobody can produce two words or two physical sounds together (i.e., simultaneously), although in sign language simultaneity is an important characteristic. (See Peng (1978) which is the first locus of this fact in writing and Peng (1994).)

I have, therefore, come to call the processes of 'sequencing' and 'linearization' the brain functions of segmentation (Peng, 1994); presumably, the process of sequencing is done in the neocortex as a whole; it is where 'concepts are elaborated', because concepts are not lateralized to either hemisphere in my framework. However, the elaboration of concepts refers to the unlocking of each corresponding sound-image in the selection of the linguistic meanings into which the original proto-meanings have changed. But the linearization must be done after the binding (or pairings) of the sequenced linguistic meanings (or concepts) to the corresponding sound-images and before the sound-images as impulses go through the looping in the extrapyramidal tract to reach the organ through the activation of the proper cranial nerves used in producing the actual physical sounds; once the actual physical sounds are articulated, they are already linearized as a continuum of sound waves.

I must add that before the process of sequencing begins to take effect in the neocortex, there must be another process called 'chunking' or 'parcelling' (suggested by Professor Roger Matthews) for handling the proto-meanings, which is tied to the sensory system – in the case of oral language, to the bulbocortical pathways. Thus, there appear to be three processes in the brain functions of segmentation: the process of chunking; the process of sequencing; and the process of linearization. Since we are concerned here with the strata of Meaning and Wording, rather than with the stratum of Sound Patterns, I shall now put the last-mentioned process aside for the time being, until otherwise called upon later.

One question that immediately arises then is this: how do the brain functions of segmentation operate? This question can be answered differently, depending on whether we are talking about a child whose language in the brain is still maturing, developmentally, or an adult whose language in the brain has already firmed up. I may even complicate the answer by adding a brain-damaged person whose language in the brain is disordered. To simplify the matter, I shall select the answer that deals with the healthy adult whose language in the brain is intact.

3. Operations of the Brain Functions of Segmentation

Given this selection, we can change (or reword) the question as follows: when do the brain functions of segmentation occur, before the mappings, during the mappings, or after the mappings? This question presupposes that the three processes of segmentation can occur independently of one another. But, in reality, if a text is to be produced, they have to occur consecutively, in the order of chunking, sequencing, and linearization, more or less as a continuation, which is *not* the same as the continuum of sound waves mentioned above, so that the text can come out smoothly. That is, these three processes are time-oriented, by which are implied two things: the time factor within each process; and the time factor of pairing what come out of the first process – that is, chunking – and the results of the second process – that is, sequencing.

3.1 First Time-Orientation

For the first implication, each process is time-oriented in the following manner: in the process of chunking, the proto-meanings are not only chunked but must also be determined as to which chunked meaning will go first for pairing and which will go next, and so forth. In other words, the proto-meanings to be chunked must undergo planning which includes what to say and what not to say; it is this sort of planning that is time-oriented.

In the process of sequencing, because sound-images are maintained in the expression plane, not in the sense of being kept in some kind of 'a drawer' or filing cabinet, they must be 'looked for', as it were, as they are impulses 'roaming' around or 'lurking' in many parts of the brain; that is, they do not stay put in fixed places or regions of the cerebrum. Thus, the second process is time-oriented in retrieving, that is, looking for each appropriate acoustic image from a pool of many for the pairing with each chunked proto-meaning, so that the proto-meaning can change into the appropriate linguistic meaning (i.e., concept) and the acoustic image can change into the corresponding sound-image of the linguistic meaning. At one and the same time, because each sound-image is made up of an impulse for a physical sound or several impulses that will become several physical sounds at a later stage, say, when they pass the extrapyramidal looping in the brainstem to reach the vocal apparatus, those impulses must be somehow arranged. Or else, the individual would have difficulty producing the sounds needed, as in apraxia of speech, or might produce nonsense syllables which are known in aphasiology as neologism or phonemic jargons. The rough arrangement of the impulses during the retrieval of appropriate sound-images is also time-oriented *par excellence.*

In the third process, linearization, all impulses of sound-images, not just the impulses of each sound-image retrieved, must be linearized properly. But such linearization must take place only after the impulses reach the brainstem (for the looping) and the cranial nerves, for instance, the VIIth, the IXth, the Xth, the XIth and the XII, are about to be activated; once those cranial nerves are activated to contract the appropriate musculature, more than one of them may take part in the production of just one sound, such as [d] or [g] in *dog*; each may require the participation of the vagus (i.e., the recurrent laryngeal nerve) for the vocal cords to vibrate and to close the velic, and the hypoglossal nerve to move the tip of the tongue to the alveolar ridge, in the case of [d], and back to the neutral position for the vowel, and then raise the back of the tongue against the velum, in the case of [g], with the glossopharyngeal nerve.

The participation of such cranial nerves is simultaneous for each sound, the result being one physical phenomenon, which is *not* the same as the characteristics of simultaneity observed in sign language; the outcome of the simultaneous participation of such cranial nerves is a sound wave or a continuum of sound waves produced by the air stream from the lungs. In real time production, however, [d] will come out first, which is following by [o] which is in turn followed by [g], thereby constituting a continuum of sound waves.

3.2 Second Time-Orientation

In the second implication, only the first and the second processes are involved; that is, each chunked or segmented proto-meaning must become a linguistic meaning (or concept) to form a linguistic sign when and only when it is mapped onto each appropriately retrieved acoustic image which becomes the sound-image in the linguistic sign. These two processes may be illustrated schematically, with simplification, as in Figure 18.7.

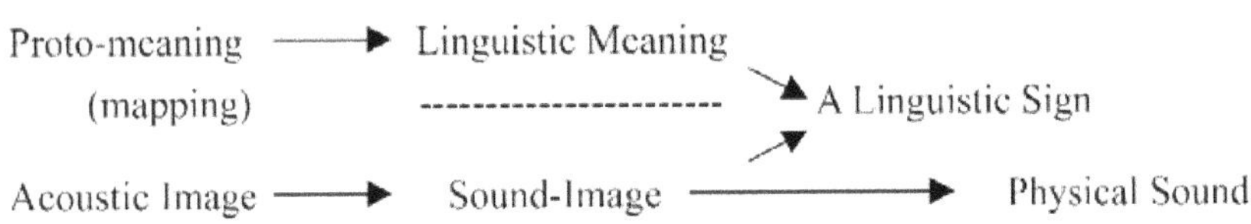

Figure 18.7 *Time-orientation*

During this selection of a proto-meaning and an acoustic image, the time needed for the unlocking (i.e., the pairing) is usually a matter of milliseconds if and when the selection is smooth; if not, phenomena such as pauses or pause-fillers – for example, *er* and *eh*, or some other substitutes – will occur. We all have the experience of 'looking for words' in the middle of a conversation. When hesitation of this sort takes place, the selection may need several seconds.

In practical terms, each process, in either implication, may be 'repeated' more than once, as a result of interruption, false start, or sheer inhibition of the excitatory motoric neurons which are emitting impulses, as in stuttering. In each of the three processes, however, there is also a significant time element involved in relation to sensory neurons in reception; many proto-meanings occur in the brain as a direct result of a sensory input, as in the example of 'a house ablaze', and that significant element of time becomes more apparent when such instances of proto-meaning are accounted for from the point of view of the hearer or viewer. It is also involved in perceptual organization (when receiving sensory impulses for reconstructing various meanings) and perceptual re-organizaiton (when receiving feedback to result in reiteration), both of which will be taken up again for more details in Chapter 19.

3.3 Contingent Negative Variation in Language Potentiation

Before I return to the example of 'a house ablaze', there is one important point which must be dealt with; namely, how language potentiation takes place. This refers to the state of brain functions when most of the linguistic signs are lined up ready to come out, each linguistic sign being the combination of a linguistic meaning (or concept) and a sound-image.

However, before the mental state of language potentiation is reached, there is an important variable that must come into the picture, which is known in the literature of neuroscience as Contingent Negative Variation (CNV); it works as a communication 'precursor' between neurons, probably from SMA (supplementary motor area) as the result of anticipating a response to a sensory input for a perceptual task. Two forms of CNV have been identified so far: expectancy wave and readiness (or Bereitschaft) potential.

The former is the development of a negative baseline shift after a 'warning' stimulus S1 and prior to the 'imperative' stimulus S2 which requires a response; the latter is a similar negativity which develops prior to a self-originating motor activity. (See Picton and Hink (1974) for more details.)

The readiness potential, however, varies with the levels of intention engaged in the activity by the individual. For instance, a person may accidently hit another person, or may intentionally assault that person. In the first case, a CNV may not develop in the brain of the person hit, as a direct result of a motor response, when accidently hit, as may be evidenced by a reflex, for example; on the other hand, a small negative shift will surely precede a purely perceptual task in the brain of the person being deliberately assaulted and vary with the amount of attention the task requires (Picton and Hink, 1974).

Such being the case, it is quite possible that the negativity occurs in the great intermediate net of neurons (i.e., all neurons minus motoric and sensory neurons), representing presumably some sustained activation in the cortical areas concerned with the task (ibid.). In this connection, it is of interest to observe that sustained sensory stimulation evokes a prolonged negative slow potential shift possibly originating in the primary sensory cortex (Keidel, 1972), and not from the SMA.

In light of the observations above, language potentiation, as it should be borne in mind, is *not* reached straightforwardly; one or more than one CNV may have come into play when the individual's brain functions reach the state of language potentiation. Because very little is known about the role of CNV in relation to the brain functions of language in general, or language potentiation in particular, I shall assume, as shown above, and continue to do so, until more is known about CNV *vis-à-vis* language potentiation, that it is reached more or less straightforwardly without recourse to CNV.

Notwithstanding the above-mentioned claim or assumption, in the example of 'a house ablaze' I am not concerned with the hearer but rather with the speaker, although the proto-meanings are the direct result of a sensory input. Under such circumstances, the three processes of segmentation for the English text are relatively simple, because the text consists of just one word, if the intonation is ignored for the time being, and its time-oriented element in wording is also simple. That is, the proto-meanings need not be chunked; when no chunking of meanings is necessary, there is no sequencing of meanings, because the proto-meanings can be directly mapped onto the appropriate corresponding acoustic image, to result in a linguistic sign as one coherent unit. In other words, no wording as a stratum is required in the English text, other than the pairing of the proto-meaning and its corresponding acoustic image, which is the basis of wording, even though the sound-image resulting from the mapping must be linearized when reaching language potentiation for expression in the cortico-bulbar pathways. In this case, there is no sequencing required prior to reaching language potentiation, because there is only one linguistic sign, although linearization is needed in the sound-images for the involvement of time.

In the Japanese or the Chinese text, however, the proto-meanings must be chunked; that is, what appears as one mass of proto-meanings in the brain, which are taken for granted in the brain of an English speaker, must be chunked into at least three 'pieces' of meaning; the chunking allows the sequencing of these three 'pieces' of meaning to take over as the continuation of brain functions of segmentation in the brain of a Japanese or a Chinese speaker. Put differently, a great deal of wording as a stratum is required in the production of the Japanese and Mandarin texts. To explain further how wording becomes involved in the brain of the Japanese or the Chinese speaker, I will now focus on the three processes of segmentation in connection with the Japanese or the Chinese case.

4. The Process of Chunking

When a person sees 'a house ablaze', the sensory system – in particular, the visual system – immediately recognizes that incident as a single whole, primarily because of perceptual organization in the brain, if and only if it occurs here and now without involving much movement of time. At that particular moment, which may be a split second or a matter of two to three seconds or more, his/her brain is faced with two things: the incident as a stimulus of 'a house ablaze', and the decision of how to deal with or describe that incident.

The incident as a stimulus is perceived in the same way by any higher organism, human or non-human, that has a brain. The perception is innate because the nervous system is equipped with the ability to respond to such an external environment requiring a proper adjustment.

The decision, however, involves proper adjustments to the external environments, the adjustments being verbalizing and/or fleeing. Either way, it must come from the individual's brain functions of memory, involving memory as content with retrieval by memory as mechanism from memory as capacity on the assumption that that person has seen the phenomenon of 'fire' (i.e., internal combustion) before; that is, he/she knows the danger of 'fire' or 'a house ablaze'.

In Figure 18.2, I deliberately chose to indicate that chunking is accomplished 'temporally' prior to the mappings of the chunked proto-meanings onto the corresponding acoustic images. The reason then was that I wanted to illustrate the neurophysiological process of (catalytic) mapping in the brain, rather than the process of chunking. Now that I have given the Figure, it is important that I also show that chunking is not necessarily accomplished 'temporally'; there is a 'non-temporal' alternative way in which chunking is accomplished more or less simultaneously with the neurophysiological process of mapping. Schematically, this 'non-temporal' segmentation of proto-meaning in pre-mapping is shown in Figures 18.8, 18.9 and 18.10 for the Japanese and the Mandarin text, albeit not needed for the English text.

Given the 'temporal' and 'non-temporal' possibilities of chunking, one question immediately arises: which alternative is more appropriate to, or represents, what is going on in the brain? My answer is that both possibilities are conceivable, depending on the type of context of situation and the amount of proto-meanings perceived by the individual, which need to be mapped onto the corresponding acoustic images, because of the movement of time. So, I will now explicate the differences between the two possibilities and the feasibility of each one of them below.

Basically, the distinction between the two possibilities lies in the amount of time that has elapsed prior to the process of chunking. The amount of time that has elapsed presupposes the amount of proto-meanings which must be chunked; that is, more movement of time suggests more proto-meanings but less movement of time suggests fewer proto-meanings.

However, time movement is not the only variable in respect to the amount of proto-meanings that need to be chunked; the brain functions of memory

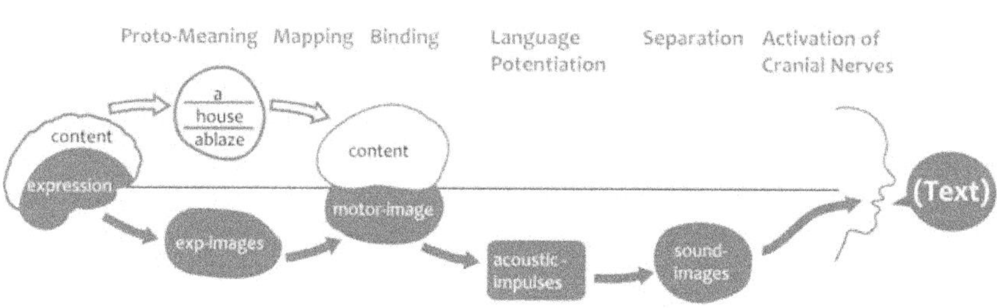

Figure 18.8

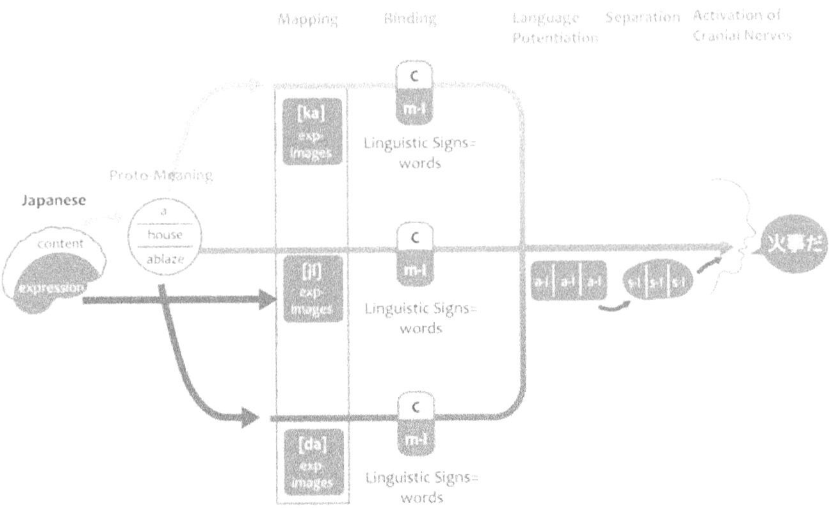

Figure 18.9

are highly relevant here. That is, the brain functions of memory can only hold a certain amount of new information for so long that even if hours have passed and the amount of information (i.e., proto-meanings, for short) is so enormous, the brain functions of memory cannot possibly contain or hold on to all the information (or proto-meanings) throughout. In other words, the brain functions of memory are not like a video camera, with a video tape, which can record and keep the events for six hours, for instance, or longer. The brain functions of memory, after receiving the information from the context of situation, will sort out the information and erase some of it after a short period of time; when the event is over, most of the vivid scene from the context of situation will be forgotten, and what is left will be maintained temporarily in the individual's content plane as background noises and may eventually disappear for good. Moreover, what is left in the brain functions of memory as content cannot be reported verbatim; it can only be summarized through the brain functions of memory as mechanism (i.e., integration).

In practical terms, the basic distinction between the two possibilities lies in the amount of proto-meanings to be processed. If the amount of proto-meanings is enormous, probably the temporal possibility will prevail, for the sorting out of the information requires planning which is time-oriented. On the other hand, if the amount of proto-meanings is not much, probably the non-temporal alternative may also play a role in the process.

Be that as it may, because of the brain functions of memory, here is what is likely to happen. Earlier, I envisioned that 'a house ablaze took place here and now', as if time were held constant. In reality, time cannot be held constant; it elapses continuously. A good example is how we describe the incident of 'a

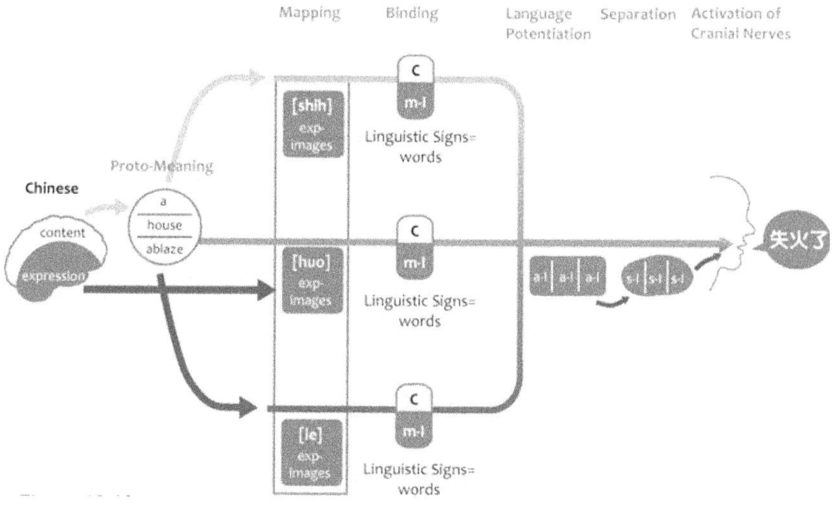

Figure 18.10

house ablaze' to our friends, after it is all over, say, in six hours, who were not at the scene or came later to observe the incident. In that case, we can be sure that each speaker at the scene, from the beginning to the end, will have accumulated lots of information (i.e., proto-meanings) in his/her brain. But we can be equally sure that no speaker in any language will report that incident as simply 'Fire!' or its equivalent in any language; nor will any speaker be able to report every single detail which he/she saw, smelled, felt, or otherwise encountered and perceived during the entire event. This limitation is a result of the mechanism of integration which is an important part of the Specific Brain Functions of Memory (Peng, 1994); it is purported to be a concept for the collective effort of Summarizing, Paraphrasing, and Inferencing.

Because of the time variable and the memory variable, the text we might expect could be something like this: 'I saw a house ablaze on the way back, and I shouted "Fire!", and people came out to save the house.' This can only be the result of the specific brain functions of summarizing, which are a part of the brain functions of memory as mechanism; to report or describe every bit of information in the events of the previous six hours would surely take another six hours. On the other hand, even if no one came out to save the house, the first two clauses are sufficient to summarize the event and clearly illustrate the increment of the amount of proto-meanings on account of the elapsing of time, which must now be chunked temporally, never non-temporally.

5. The Process of Sequencing

In either temporal or non-temporal chunking, sequencing of the chunked pieces of proto-meanings is required, which is to say that they must be temporally arranged in the brain, while undergoing the neurophysiological process of mapping. It is in the arranging of proto-meanings into some kind of a sequence, either pre-mapping (in the case of temporal chunking) or post-mapping (in the case of non-temporal chunking), that meanings are realized in wording as brain functions. At the same time, however, the neurophysiological process of mapping is also taking place in the brain. I shall call this simultaneous processing of mapping proto-meanings onto the appropriately retrieved acoustic images, in connection with the process of chunking and the process of sequencing, respectively, the highest brain functions for the realization of meaning in wording.

In the case of pre-mapping segmentation, the process of sequencing is, as I said earlier, anticipated by the process of chunking; the two processes constitute a continuation of the specific brain functions of segmentation (Peng, 1994), that is, they are 'superimposed' by mappings which are also temporally processed.

In the case of post-mapping segmentation, on the other hand, the process of sequencing is *not* anticipated by the process of chunking; thus, the two processes do *not* constitute a continuation of the specific brain functions of segmentation (Peng, 1994), although they are now interpolated by mappings which, nonetheless, are *not* temporally processed; the reason is that the acoustic images are 'lurking', as it were, in the brain waiting to be 'unlocked', without being linearized in any way. I am of the opinion that each acoustic image is like a thinly veiled whole that is assembled from the decomposed elements – like a Chinese character, figuratively speaking – which has a 'shape' but not linearized within itself, before a chunked piece of proto-meanings is mapped onto it.

The impulse(s) of an acoustic image is (are) arranged during the catalytic mapping, that is, when a linguistic meaning is mapped onto it which then becomes a sound-image. The reason I have proposed is that acoustic images as a whole do not stay put nor are they locked and fixed in static positions in the brain, waiting 'idly' to be 'picked up'; rather, they are impulses which move around from one region of the brain to another, and therefore must be 'caught'. This is what I think neurosurgeons mean when they claim they have 'arrested' language in epilepsy surgery (Ojemann *et al.*, 1989) when in fact they simply 'catch' a lurking acoustic image or a sound-image.

The pre-mapping segmentation, thus, refers not so much to the process of sequencing as to the process of chunking and the temporal arrangement of proto-meanings for pairing the chunked proto-meanings with their corresponding acoustic images as a continuation of the brain functions of segmentation; the results are sequenced linguistic signs each of which consists of a concept (C) and a corresponding sound-image (S-I). The post-mapping segmentation, by contrast, refers to the sequencing of linguistic meanings –

more precisely, the linguistic signs coming out of the catalytic mappings as the 'products'. It may be said, as a consequence, that in either the pre-mapping segmentation or the post-mapping segmentation, it is the sequencing of linguistic meanings that may be regarded as wording *per se*.

Here, a crucial distinction may be drawn between wording, as it is defined above, and lexicogrammar, as it is understood elsewhere. So far, the distinction has been ignored because in systemics wording and lexicogrammar are synonymous; so are meaning and semantics. But, in my neurolinguistics, I have come to realize that the synonymity seems unattainable. Two reasons will suffice to illustrate the need for a distinction.

First, wording as a stratum is in the individual aspect of language, whereas lexicogrammar as a stratum is best restricted to the social aspect of language. It is totally impossible to describe or designate certain impulses as 'nouns' or 'verbs' or as 'Subject' and 'Predicate' or whatever linguists are fond of doing. Impulses are universal, be they from a squid or a monkey or a cat or a human being. However, there are differences which lie in four areas of brain functions:

1. the patterns of circuitry (i.e., the interconnected network) in which impulses are transduced, such as aborization and myelination;
2. the degree of complexity (or sophistication) of the synaptic organization of the brain in each species, such as in relation to neurotransmitters and CREB proteins (cf. Shepherd, 1998);
3. the complexity of the neuronal organization in the nervous system in respect to the three groups of neurons, that is, motoric neurons, sensory neurons, and the great intermediate net of neurons, that is, different proportions in different species (Nauta and Feirtag, 1979);
4. the patterns of signalling for the transduction of impulses, such as in respect to binding, coherence, adjustments in the midbrain and the thalamus, and perceptual organization and re-organization.

Second, in linguistics there was a time when grammarians and computer programmers were 'indistinguishable', the reason being that linguists in the 1950s imported *en masse* ideas from computer science and modelled their theory of linguistics on the computer for what was called computational linguistics and machine translation; that trend was in vogue during the Cold War of the 1950s, 1960s and 1970s; even when the Cold War ended in the 1980s, lexicogrammar or syntax in linguistics was still greatly influenced by the computer. To this date, the trend continues, because linguists (or grammarians) still have the computer in mind when they theorize on syntax or lexicogrammar.

For these reasons, lexicogrammar may be useful for data-processing but has no representation or bearing in the brain, which is to say there is no grammar in the brain. On the other hand, wording which is based on the transduction of signals in the nervous system has no place in the computer because there are no neurotransmitters, nor is there CREB protein, in the computer.

If linguists want to model their theory of language or linguistics after the computer, they have a perfect right to do so. However, when they start to claim that what they have described in their theory as syntax or lexicogrammar represents or resembles how the brain works for human language to 'generate' sentences, then somebody has got to pull the plug and halt the claim. This monograph is intended to play that role, because the brain does not function like, nor is it, a computer. It is an insult to downgrade the brain functions of language to the level of the computer generating an infinite set of sentences which is then claimed to be what language in the brain is supposed to be.

6. The Process of Linearization

I have mentioned before the process of linearization as a part of the brain functions of segmentation, suggesting that it presumably takes place towards the end of the cortico-bulbar pathways. I should now add that this process of linearization is involved in two places: during the mapping of each concept onto its corresponding sound-image (cf. unlocking); and when each sound-image leaves the corresponding meaning behind after the mental state of language potentiation and enters the brainstem during the looping.

I have also said that when the sound-images of a sequence of linguistic signs, as impulses, enter the brainstem, there are no meanings as impulses in or attached to those sound-images, because the linguistic meanings have been left 'behind'; thus, the impulses must be strictly ordered linearly when they are on their way to the extrapyramidal loop in order to return to the cerebral (motor) cortex; after that, they go through the pyramidal tract to reach the synapses of the various nuclei of the cranial nerves in the brainstem in order to arrive at the vocal apparatus for the production of the actual sounds, one at a time. There is no other way in which the sounds can come out of the speaker's mouth.

In the case of [fáyr], however, the VIIth (facial) cranial nerve will have to work hard by putting the lower lip against the upper teeth. At the same time, the recurrent laryngeal nerve of the vagus must open the vocal cords in order not to let them vibrate because of the air stream passing through the glottis. But, immediately after that, when the facial nerve releases the lower lip and drops the mandible to reach the neutral position for vocalization in order to set the stage for [a], the recurrent laryngeal nerve must be activated again to close the vocal cords slightly so as to allow them to vibrate on account of the air stream passing through the glottis. In the course of such activations of the VIIth and Xth cranial nerves, the IXth and the XIth cranial nerves (glosso-pharyngeal and accessory, respectively) close the velic and move the larynx while the XIIth (hypoglossal) cranial nerve moves the tongue upward and forward from the [a] position to the [y] position, and then curls the tongue tip to form the retroflex shape of [r]. In other words, all these cranial nerves are activated in synchronization with the basic brain functions of the centre of respiration (in the floor of the fourth ventricle), or else [fáyr] will not come out of the speaker's mouth.

Such being the case, the only place and time when meaning can still be manipulated is the state of language potentiation where the sound-images as impulses are only 'loosely' linearized. In the absence of CNV, I am more inclined to suggest that this manipulation of meaning may depend on or have something to do with morphological derivation for most languages and morphological inflection of languages which have that system; neuro-anatomically, it most likely involves the great intermediate net of neurons including the extrapyramidal system and the pyramidal system which have a recurrent pathway going back to the thalamus that leads back to the motor cortex in the cerebrum which also reciprocates fibres to the thalamus (cf. Carpenter, 1976).

It is this 'loop', the cortico-striato-pallido-thalamo-cortical loop, within the great intermediate net of neurons, that enables the individual to manipulate meaning at the 'last minute', as it were, because thinking takes place in the midst of the manipulation of varying meanings during the 'looping'.

The manipulation, however, is *not* mandatory; if the speaker feels each sequence of linguistic signs is in order, he/she simply lets the sound-images in the sequence enter the brainstem, while leaving the corresponding meanings (i.e., concepts) behind as he/she produces the sound waves. In that case, the outcome may not be right as in foreigner's talk. Of course, thinking also takes place when each sequence of linguistic signs is in order. When and only when the speaker feels the need to adjust the meanings and the corresponding sound-images at the last minute will manipulation occur, which includes false start, errors, hesitation pauses, additions and the like, at which time thinking must be at work, too.

At one and the same time, moreover, the 'loosely' linearized impulses of the sound-images during the state of language potentiation can be and are adjusted for what linguists call morphophonemic alterations; every human language is known to have such alterations, arising from historical changes; for example, *wife/wives*, where [f] is changed to [v] which is voiced, because of the plural suffix that has the [z] sound which is also voiced. The same is true in Japanese and Taiwanese, for instance, [siro-i] 'white' and [sira-kawa] 'White River' in Japanese where [o] is changed to [a] and *siòng* 'to aim for' and *sióng-chhin* 'marriage interview' in Taiwanese where the third tone [`] is changed to the second tone [´] for a tone sandhi. I am inclined to believe that morphophonemic alterations are adjusted in conjunction with the 'last minute' manipulation of meaning in morphological derivation and inflection on the basis of the brain functions of memory.

This is not to say, however, that I advocate the existence of morphophonemes and the like in the brain; I used such linguistic terms as derivation, inflection, morphophonemic alterations just to facilitate my explication to linguists of the brain functions of linearization of impulses in the sound-images during the state of language potentiation. In terms of neurophysiological properties, [f], [v], and [z] in English or [o] and [a] in Japanese or [`] and [´] in Taiwanese, are just impulses which linguists for the sake of convenience designate as morphophonemic alterations, suffix, and tone sandhi in their creations of morphophonemics, grammar and phonemics to facilitate discussion among themselves.

The last-minute manipulation of meaning may be jeopardized. The evidence I propose is the symptom complexes of 'aphasia' caused by subcortical lesions in structures like the thalamus or the basal ganglia or even the internal capsule (Peng *et al.*, 1986; Murdoch, 1987; Damasio *et al.*, 1982; Kennedy and Murdoch, 1989). When any such subcortical structure is lesioned because, for instance, of infarction or haemorrhage, language disorders of one kind or another are bound to occur as sequelae. Literature in this regard is abundant. Whether or not such symptom complexes can be called 'aphasia' is a different story, however.

Once the impulses of sound-images leave the linguistic meanings 'behind' and enter the brainstem, the various nuclei of the cranial nerves involved in the vocal apparatus take over to handle the actual articulation of sounds by way of the various motor units in the vocal apparatus. A motor unit consists of a lower motor neuron, its axon, and 10–400 muscle fibres innervated by the cell.

Between the cerebral cortex and the nuclei in the brainstem there are two systems which are relevant to the process of linearization; namely, the pyr amidal system and the extrapyramidal system. Some people think that the pyramidal system is strictly for grammar (in the sense used in linguistics). But, as I have already mentioned above, wording is not synonymous with lexicogrammar, because there is no lexicogrammar in the brain, and therefore although the pyramidal system is significant in and associated with the corticobulbar pathways, wording is not solely handled by this system, not to mention that wording is also relevant to the sensory system.

What I want to stress here is the role played by the extrapyramidal system in the process of linearization; many people seem to confuse the process of linearization, which pertains to the impulses of sound-images, with the process of sequencing, which pertains to the pairings of concepts and sound-images and the sequencing of the resultant linguistic signs. Care must be taken to avoid such confusion.

The extrapyramidal system is of relevance here in that when it is disordered, as in PD, the patient can hardly talk, because of dystonia and/or hypertonia, not to mention gait disturbances, rigidity of the limbs, resting tremor, dyskinesia or bradykinesia and mask face. The patient's language is of course disordered (Peng *et al.*, 1992; Peng and Huang, 1996). The important point here is that the disease also disorders the process of linearization, to the extent that when the patient is off medication, he/she cannot talk, that is, mute, in a later stage; presumably the impulses of sound-images are 'blocked' by the disordered extrapyramidal system, for the lack of dopamine, a neurotransmitter that is vital to the functioning of the system, and therefore cannot enter the brainstem for the activation of the relevant cranial nerves.

To these two systems must be added the cerebellum that is also an important subcortical structure for the cerebello-cerebral circuit which plays a significant role in the process of linearization and intonation (Chiu *et al.*, 1996). But both the extrapyramidal system and the cerebello-cerebral circuit have anatomical connections with the thalamus (Allen and Tsukahara, 1974; Schmahmann, 2003). Thus, like the striatum in the striato-pallido-thalamic connection, the cerebellum has the cerebello-ponto-thalamo-cortical route for which the impulses of sound-images may be re-routed back to the cerebrum via the superior cerebellar peduncle, albeit less effective in making adjustment for meaning.

The discussion presented depicts the cortico-bulbar pathways in connection with the cerebello-cerebral system and the peripheral nervous system of the vocal apparatus. It may, therefore, be stressed that the extrapyramidal system (the cortico-striato-pallido-thalamo-cortical loop) probably initiates the transmissions of the acoustic images onto which the proto-meanings have been mapped in the cerebral cortex that has thereby transduced the coherent images of the resultant linguistic signs to the state of language potentiation in anticipation of separation; in the course of the separation of concept and sound-image in each linguistic sign, the cerebello-cerebral system adds fine-tuning to the impulses of the sound-images when they leave the corresponding meanings (i.e., concepts) behind and enter the brainstem, so as to 'stablize' or 'improve the quality of' sound production as the impulses come down to the cortico-bulbar pathways, that is, as they reach the appropriate cranial nerves for sound production. Even if and when those sound-images do not come down to the cortico-bulbar pathways for sound production, and stay in the extrapyramidal looping for inner speech, the role of the cerebello-cerebral circuit cannot be underestimated, as it certainly modulates the looping for quality improvement in thinking.

In this connection, I must add that in the case of the cerebellum, the 'stabilization' owes much to the cerebello-cerebral circuit, because each cerebellar hemisphere receives imputs primarily from association areas of the cerebral cortex (Allen and Tsukahara, 1974; Schmahmann, 2003). Also note that only 0.5×10^6 cortico-spinal fibres leave the cerebral cortex, giving off collaterals to the brainstem nuclei relaying the cerebro-cerebellar information, whereas 20×10^6 cortico-bulbar fibres innervate the same relay neurons, apparently providing a more significant input to the cerebellum than the PT (pyramidal tract) collaterals (Allen and Tsukahara, 1974). Moreover, of the relay nuclei projecting to the cerebellum, the pontine grey is numerically most significant with 21×10^6 in contrast to 0.5×10^6 for the inferior olive nucleus in the medulla oblongata (ibid.).

As a result, there have been reports that the cerebellum may play a much more significant role in the brain functions of memory. If so, the brain functions of memory will have to incorporate the role played by the cerebellum in relation to chunking and sequencing, not just linearization.

7. Context of Situation as a Stratum of Language in the Brain

In the course of this exposition, I stated earlier that language in the brain is memory-governed and meaning-centred. But I have concentrated on the latter in this chapter, because the brain functions of memory are briefly described in Part III. However, I should add here that since language in the brain is memory-governed, this theoretical construct implies that the four strata of the individual aspect of language are memory-governed. For that reason, context of situation is an integral part of the individual aspect of language.

In the individual aspect of language, it must follow, context of situation is *not* something 'out there' but 'something that is maintained in the brain', permanently as the sources of experiences (i.e., background noises) or temporarily as the source of information in the content plane. Such experiences or information thus become proto-meanings, like 'a house ablaze', which may or may not be immediately relevant to the individual's language in the brain. For instance, if the individual shouts [fáyr], then the proto-meanings are relevant to the individual's language in the brain as behaviour; on the other hand, if the individual sets the house on fire and simply flees, without saying a word, then the proto-meanings of what he/she did are irrelevant to the individual's language in the brain as behaviour but become only meaning potentials which may be kept in the individual's brain functions of memory (as background noises) for a later use, that is, when he/she is caught for interrogation.

To justify the claim that context of situation is an integral part of language, I will extend the example of 'a house ablaze' by changing the context of situation to see what will happen.

Suppose I change the context of situation to a battlefield (or a hunting ground). What will happen if and when a commander wants to order a group of soldiers to shoot the enemy or a predator wants to catch a prey? I will illustrate the battlefield context of situation below.

In this context of situation, non-human animals cannot do anything about it, but humans can; they also have a choice, either using guns or charging. When using guns, however, the commander must give an order which comes out as a text. In English, the text is *Fire,* again; in Japanese, the text becomes *ute*; in Mandarin Chinese, the text changes to *K'ai Ch'iang,* (lit.) 'Open the gun'.

Ostensibly, then, the two contexts of situation – 'a house ablaze' and 'a battlefield' – seem to have nothing to do with language, if language is taken to refer to the social aspect of language; but, at least, they assist in the forming of meaning. However, in the individual aspect of language, each of the two contexts of situation is an integral part of it, which contributes differently to the forming of proto-meanings in the brain.

Of course, there is room for argument as to whether the proto-meanings in the two contexts of situation are similar, let alone the same, or not, just because the two texts in English have come out the same, that is, *Fire.* The reason is that in Japanese or Mandarin Chinese, two different texts must be produced in each language for the two contexts of situation. Thus, what I am interested in is this, regardless of which language produces the text: in the context of 'a battlefield', the proto-meanings which are biologically based must be formed in the brain before and not after the 'shooting' begins; in the context of 'a house ablaze', on the other hand, the proto-meanings which are also biologically based can only be formed after the house has already been set ablaze and not before, unless the speaker wants to joke about it; in that case, it is an entirely different 'ball game' because the context of situation has already been tampered with.

The consequence of the difference in the contexts of situation lies in the fact that in the case of 'a battlefield' the shooting event is the effect of the text, whereas in the case of 'a house ablaze,', there is *no* direct effect of the text, until someone else comes to the rescue. Moreover, in the former, nobody attempts to eliminate the context of situation; in the latter, however, either the speaker or someone else who has come to the rescue will attempt to eliminate the context of situation or change it.

Given the previous Figures, it should be clear that the context of situation is directly linked to the individual aspect of language; it becomes a part of the brain functions controlled by the individual's nervous systems, the fundamental functions of which are to enable the individual to maintain proper adjustments to the internal and the external environments.

In the same vein, then, meanings or meaning potentials, derived from the context of situation, are not referents out there but something in the form of impulses already maintained or being kept in the brain, as were amply illustrated above, because meaning is a stratum of language in the brain.

In the case of 'a house ablaze', for instance, if the individual decides not to shout [fáyr] but to flee, the impulses of the proto-meanings are either temporarily or permanently maintained in the individual's brain, which thus become meaning potentials (or background noises) in his/her memory as content. Put differently, meaning potentials are part of the individual's memory as content, until the individual decides to make use of the meaning potentials from his/her memory as content on another occasion, say, a year later, to tell the story of 'a house ablaze' to his/her friends, unless they have been forgotten entirely. Then and only then will the meaning potentials (from memory as content) become proto-meanings which can change to linguistic meanings by going through the brain functions of segmentation for both chunking and sequencing, and then for linearization, before an appropriate text in any language can come out of the individual's mouth.

If meaning potentials are part of the individual's memory as content, when such meaning potentials become proto-meanings which can be arranged by way of chunking and sequencing and must also be mapped onto their corresponding acoustic images, then wording must be a part of the brain functions of memory, too; that is, wording pertains to the brain functions of segmentation minus linearization, and therefore is a part of the brain functions of memory as mechanism.

The Sound Patterns of oral language (or the Sign Patterns of sign language) are also part of the brain functions of memory as content but pertain to the brain functions of memory as capacity rather than to the brain functions of memory as mechanism unless they are activated to participate in the brain functions of segmentation for linearization; that is, they must be learned through mimicry (from childhood, in the case of the individual's first language) and vary in size from individual to individual in terms of the brain functions of memory as capacity. Even within each individual, there are vast differences between production and reception in the numbers of sound-images (i.e., vocabulary items); that is, every individual's reception in the number of sound-images is greater than his/her production in the number of sound-images.

These biological foundations of the four strata of the individual aspect of language can be depicted schematically in relation to the central and the peripheral nervous system and the brain functions of segmentation as in Figure 18.11.

In light of the existence of language in the brain, I should conclude this chapter by saying that wording is *not* 'neutral'; rather, it is quite 'personal' in that it varies from one individual to another, although proto-meanings may be quite universal. However, because the experiences of individuals differ considerably even between brothers or husband and wife, linguistic meanings will also differ from one person to the next depending on the individual's background. That is why I have said that the meaning the speaker constructs is nine times out of ten *not* the same as the meaning the hearer reconstructs. It is on the basis of such differences that language in the social aspect can change, because the individual aspect of language changes (Peng, 1976, 1979).

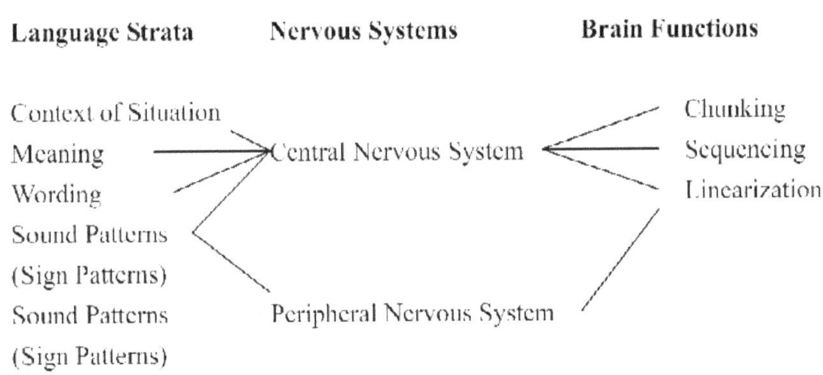

Figure 18.11

If this conclusion is reasonably sound and valid, linguists should take note not to model their theory of language on the computer, using the software of the computer as a model. Whatever software program, as in the late 1950s, and the 1960s, for instance, Chomsky's *Syntactic Structure*, that was created by linguists then for language was not a wording of human language; rather, it was an artifact that could not represent and has no bearing on human language in either aspect, any more than an aircraft design could be claimed to represent human language.

Finally, mention should also be made that in neither the social nor the individual aspect of language is there a psychological process in the brain;

whatever a human does in his/her language as behaviour is purely neurophysiological, the main manifestation of which can only be social because it occurs in a social context of situation. Thus, the individual aspect of language is the highest of all brain functions, in relation to Saussure's *langue* and *parole*, because it is behaviour based on the two nervous systems for the interplay of their various functions.

19 The Reconstruction of Meaning: Coupling of Expression and Content

Having demonstrated the production of language in the brain, I must now demonstrate the reception of language in the brain. To do so, I shall rely on, expand, and modify what I have said in 'Language disorders and brain functions' (Peng, 1994). In that article, I also stress the connections between the social aspect of language, as espoused in the Hallidayan theory, and the individual aspect of language, as proposed by me, to promote briefly for the first time the brain functions therein with respect to language disorders. For this chapter, I shall therefore concentrate on the individual aspect of language, stressing the brain functions involved for reception which will invariably touch on production as well, because the brain functions for production have already been presented. However, as there is only one brain which enables the individual to have both production and reception in his/her behaviour, some of the brain functions mentioned in this chapter will pertain to both production and reception.

1. Wording in Reception for Reconstructing Different Shades of Meaning

In Chapter 18, I described the Stratum of Wording in production in three ways: chunking of proto-meanings; the time factor involved for sequencing the proto-meanings already chunked in anticipation of the sequencing of the number of acoustic-images needed for catalytic mappings; and linearization as a result of unlocking each corresponding acoustic image in the selection by the linguistic meanings into which the chunked proto-meanings are bound to change subsequently. The role of wording in production is thus obvious: it changes certain proto-meanings from thought, an inchoate mass of impulses, into subsequent but definitive or specific linguistic meanings.

Wording in reception, however, is different in two ways: the role of wording in reception is to reconstruct, not construct, meanings; and as the incoming auditory stimuli are in some way linearized, the sequencing of the impulses is pre-determined, even though the acoustic images are the results of recombination (or binding) of decomposed auditory impulses from the brainstem, or the thalamus in particular. Thus, the reconstruction of meanings takes place after the acoustic images have already been formed as a result of the subsequent process of coupling with their corresponding meanings to change into the sound–images and the corresponding linguistic meanings, respectively. In that case, the process of coupling presupposes the selection of linguistic meanings from Thought, which must also undergo chunking in order to allow for the coupling of chunked pieces of proto-meaning with their corresponding acoustic images. What follows is the perceptual organization (or re-organization) which gives rise to a percept (or a series of percepts). This process of coupling may be schematically illustrated, with simplification, as in Figure 19.1.

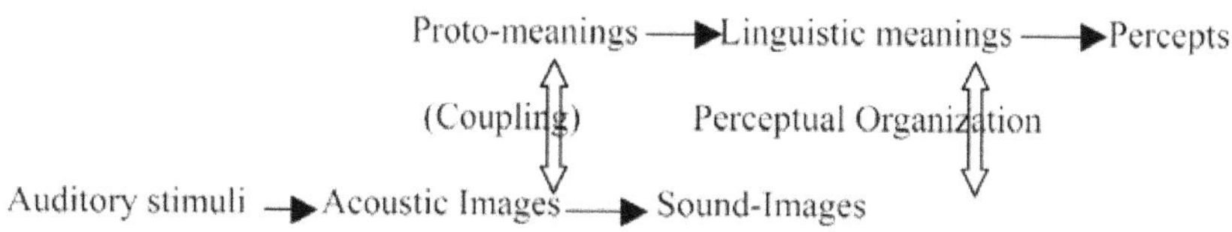

Figure 19.1 *Time-orientation*

However, when the process of coupling takes place, there may be more than one corresponding meaning with each acoustic image. Unlike the process of catalytic mappings in production, which permits a one-to-one mapping of proto-meanings and their corresponding acoustic images, the process of coupling in reception allows for a one-to-many coupling of acoustic images and their corresponding proto-meanings. That is why I have said that ambiguity is a decoding problem and not an encoding one (Peng, 1992a). For instance, as in punning, when a train is coming into the railroad station, someone may jokingly say, 'Here he comes, because it's a [mÉyl t^hrÈyn]'. The hearer will have to be able to couple the acoustic images with the proto-meanings of both *male* and *mail* almost simultaneously in order to appreciate the joke. If he/she is unable to do so, (that is, if only one proto-meaning, more likely *mail*, is selected for coupling, because the hearer is not a native speaker of English), he/she will not appreciate the joke.

Before the process of coupling can take place, there are many more brain functions of memory which go through the hearer's brain for reconstructing meanings from the speaker's utterances. Although I cannot describe all those intriguing brain functions in one monograph, this chapter depicts the complexity of such brain functions involved and, at the same time, describes in some detail, with appropriate examples, how such brain functions work.

2. The Hierarchy of Brain Functions

On the basis of the descriptions of the Individual Aspect of *Parole* in Part III, I have posited in Peng (1994) four layers for all brain functions. I call them: Basic Brain Functions, Higher Brain Functions, Specific Brain Functions, and Highest Brain Functions (or Brain Functions of Language) as part of the Individual Aspect of Language, that is, Language in the Brain. These brain functions described below are intended for humans and overlap to a large extent with the brain functions of memory presented earlier. The distinction, however, is in the way in which such brain functions are looked at and described: the brain functions of memory are looked at and described categorically whereas the four layers of all brain functions are looked at and organized hierarchically in anticipation of the connections with the common nervous functions which are based on the peripheral nervous system because of interdependencies.

2.1 Basic Brain Functions

Each organism has a nervous system whose basic function is to enable the organism to maintain proper adjustments to the internal and the external environments. The proper adjustments to the internal environment, for instance, can be achieved by any non-human primate, such as the proper adjustments to hunger, thirst and pain. In like manner, the proper adjustments to the external environment can also be effected by any non-human primate through the five senses, among others; for example, attention, reflex and the limbic system. I have already mentioned 'a house ablaze' to illustrate proto-meanings in reception through one of the five senses. The realization of such adjustments to the external environment relies naturally on the organism's intact motor activities.

Each of these basic functions is, of course, controlled by the central nervous system through the peripheral nervous system. And where they are located in the brain and how they are transmitted through the peripheral nervous system are well documented. I have also briefly recapitulated and elaborated them in Part III and Part IV (e.g., in relation to phantom limbs).

The problem that needs to be raised here is this: do those basic brain functions include or pertain to language in the brain or not? Put differently, if language is believed to be part of higher brain (or cortical) functions, as has been so claimed by most, neuroscientists in particular, are such higher brain functions on a par with those basic brain functions that enable the individual to maintain proper adjustments to the internal and the external environments or are they brain functions of a different kind?

I will address myself to this crucial question below. To do so, I shall compare human and non-human primates.

2.1.1 Human and Non-human Pathways

Since we now know that the vocal apparatus in non-human primates is different from the human vocal apparatus, the cortico-bulbar pathways in non-human primates and those in humans are employed differently for transducing the impulses from the expression plane in production, because of the evolutionary changes mentioned in Part III; that is, non-human primates have their own vocalizations and we have our own vocalizations, even though both may be equally versatile with different complexities because each species maintains its own kind of background noises in the content plane. The bulbo-cortical pathways are a different story. That is to say, the bulbo-cortical pathways are more similar to each other between humans and non-human primates (or even between humans and lower forms of mammals, say, dogs and cats) than the cortico-bulbar pathways between them.

The main reason for the similarity is because auditory reception has no anatomical restriction among most mammals, although visual reception and olfactory reception may differ. For instance, cats and dogs can run easily at night in darkness but humans cannot; and a dog's olfactory system is 10,000 times more powerful than that of a human. Consequently, when any auditory stimulus enters the bulbo-cortical pathways, it is received and transmitted in very much the same way by humans and non-human mammals from the brainstem to the cortex. This stage of reception up to the nuclei of the vestibulo-cochlear (VIIIth) nerve is called the brain functions of Recognition, starting with the initial contact of the peripheral nervous system with the stimulus, which is then followed by the brain functions of Identification. So, let me examine the similarity and dissimilarity more closely below.

2.1.2 Bulbo-cortical Pathways in Humans and Non-human Primates

By bulbo-cortical pathways, of course, I mean all sensory connections from the brainstem to the cortex, save for the olfactory system whose nuclei are directly under the olfactory bulbs buried inside the cortex rather than in the brainstem, and the visual system even though its pathways (retino-thalamo-cortical) go through the brainstem.

The functions of such afferent connections, therefore, are to provide the cerebrum, especially the neocortex, with the necessary information from the external and the internal environments. As a result, an individual organism can then make the proper adjustments (i.e., decision) by sending out the needed efferent impulses through the cortico-bulbar pathways for the production as behaviour in order to maintain proper adjustments to the environments.

In the neocortex, however, there are tremendous differences between humans and non-human primates. In other words, the fact that the bulbo-cortical pathways in humans and non-human primates are very similar in terms of reception and its transmission of impulses is not tantamount to saying that such impulses are processed similarly by the human and the non-human cerebrum. Quite the contrary, it is the process in the cerebrum, coupled with its connections with the extrapyramidal tract, the cerebello-cerebral circuit, and the Papez circuit, in connection with the anatomical differences in the vocal apparatus, that makes the most clear distinction between human and non-human primates in terms of language in the brain. Put differently, an ape or a monkey or even a dog may be able to hear a sequence of sounds or words in a human language in very much the same way as a human would hear the same sequence of sounds or words in a language he/she does not know, because the sounds are simply noises. However, they are not indistinguishable from other noises.

The first process the cerebrum (or neocortex) undertakes upon receiving the impulses from the brainstem, where the initial contact is processed, is to distinguish one kind or one sequence of noises from another kind or another sequence of noises. Since non-human primates cannot use the cortico-bulbar pathways for the vocal apparatus to create a wide variety of acoustic images in the cerebrum, the distinction is made on each sequence or segment (i.e., chunked noise) as a decomposed whole – for a sort of perceived 'general impression' – rather than for minute details. Such a distinction, that is, the ability to differentiate one kind of noise, that is, pitch, loudness, quality, speech, timbre, etc., from another, can be done very easily by all mammals, I believe, because it is processed by the basic brain functions on the basis of the common nervous functions. The same is true of making distinctions among different colours of objects, shapes of such objects, configurations of signs, and movements of such objects and signs. The distinctions of olfactory functions or gustatory functions (as in taste buds) are also processed by the basic brain functions.

The important point here is that each sequence of sounds or words must be further divided into smaller chunks (technically called constituents or segments) by a process called segmentation that is extremely crucial in the demarcation of how much one species or even one member of a species can have a language in the brain. This process of segmentation in reception is similar, albeit not identical, to the brain functions of segmentation discussed in connection with production above. It is within this process of segmentation that the brain functions of Identification and Coupling take place. In general, I can say that while the human brain is able to make the segmentation fairly easily and in great detail, the non-human brain finds it extremely difficult, although it can be done to some extent by the non-human primate brain, as is evidenced by Koko's ability to understand Patterson's English while responding in ASL. The reason lies in the differences in the cortico-bulbar pathways and their connections to the vocal apparatus, which I have already discussed in great detail above.

What I am saying is that the segmentation of the impulses transmitted to the neocortex through the bulbo-cortical pathways depends to a great extent on the functions of the cortico-bulbar pathways. That is to say, unless the cortico-bulbar pathways can function to 'imitate' (i.e., mimic) the impulses received by the neocortex, there is no way in which the process of segmentation can take place in the brain to segment each sequence of sounds received. I thus claim that while the human brain can make the functionally connective loop, which is presented below, the non-human brain cannot do so, because of the anatomical restriction in respect to the cortico-bulbar pathways mentioned earlier. In other words, the impulses transduced from the bulbo-cortical pathways to the neocortex must be 're-transduced' through the cortico-bulbar pathways to the vocal apparatus for the production of, that is, mimicking, what may at first be heard simply as noises.

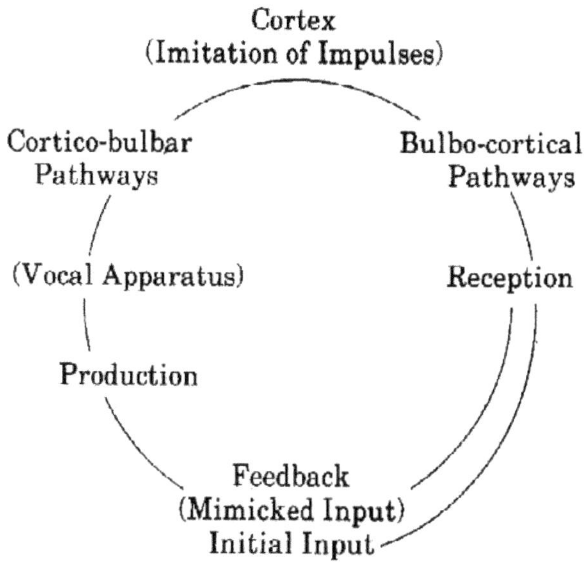

Figure 19.2 *Functionally connective loop for the segmentation of impulses*

Before the 're-transduction', however, the impulses must undergo Identificaton with the existing impulses (i.e., acoustic images) in the expression plane, so as to couple with their corresponding meanings. The question is where the brain function of identification takes place. Answer: in the connective loop. I have not indicated the details of the bulbo-cortical pathways, but I can say for sure that it takes place in the thalamus within the bulbo-cortical pathways.

Recall that the thalamus is the 'super relay station' involved in not only the bulbo-cortical pathways and the spino-cortical pathways but also the extrapyramidal loop, the cerebello-cortical circuit and the Papez circuit. I should add that all sensory impulses from the five senses must go through the thalamus which has fibres that reciprocally connect the thalamus and the cortex, thereby constituting the thalamic radiations (Carpenter, 1976: 462). I have already briefly described the adjustments of impulses for visual and auditory stimuli in the lateral geniculate body and medial geniculate body, respectively, which are part of the thalamus. The same goes for olfactory stimuli which send projections to both the thalamus and the limbic system as relay stations to the frontal cortex which reciprocates fibres back to the thalamus and the limbic system (Freeman, 1991).

On the basis of such anatomical evidence, there is no doubt that during the adjustments of auditory impulses in the medial geniculate bodies, after they have passed through the inferior and the superior colliculi in the midbrain, as part of the functions of the bulbo-cortical pathways, the brain function of identification takes place. It identifies any incoming (i.e., afferent) impulse with the pool of existing impulses (or acoustic images) in the cerebral cortex (which are part of the background noises in the expression plane) maintained in the brain functions of memory as content.

Once each impulse is so identified, it goes through the process of coupling with the corresponding meaning in the content plane. The coupled meaning in reception becomes a linguistic meaning (or concept) and the corresponding impulse becomes a sound-image. The concept, together with its corresponding sound-image, constitute (or are organized into) a linguistic percept in the brain for reception, which is the analogue of a linguistic sign in production. It is in the process of coupling that the perceptual organization also takes place in order to constitute a linguistic percept.

Here, an important difference between reception and production is worthy of mention; that is, while for reception a linguistic percept does not go any further for separation in the brain, for production a linguistic sign must go one step further to undergo separation in order to allow the sound-images as impulses to go through the extrapyramidal loop so as to come out as a text (in physical sounds) unless the speaker decides not to say anything. In that case, a linguistic sign may temporarily become a linguistic percept in the cerebral cortex until the speaker changes his/her mind to produce the original linguistic sign as an utterance.

On the other hand, if and when an incoming impulse fails to be so identified, that is, there is no existing impulse that matches it, it does not go through the process of coupling, because there is no corresponding meaning for coupling, and therefore it will be treated as 'a noise' (or 'a nonsense syllable' for a series of incoming impulses). Of course, we can also regard the notion of 'a noise' as a concept (i.e., 'nonsense'), in which case, the incoming impulse will couple with such a concept of 'noise' for a perceptual organization and the resulting percept will be 'filed under nonsense'.

The connections of reception and production in respect to oral language and sign language (or Braille) may be summarized in Figure 19.3. The sensory function is intended to subsume the brain functions of recognition (i.e., initial contact), identification and coupling (including perceptual organization). The brain function of coupling, however, is explained in greater detail further below.

2.2 Higher Brain Functions

The above differentiations of the pathways and the cross-modal connections of the nature of sign language production suggest that the brain functions of both human and non-human primates have something in common, although I am not claiming that their brain functions in the neocortex are similar. The common element is the process called segmentation which segments meaning in or from the content plane.

I have already described this process in some detail in connection with production in Chapter 18. In reception, I believe that this process is similar or related to that in production, although I am not saying that the process of

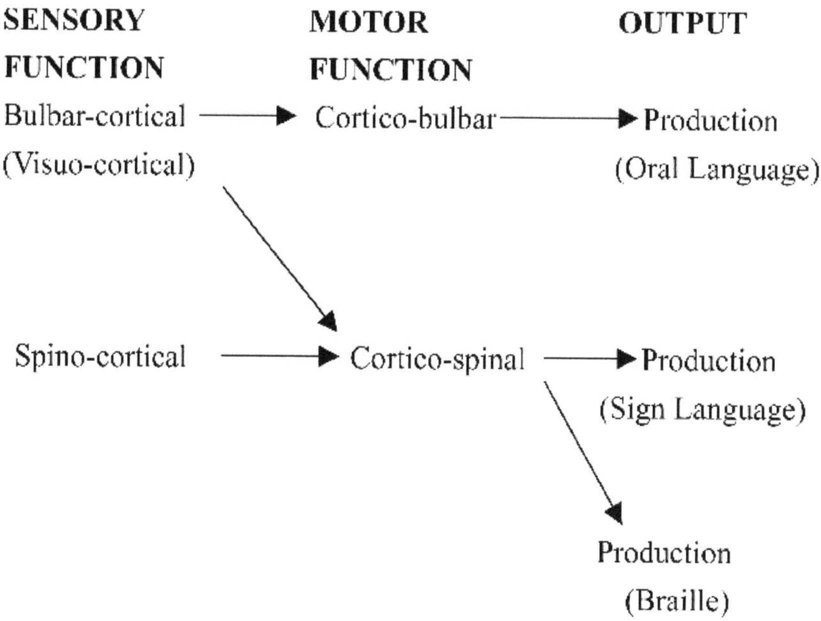

Figure 19.3 *A simplified illustration of the connection of reception and production in respect to oral language and sign language*

segmentation in reception is the same as the process of segmentation already described in production.

Recall, however, that I have said that in the case of oral language, segmentation in production is impossible for non-human primates, because of the restriction of their vocal apparatus to create in the brain a sufficient number of acoustic images comparable to those in humans, although a limited number of acoustic images comparable to their vocal apparatus are available to them. But I must now qualify this statement by saying that segmentation in production is possible for them in the case of sign language (in contrast to the fact that segmentation is essential, not only possible, in the case of humans for both oral and sign language). In the main, it pertains to both the higher brain functions and the specific brain functions which will be described later.

What is this process called segmentation, then, in relation to reception, now that we know what it is in relation to production? In this regard, I should say that it usually starts with the distinction of same/different through mimicking. For instance, when learning a new language as behaviour, mimicking can be 'upgraded' to become the specific brain functions, by way of what I have called function enhancement in the brain functions of memory as mechanism, so that the new language can be learned as new behaviour; that is to say, the new language as new behaviour can be maintained in the content plane and the expression plane on account of memory as content and memory as capacity.

I should for the time being add that the process of segmentation in reception is the biological foundation (or neural substrate) of Context of Situation, Meaning, Wording, and Sound Patterns (and to some extent of Sign Patterns) and belongs to both the higher brain functions and the specific brain functions. It belongs to the former when learning new things; it belongs to the latter when dealing with familiar things. Either way, it cuts up the 'outside world' for meaning and wording, in anticipation of coupling, and then linearizes the output – that is, the cut up 'outside world' – and confirms the linearized input from the cerebral cortex. The input is temporarily determined, in accordance with the incoming stimuli, for integration (in particular, summarizing and inferencing) which I have already discussed in connection with production.

There are, of course, many more higher brain functions than the process of segmentation, which are relevant to language as the highest of all brain functions. Such higher brain functions pertain to meanings in language, for instance, space orientation, abstract notion of kinship relationships, and complicated arrangements of objects, patterns, designs, etc. These higher brain functions can also be upgraded by the mechanism of function enhancement to the status of specific brain functions for the enhancement of meaning, such as connotation, colour-coded objects or paths, inference, among others; the upgrading of function status for the enhancement of meaning is more common in reception than in production of language and more so in non-language materials. For instance, if a person sneezes, his/her sneeze is a non-language material in production, but it will *not* be processed by the hearer as simply a noise or a nonsense syllable in his/her percept. The evidence is that the hearer qua speaker will more often than not respond with '(God) Bless You!' suggesting that the hearer has upgraded the input to the status of a meaning comparable to 'catching a cold' or something to that effect. Such an upgraded percept in hearer's brain was, of course, hearer's own reconstructed meaning and not the proto-meaning intended by the 'sneezer' in the first place. No 'sneezer' would intend to catch a cold in order to sneeze; nor would any individual intend to sneeze in order to catch a cold.

2.3 Specific Brain Functions

So far, I have confined the discussion to the basic brain functions and the higher brain functions of the nervous system by comparing the human and non-human primates in relation to their cortico-bulbar pathways and the bulbo-cortical pathways, on the one hand, and by focusing on the differences between the cortico-bulbar and the cortico-spinal pathways, on the other. In so doing, I have also touched on the new but extremely important mechanism of function enhancement. This notion has enabled me to differentiate in some detail meanings in reception from meanings in production with respect to segmentation which pertains to coupling and mapping, respectively.

In this connection, I have mentioned mimicking which is needed for the process of segmentation in both reception and production; after sensory impulses have passed through the bulbo-cortical pathways, they undergo the process of segmentation through mimicking; when a new language is being learned as behaviour, for instance, mimicking is essential, which triggers the process of segmentation in both reception and production. In order to explain the specific brain functions in greater detail, I should now introduce another important distinction in production that exists in what I have called motor function and motor activity on which body movements are based.

Superficially, both motor functions and motor activities in relation to the production of sounds make use of the cortico-bulbar pathways to innervate the musculature of the vocal apparatus. The distinction, however, is that motor functions are part of language behaviour involving its expression plane, whereas motor activities are not, because acoustic images from the expression plane must be mapped onto their corresponding meanings in oral language behaviour. The same is true of sign language behaviour, which is also based on motor functions in production and not on motor activities. The distinction between motor function and motor activity in either oral language or sign language, in relation to mimicking, may be summarized in Figures 19.4 and 19.5.

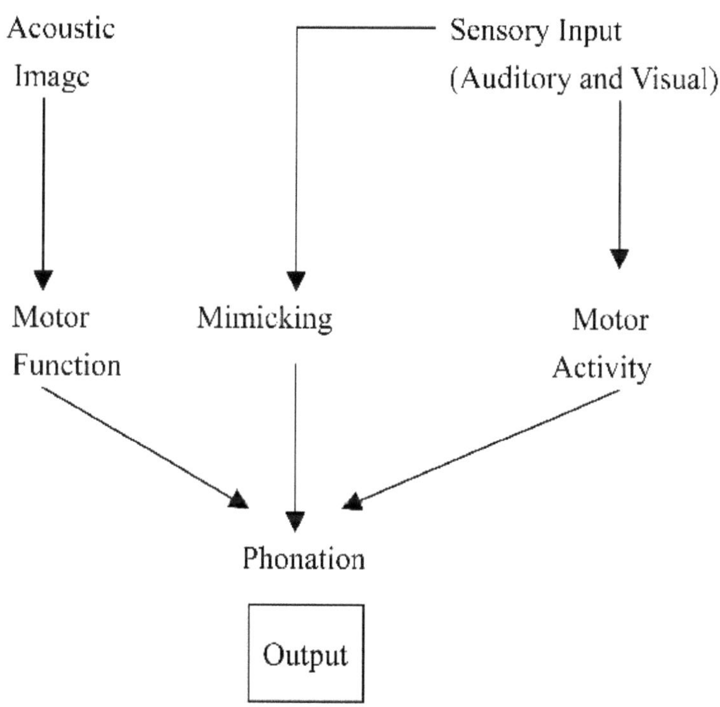

Figure 19.4 *A schematic illustration of the differences among motor function, mimicking, and motor activity in respect to phonation via the cortico-bulbar pathways*

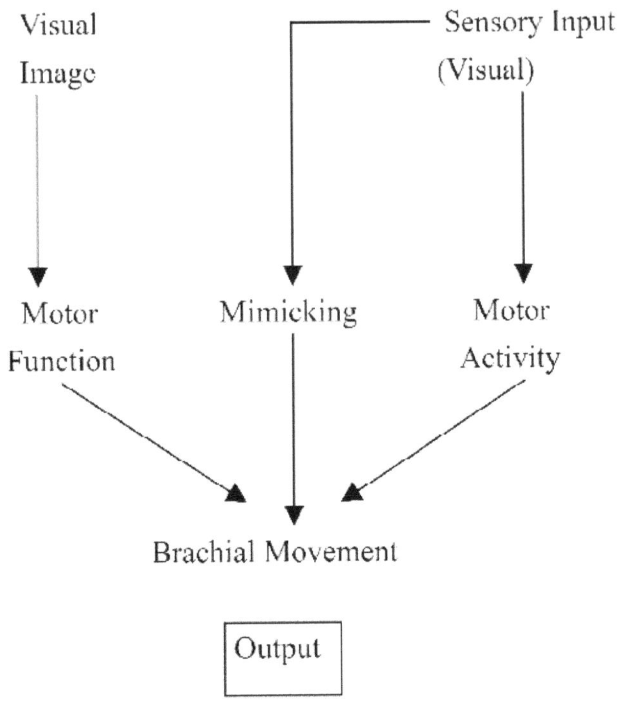

Figure 19.5 *A schematic illustration of the differences among motor function, mimicking, and motor activity in respect to brachial movement via the cortico-spinal pathways*

If these distinctions are sufficiently clear, it should be easy to understand that motor functions are specific brain functions which are actually 'upgraded' higher brain functions; likewise, mimickings are higher brain functions which are in turn 'upgraded' basic brain functions, while motor activities are plain basic brain functions. Put differently, all motor functions may in one sense be defined as motor activities upgraded twofold, in developmental terms, to carry out or to be intended for the catalytic mappings of meanings upon the corresponding acoustic images, thereby becoming specific brain functions (i.e., handling familiar impulses), because a language has already been learned by way of the brain functions of memory. Likewise, all mimickings may be defined as motor activities upgraded onefold, in terms of 'training' or 'teaching' involving the mechanism of repetition, rehearsal and reinforcement, thereby becoming higher brain functions in the course of learning or experiencing a new language as behaviour.

Such being the distinction of motor functions and motor activities, the same can be said of sensory functions and sensory activities, except that there are no mimicking to form a trichotomy; that is, every sensory input becomes either a sensory function or a sensory activity. In other words, mimicking is the sender's motor prerogative which presupposes the presence of a sensory stimulus without which, auditorily or visually, there is simply no mimicking at all; what the receiver gets in his/her sensory system is either an input that becomes a sensory function (for which he/she has to reconstruct meaning) or an input that becomes a sensory activity (for which he/she need not but may reconstruct 'meaning', as in a response to sneezing). The former (i.e., sensory function), of course, is an upgraded basic brain function, while the latter (i.e., sensory activity) is a straightforward basic brain function. If the receiver of an input that is a sensory activity, such as a sneeze, decides to respond with 'God Bless You', that input has already become a sensory function.

In reality, however, the situation is much more complicated than what I have depicted above. For instance, when you hear a bee buzzing, does this noise become a sensory function or a sensory activity in your brain? On the other hand, if you hear 'Watch out!' simultaneously, the buzzing immediately becomes a sensory function in your brain for sure, because your brain has to reconstruct the meaning of the noises for you, so that you will be able to take a proper adjustment to the external environment, not the text 'Watch out!' but to the bee buzzing around you, in order to avoid being stung by the bee.

Such being the case, it is possible to have a motor function from a sender but, since the output is an input to a receiver, it may become a sensory activity, rather than a sensory function, to the receiver; the input is just a nonsensical noise, for which the receiver cannot reconstruct any meaning. A good example is when two monolinguals speaking two different languages attempt to 'communicate' with each other. In that case, each person can only attempt to resort to gesticulation, in relation to the context of the situation, hoping that the other person will catch some of the gestures employed as sensory functions in order to make some adjustments to the external circumstances.

Theoretically, of course, a motor function should be heard or received and become a sensory function, just like a motor activity should be heard or received and become a sensory activity. However, because of the stratum of context of situation, comprising the three elements of Environment, People and Code, corresponding roughly to Halliday's Field, Tenor and Mode, respectively, in the social aspect of language, the correspondences of motor function/motor activity and sensory function/sensory activity are not always one to one.

The following illustration depicts all possible correspondences between the motor system and the sensory system in respect to brain functions.

2.4 Kinds of Specific Brain Functions

So far, I have concentrated on the motor and the sensory system to illustrate what I mean by specific brain functions which are more often than not upgraded basic brain functions. If the upgrading is onefold, the upgraded resultant brain functions are higher brain functions, becoming what I have already indicated; namely, the process of segmentation (when learning new things), space orientation, abstract notions of kinship relationships, and

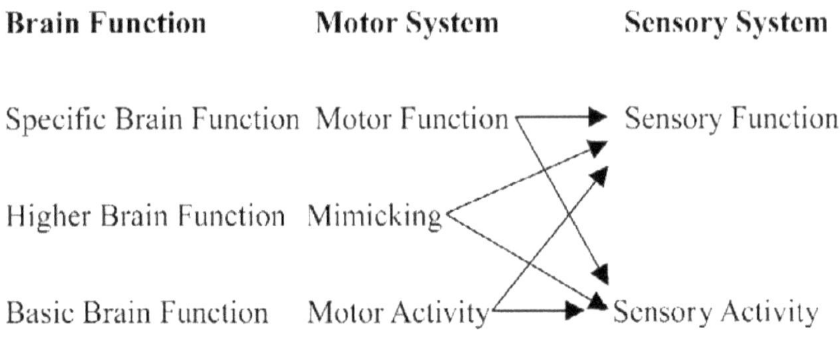

Figure 19.6 *An illustration of all possible correspondences in brain functions between the motor and the sensory system in a dyad*

complicated arrangements of objects, patterns and designs (as in WASIS for an IQ test or Wisconsin Card Sorting Test used to test brain-damaged patients by psychologists, and the like). If the upgrading is twofold, the upgraded resultant brain functions are specific brain functions and become what I want to indicate here.

I have already shown the process of segmentation (when dealing with familiar things, for improvement, for instance) to be one such specific brain function. I have also discussed further the relation to production in Part IV. There are, of course, other kinds of specific brain functions. Although I cannot name them all, because brain functions are so enormously complex and so intrinsically interrelated and interdependent that they cannot be taxonomically simplified to a mere clear-cut classification. I shall identify a few more and recapitulate those which have been indicated with some elaborations, together with motor and sensory functions shown above. In general, there are two major but interrelated types; namely, the Specific Brain Functions of Segmentation and the Specific Brain Functions of Memory.

The former includes the following minor types of specific brain functions:

1. for the categorization of meaning;
2. for the reception of meaning;
3. in the 'chunking' of meaning in wording;
4. for the interpretation of linguistic meanings from wording;
5. for phonation;
6. for audition;
7. motor functions (as defined above); and
8. sensory functions (as defined above).

These minor types of specific brain functions are the elaborations of the brain functions of segmentation described earlier; namely, chunking, sequencing and linearization.

The last mentioned, on the other hand, includes two very important mechanisms each of which has been briefly explicated above. I have come to call them Function Enhancement and Integration. I shall in the following elaborate these two types of specific brain functions with examples, when appropriate, in connection with the brain functions of memory, as language in the brain is memory-governed, meaning-centred and multifaceted.

2.4.1 *Categorization of Meaning*

This specific brain function is tied to the brain functions of memory and subsumed by the brain functions of chunking. Since nobody can reproduce what has been heard, seen, touched, smelled or tasted in its entirety, because of the enormity of context of situation and the time factor involved after an event has taken place, the brain has the ability to categorize proto-meanings from the content plane: what are more important or less important to the individual before or even as a part of the process of chunking for catalytic mappings are categorized into different meaning groups; the individual can then select those categories of meanings for mappings, which are best suited for the individual's adjustments to the environments when he/she has to report orally or manually regarding the event through the brain functions of segmentation.

The brain functions of memory which are best suited under such circumstances are probably the mechanisms of Retrieval, Repetition, Summarizing, Paraphrasing or Inferencing (for the effect of function enhancement on the part of the hearer). A good example is a criminal case, either in a hit-and-run traffic accident or a house set on fire, when police begin to ask those who were at the scene.

2.4.2 *Reception of Meaning*

When police have heard the oral report or description of what happened, it will be very unlikely that they will take what they have received literally, through the processes of recognition, identification and coupling; more likely they will analyse (or sort out) the meanings of what they have reconstructed, through coupling, by categorizing them (as defined above), in combination with what they saw upon arrival; the reception of meanings must rely on the mechanisms of Function Enhancement and Inferencing, in order to determine the true meanings or a sequence of the true meanings of what the context of situation was like when the event took place.

The analysis in the reception of meanings includes categorization, function enhancement and inferencing, all of which require the time factor, which is to say that the true meaning cannot be arrived at on the spot or instantaneously. That is, the meanings initially received through coupling may be inaccurate or false, and therefore must be supplemented or changed and modified by new information that comes in or is received later through further function enhancement and inferencing.

2.4.3 'Chunking' of Meaning in Wording

The report received is of course not accepted as a whole, which is most likely written to facilitate or help the brain functions of memory, so as to counter Forgetting in the brain functions of memory as capacity. The written record serves as a 'crutch' to retrieve memory as content in order to facilitate the mechanisms of Repetition, Recall and Reinforcement. The aim is to handle the goings-on of the here-and-now by relying on the mechanisms of Problem-Solving regarding memory as content in the past, Decision-Making of memory as content in the present, Judgement of conflicting memories as content in the past and the present, the Ability to orient in time and space, and the Ability to think.

2.4.4 Interpretation of Linguistic Meanings from Wording

The actual intepretation of the event as part of the context of situation is to rely on the mechanisms of Judgement of conflicting memories as content in the past and the present to derive the true meanings of what happened at the scene of the accident. Since the reports given by people at the scene may not all be 'unanimously correct', more often than not several possibilities or hypotheses are posited to weigh the validity or 'trustworthiness' or pros and cons of each.

2.4.5 Phonation

When an interpretation is reached, and believed to be compatible with the true meaning of the event, it can be orally transmitted to the headquarters or written down as a case report. In the case of oral transmission, it involves phonation which should not be taken at face value as just the vibration of the vocal cords. Imagine the brain functions of reading a written record aloud or testifying in court as a witness for the event. They are much more than a simple vocalization of written words; they involve the capacity of Replication so as to retrieve impulses from the content plane subserved by the brain functions of memory as content in order to present the findings (i.e., final interpretation of the case) orally; if a written case report is read, the Retrieval of impulses from the content plane must transfer them from the visual system to the aural–oral system.

2.4.6 Audition

When police have heard different oral reports from people at the scene, the audition is much more than the reception of sounds or the vibration of the eardrums. It is even more complex when phonation is also involved. Imagine a bilingual interpreter acting between police and foreigners at the scene. If sign language is a medium of interpretation in court between the judge and a deaf defendant, the brain functions of audition will be extraordinary. It involves two different content planes and two different expression planes for the interpreter when sign language is involved or when two oral languages are involved.

Whether two oral languages or one sign language and one oral language, the brain functions of audition can vary significantly depending on whether the interpreter's job is simultaneous, as in the United Nations, or sequential, as in a court hearing. In the case of simultaneous interpreting, the visual system is overtly involved when one of the languages is a sign language. In that case, the interpreter's switching from the oral language or the sign language, when receiving it from the brain functions of audition or visualization, will have to facilitate the brain functions of memory as capacity; that is, the interpreter has to rapidly or even simultaneously transmit the incoming impulses to the temporal or occipital lobe through the adjustments mentioned earlier in the brainstem and then change code from one expression plane to the other for the production of the other language. Such being the process involved, all the mechanisms of memory, such as chunking, sequencing, and linearization, will have to take part. The switching from oral language to sign language or vice versa is even more involved, be it simultaneous or sequential, because it includes not just audition but also visualization using different pathways.

2.4.7 Motor Functions

In the distinctions of motor functions and motor activities presented above, motor functions are succinctly depicted as if they simply took over acoustic images or visual images and transferred these impulses to phonation or brachial movement. However, I should add now that they involve planning, which is time-oriented, and CNV, which evokes expectancy wave and/or readiness potentials to 'alert' or even 'warn' the sender to get set, albeit briefly in milliseconds, as in fencing, for his/her motor functions. Thus, motor functions in both oral language and sign language are important brain functions just the same, involving not only the expression plane but also the content plane.

2.4.8 Sensory Functions

Likewise, in the distinctions of sensory functions and sensory activities, sensory functions are depicted as though they only received impulses from motor functions, whereas in such distinctions, acoustic images were depicted only as sensory input. In reality, however, sensory functions and motor functions are tied together in a connective loop, as has been succinctly described. In other words, the relationships between motor functions and sensory functions are such that you cannot have one without the other, if the individual is 'normal'; if one of the senses is impaired, as in deafness or blindness, the pathways making up the connective loop will be broken or at least impaired, leading to language impairment in either expression plane (as in deafness, when oral language as behaviour is no longer possible) or content plane (as in blindness, when signing or gesticulation is impossible, and therefore the stratum of meaning is partially impaired).

2.5 The Highest Brain Functions

Earlier I quoted US President Harry Truman's famous statement, 'If you can't stand the heat, get out of the kitchen' to illustrate the effect of function enhancement in reaching the 'true meaning' or an enhanced meaning other than the linguistic meanings which are mapped onto their corresponding sound-images. I have in keeping with common practice called such enhanced meanings inferences. In order to conclude this chapter, I shall now describe how inferences can be achieved in the brain; at the same time I shall emphasize that the highest brain functions are based on all the other brain functions, or even the common nervous functions, because language in the brain or the individual aspect of language is behaviour resulting from such highest brain functions.

If this famous statement is repeated verbatim, the context of situation will have to be so adjusted or simulated that it would look superficial. However, the statement can be modified, or the wording (i.e., sequencing) changed, to still enable the reader/hearer to couple it with the original inferenced meaning President Truman had in his mind. For instance, here are two modified versions written by a columnist, Mr Max Lerner, for *The Japan Times* some years ago.

1. The Russians couldn't stand the heat of the world opinion, and they got out of the kitchen.
2. I got the feeling that these young people – and millions like them across the country – won't get out of the kitchen, however hot the fire.

But if the reader/hearer's brain cannot couple the modified versions with their corresponding meanings which include the original meanings as part of his/her experiences or thought (i.e., context of culture), he/she will not be able to reconstruct the appropriate inferenced meaning close to President Truman's original meaning. The reason is simple: he/she does not have in his/her content plane (i.e., the inchoate mass of impulses that constitute his/her thought based on experiences or context of situation) the needed corresponding impulses, no matter how good his/her English may have been. Here is a good example from *The Japan Times* (Reader's Council).

> I found in Mr Max Lerner's column ... 'The Russians couldn't stand the heat of world opinion, and they got out of the kitchen'. I couldn't understand the phrase in bold type, nor did I find it in any dictionaries, leaving it unsolved to my 'frustration'. On ..., I found again the same phrase by the same writer in his column, such as 'I got the feeling that these young people – and millions like them across the country – won't get out of the kitchen, however hot the fire'. I can manage to guess the meaning, but I am afraid I can't get at the true meaning.

In answer to the reader's inquiry, the Editor of *The Japan Times* provided the following opinion:

> US President Harry Truman once said: 'If you can't stand the heat, get out of the kitchen'. He was talking about the need for a politician to be unaffected by attacks on him by the press. He meant by this piece of advice, 'If you are affected too much by the criticism of the press, then you shouldn't be in politics in the first place, because it is natural for the press to attack politicians'. Generally speaking, 'to get out of the kitchen' would mean to remove oneself from a difficulty or intolerable situation.

Notice that in Mr Truman's original statement (or its modified version in Mr Lerner's column), there are no such words as 'politician', 'the press', 'politics', 'criticism', 'attacks' and the like. Yet, the meanings implicit in his brain were precisely the constructed (or true) meanings he (or Mr Lerner) had in mind, which all Americans as the hearers then (or the readers of the newspaper, who were native speakers of English) caught (i.e., reconstructed) as the true meaning immediately, that were missed by the Japanese reader. Notice also that his English was pretty good, for he could manage to guess (i.e., reconstruct) the (linguistic) meaning on the basis of retrieval from his memory as content of English by consulting his dictionaries, using the mechanism of reinforcement, but still he could not get at the true meaning, when reading the newspaper.

2.5.1 The Highest Brain Functions as Context of Culture

What are then the differences between the reader and the editor? Ostensibly, the answer may be that the reader did not have enough knowledge of English. But this answer is too simplistic. The real answer has to be that the reader had not had the needed brain functions of memory as content, so much so that his brain functions of memory as mechanism could not integrate his brain functions by upgrading what he read to each of the higher statuses in order to reach the highest brain functions for inferencing the 'true meaning' he wanted to reconstruct.

Notice that the statements presented were written, and not spoken, statements. Therefore, when he read Lerner's modified versions of the president's original statement, there were no brain functions of audition in operation; rather, it was the reader's brain functions of visualization that were at work. Here is what happened to his brain:

1. The Common Nervous Functions started with his retinae for the initial contact in recognition; they had to be functional, because the reader was not blind and therefore was not using his fingers to 'read' the Braille.
2. The two optic nerves served the purpose of his Basic Brain Functions to connect the impulses from the two retinae to the lateral geniculate bodies in his two thalami for the adjustments needed.
3. His two superior colliculi also helped in identifying the incoming

impulses with the visual images in his expression plane as part of his Higher Brain Functions, a job that was partially done when the visual images went up to the optic radiation to reach his occipital lobes, for he was able to find the visual images in his brain, that is, he could read the words printed; written English was not something new to him. However, Lerner's statements were new to him.

4. On the other hand, the visual images so identified could not be coupled with the appropriate corresponding 'true' meanings in his content plane within his Specific Brain Functions because what he read was partially familiar (English words) but partially new (Lerner's statements), thereby making him say, 'I can manage to guess the meaning, but I am afraid I can't get at the true meaning'.
5. Observe that he did utilize the mechanism of Reinforcement. That is why he said, 'I couldn't understand the phrase in bold type, nor did I find it in any dictionaries, leaving it unsolved to my "frustration".' Put differently, his Highest Brain Functions, despite his efforts to make use of the mechanism of reinforcement in his brain functions of memory as mechanism, were not properly operative, because his specific brain functions of segmentation were not sufficient to overcome the newness of Lerner's statements; that is, he was only able to couple the incoming familiar visual impulses with the linguistic meanings of the words he read, even though he has plenty of specific brain functions at his disposal, which is to say that he lacked certain highest brain functions in his context of culture with respect to English, for he was able to write that letter in English to the Editor.

2.5.2 The Highest Brain Functions and Inferences

Given the illustrations of *male/mail* for punning and President Truman's famous statement, it can be said clearly and with certainty that language in the brain is memory-governed, meaning-centred and multifaceted. It is not enough to be able to match words, written or spoken, with their linguistic (or dictionary) meanings in the brain; the individual must also be able to instantaneously enhance the linguistic meanings, when speaking or hearing, to include different shades of meaning as enhanced meanings or inferences. The highest brain functions play such a role on the basis of the other brain functions and the common nervous functions.

In the case of puns, the highest brain functions must adjust both catalytic mappings and couplings. In catalytic mappings, the speaker intentionally plays on the possibility of more than one chunked proto-meaning being mapped onto one acoustic image (but two visual images); this possibility, many-to-one mapping in punning, from the content plane to the expression plane, is known in linguistics as homophones (but not homographs). In coupling, however, the hearer has to match the sounds heard (only one sequence of sounds, that is, [mÉyl t^hrÈyn]) with more than one chunked proto-meaning to come up with two possible linguistic meanings in two linguistic signs in the brain, one-to-many coupling, from the expression plane to the content plane, in order to be able to appreciate the joke.

In the case of the famous statement, it is not just a matter of many-to-one mappings or one-to-many couplings; rather, it involves the search of many seemingly unrelated linguistic signs (or words) from the pool of impulses called thought for both mapping and coupling. For instance, in Truman's statement, 'politician', 'attacks', 'press', 'criticism' and the like were not even included (i.e., uttered) and yet the hearers (the Americans during Truman's re-election campaign) were all able to relate the 'true meaning' from those 'unspoken' words (or linguistic signs) to the 'linguistic meanings' from those 'spoken' words (or linguistic signs). This ability of arriving at 'true meaning' from 'linguistic meaning' or relating 'linguistic meaning' to 'true meaning' is none other than a part of the highest brain functions and is the crux of inference or of the mechanism of integration in the brain functions of memory. Language in the brain is incomplete without this ability. None of the contemporary theories of linguistics, including Saussure's, or even the semiotic theories, has this ability included, for they are based on mechanistic or one-to-one semantic association models.

2.5.3 Inferences in Child Language

What if interactions take place between a child of, say, one year of age or so, and two adults one of whom is the mother? Here is an example from Snow (1978):

C: Badaid.
E: Where's your bandaid?
C: Bandaid.
E: Do you have a bandaid?
C: Bandaid.
E: Did you fall down and hurt yourself? (Mother entered)
C: Bandaid.
M: Who gave you the bandaid?
C: Nurse.
M: Where did she put it?
C: Arm.

For this example, Snow points out that the mother and the child continue an extensive conversation about their visit to a doctor's office. But I must add that there is no denying that the child had only a limited vocabulary and its experiences were much more extensive, so much so that its proto-meanings were categorized differently from the way in which an adult's proto-meanings from the same context of situation would be categorized. An adult who did not share the child's experiences and did not realize the differences in the child's own idiosyncratic categorization of proto-meanings, as E in the example, would have difficulty interacting with the child, because the adult would not be able to inference (not infer) the 'enhanced' meaning(s) the child wanted the adult to 'guess'. That was what happened in the example.

Since the mother shared the same experiences with the child, as they visited the doctor's office together, the mother knew what questions the child could answer and the child knew what questions the mother was likely to ask, all of which were maintained in the mother's and the child's respective brain functions of memory; consequently, their interactions went smoothly. However, E did not have access to the child's recent experiences with that visit, hence E could not carry on the interaction with C, because C kept wondering why the utterance 'bandaid' did not make sense to E, when it did perfectly to M, and E kept fishing for the 'true meaning' of C's 'bandaid'; that is, E was inferencing (not inferring), by way of reconstructing, repeatedly the wrong meaning of C's proto-meaning of 'bandaid'. These interactions illustrate vividly the differences in the highest brain functions of language among those three individuals.

More examples can be found in the literature regarding the highest brain functions and inferences; for example, metaphors, analogies, proverbs, jokes, fables, riddles, supernatural stories, and the like. These materials should be taken into consideration seriously from the point of view of the highest brain functions as an ontological issue of language in the brain.

PART VI SUMMARY AND CONCLUSION

20 My Realization: An Overview

1. Summary

I started out in this monograph with a serious question of: 'What is language?' Although this question cannot be answered in just one monograph, in the course of the exposition three general historical perspectives of what different people think of language are critically assessed, so as to categorize the crisis the varying investigations of language in different disciplines are currently facing. To remedy such a crisis, I presented a mild proposal, combining Saussure's core distinction of *langue* and *parole* into a new core distinction which rests on my theoretical construct that language has two faces, Individual and Social, like the two faces of Janus, one looking inward to the nervous system while the other looking outward to society.

The reason is my realization that language is behaviour, not at all a thing or an organ or a set of rules, and that looking at human behaviour in general from wthout requires a deep understanding of each individual's brain functions from within the nervous system, especially the individual's brain functions of memory. The realization is based on my conviction, after many years of teaching linguistics at a university, that all human behaviours are memory-governed, because memory is experience-based and time-sensitive. Thus, I moved into neuroscience in 1977. This monograph is but the first fruitful result of such a realization on a large scale.

I have subsequently found through my experiences as a professional linguist and a behavioural neuroscientist that it is a serious mistake that linguists have shunned memory all along and that they have shifted the notion of what language is many times: from language being letters or texts to a system of arbitrary vocal symbols to an infinite set of sentences and to a system of making meanings through choice. The uncertainty is precisely derived from the failure to recognize the important fact that language has two aspects: Individual Aspect and Social Aspect. My mild proposal depicts that fact.

In terms of this mild proposal, I have described in some detail what language in the brain looks like, which does not include the peripheral nervous system; when the perpheral nervous system is taken into consideration, the concern will be with the individual aspect of language which is mentioned in passing but not accounted for in earnest. The full account of the individual aspect of language will be presented in a future publication, *The Central and Peripheral Nervous Systems Control of Language*.

The consequence of such a failure to recognize the distinction of the two aspects of language is the rampant pursuit of various theories of grammar or grammatics without being aware that grammar is an epistemological artifact conveniently created by linguists and not an ontological given in language: there is no grammar in the brain. When the core distinction of the individual and the social aspect is taken into consideration in connection with Saussure's core distinction of *langue* and *parole*, it becomes clear that the assertion of grammar being a module serving as the interface between semantics and phonology, *à la* Saussure's idea of language being the intermediary of Thought and Sound, is a misconception, and that the notion of language being rule-governed and innate is nonsense.

2. Conclusion

As a result of the mild proposal, I have reached several conclusions regarding the current situation several disciplines are facing about language; that is, the futile pursuit of the answer to the question of 'What is language?' by way of the approach to mechanistic grammatics and the wrong claim of the origin and evolution of language. The conclusions I have reached, therefore, constitute my two departures from the traditions in linguistics and neuroscience; such departures are likely to irk many traditionally minded colleagues who do not agree with my approach. However, to those who agree with my approach, which is not confined to the critical assessments of other approaches but, rather, has to do fundamentally with the deep-rooted misconceptions of what language is thought of by many investigators and what the brain functions of memory are like to them, my conclusions will most certainly be welcome.

What is my approach then, given the critical assessments of others and the complexity and difficulty involved in unravelling the brain functions of memory and their disorders known as dementia which is a form of language disorders? Simply put, my approach is to undertake the painstaking job of describing as accurately and clearly as my ability will permit the interrelationships and interdependencies of varying brain functions with a focus on the brain functions of memory when such brain functions manifest themselves in behaviours, language behaviour in particular, which are meaning-centred and multifaceted.

In this focus, the interrelationships as well as the interdependencies of varying behaviours and brain functions will be my targets. The following are the conclusions I have drawn in the course of my exposition.

First, all behaviours of animals, especially mammals or any animal that has a brain, are modulated by two planes, called the content plane and the expression plane, each one of which is an inchoate mass of impulses but varies from one species to another in its size and complexity. In the case of humans, these two planes may constitute Thought and Sound/Gesture, respectively. These two planes have become an important theoretical construct in my framework of the individual aspect of language, in terms of which many neural activities and the disorders thereof have been explained and demonstrated in both production and reception.

Second, in this connection, because of the interdependencies of varying brain functions, I have introduced the important time factor into such interdependencies and claim that memory and cognition are actually heads and tails of the same coin: memory deals with the past and the past in the present, never with the future which can only be talked about, while cognition handles the goings-on of the here-and-now. As such, the brain functions of memory constitute a tripartite system, consisting of memory as content, memory as capacity and memory as mechanism. That is, language in the brain is memory-governed, meaning-centred and multifaceted.

Third, such being the case, without the brain functions of memory there is no thinking which takes place in the extrapyramidal loop, because the impulses from the expression plane go through the looping to involve the cortex at least twice. In so doing, I have postulated two processes in production, that is, catalytic mapping and separation, and three processes in reception, that is, recognition, identification and coupling. The result of catalytic mapping is language potentiation for the construction of meaning on the part of the speaker/signer. The result of coupling is perceptual organization for the reconstruction of meaning on the part of the hearer/viewer.

Fourth, in the course of catalytic mapping and/or coupling and during language potentiation and perceptual organization, the cerebello-cerebral circuit and Papez circuit must take part in the construction and/or reconstruction of meanings. These two circuits influence both active and passive behaviours in the manifestation of such behaviours and are in turn influenced by external and internal environmental factors.

Fifth, the process of separation allows the impulses of the expression plane to enter the extrapyramidal loop in order to come out as physical sounds or body movements (in sign language), while leaving the impulses of the content plane (i.e., meanings) behind. Physical sounds or body movements have no meanings in and by themselves, because the speaker/signer constructs meanings which do not come out with physical sounds or body movements.

Sixth, the process of coupling, on the other hand, puts the incoming impulses of physical stimuli back to the expression plane for the purpose of the hearer/viewer's reconstruction of meanings. The meanings the hearer/viewer reconstructs in interactions are nine times out of ten different from the meanings the speaker/signer constructed. I have in this connection given two examples in Chapter 13 where I claim that unless the focus is shifted each time, that is, from a vase or two faces looking at each other, in one example, and from one box or the other, in the other example, nobody can see the two visual percepts together (i.e., simultaneously). The same goes for auditory percepts, which are even more complex.

Seventh, on the basis of the aforementioned, I conclude that the cherished notions of cerebral dominance and cerebral laterality are more fiction than fact, because language in the brain is not lateralized to one hemisphere (left or right) as an exclusive specialization; rather, the whole brain is responsible for it; nor is it a species-specific ability for humans. It is the wrong view of language that has excluded other animals from having their own languages, thereby leading to the erroneous claim of cerebral dominance for language in humans. In other words, every species has its own language; we just do not know what their languages are like; 'do not know' is not equivalent to 'does not exist'.

Eighth, the claim of FOXp2 as the language gene in chromosome 7 is a farce for sensationalism. The proponents and their supporters have never presented nucleotides as evidence as to whether such nucleotides are abnormally repeated in the affected individuals or not; nor have they ever identified the repeats of the bases in any expansion beyond the normal range, because they cannot; their claim is nonsense and the so-called language gene is a fiction. And the recent substitute of language template for the fictional ideal speaker/hearer, in keeping with the idea of a language 'gene', to uphold language innateness is indefensible and therefore false.

Ninth, the bridging of the two aspects of language is essential eventually, if we are to come to terms with reality, rather than beating around the bush by philosophizing the issues involved. The social institutions (Peng, 2003) are the place where the union can be formulated.

Tenth, language disorders must be included in the quest for the answer to the question of 'What is language?' The language behaviours of people with language disorders play a vital role in the bridging of the two aspects of language and should be considered as such.

3. Epilogue

Last but not least, the name Cajal, interestingly enough, has been erroneously referred to as the last name of Santiago in the medical literature, a wrong tradition that I follow in this monograph nevertheless, because any change in this tradition would be 100 years or so too late. The error, as was pointed out by Professor J. Peter Maher, is that Cajal was not his family name; rather, it was his mother's name. Ramón was his father's name which should have been identified as his family name in the literature.

In the Spanish system, there is no last name, only first, second, and third name. Thus, Santiago Ramón y Cajal literally stands for 'Santiago the son of Ramón and Cajal'. The 'y' in Spanish is equivalent to 'and' in English, indicative of the union of father's name and mother's name. In all medical dictionaries and literature in English, his mother's name, Cajal, has been identified mistakenly as his last name and taught as such.

While I cannot change the wrong tradition in respect to the name Cajal, I must insist on the two departures I have taken in this monograph. The hope is that other like minds will join forces with me to correct the serious mistakes, which have been pointed out, for the betterment in both the science of language and neuroscience. Language in the brain is much more complicated and complex than has traditionally been believed. If this monograph can serve as the impetus for correcting the mistakes, its objective will have been accomplished.

References

Aarsleff, Hans 1970. 'The history of linguistics and Professor Chomsky'. *Language Sciences* 46: 570–85.

Aarsleff, Hans. 1971. Cartesian linguistics: History or Fantasy. *Language Sciences* 17: 1–12, October.

Aglioti S., Bonazzi, A., and Cortese, F. 1994. 'Phantom lower limbs as a perceptual marker of neural plasticity in the mature human brain'. In *Proceedings of the Royal Society of London*, Series B: Biological Sciences. 255 (1344): 272–8, March 22.

Aglioti, S., Cortese, F., and Franchini, C. 1994. 'Rapid sensory remapping in the adult human brain as inferred from phantom breast perception'. *Neuroreport* 5 (4): 473–6. January 12.

Aglioti, S., Smania, N., Atzei, A., and Berlucchi, G.. 1997. 'Spatio-temporal properties of the patterns of evoked phantom sensations in a left index amputee patient. *Behavioral Neurosciences* 5: 867–72. October.

Alexander, G. E., Delong, M. R., and Strick, P. I. 1986. 'Parallel organization of functionally segregated circuits linking basal ganglia and cortex'. *Annual Reviews of Neuroscience* 9: 357–81.

Allen, G., I. and Tuskahara, N. 1974. 'Cerebrocerebellar communication systems'. *Physiological Review* 54: 957–1008.

Amaducci, A., Rocca, W. A., and Schoenberg, B. S. 1986. 'Origin of the distinction between Alzheimer's disease and senile dementia: How history can clarify nosology'. *Neurology* 35: 1497–9.

Baddeley, A. 1986. *Working Memory*. Oxford: Clarendon Press.

Barr, M. L. 1974. *The Human Nervous System*. Second Edition. New York: Harper and Row.

Berlucchi, G., and Anglioti, S. 1997. 'The body in the brain: neural bases of corporal awareness'. *Trends in Neurosciences* 20 (12): 560–4. December.

Bower, J. M, and Parsons, L. M. 2003. 'Rethinking the 'Lesser Brain'. *Scientific American* 41–47, August.

Bracken, H. M. 1970a. 'Chomsky's language and mind'. *Dialogue* 9: 236–47.

Bracken, H. M. 1970b. 'Chomsky's variations of a theme by Descartes', *Journal of the History of Philosophy* 18: 181–92.

Brown, R. 1965. *Social Psychology*. New York: The Free Press.

Carpenter, M. B. 1976. *Human Neuroanatomy*. Seventh Edition. Baltimore: The Williams & Wilkins Company.

Cassirer, E. A. 1945. 'Structuralism in modern linguistics'. *Word*. 1 (2): 99–120.

Chan, J. L. and Ross, E. D. 1988. 'Left-handed mirror writing following right

anterior cerebral artery infarction: Evidence for nonmirror transformation of motor programs by right supplementary motor area. *Neurology* 38: 159–63.
Chiu, M. J. Chen, R. C. and Tseng, C.Y. 1996. 'Clinical correlates of quantitative acoustic analysis in ataxic dysarthria'. *European Neurology* 36: 310–14.
Chomsky, N. 1957. *Syntactic Structure.* The Hague: Mouton.
Chomsky, N. 1965. *Aspects of the Theory of Syntax.* Cambridge, Mass: MIT Press.
Chomsky, N. 1966. *Cartesian Linguistics.* New York: Harper and Row.
Chomsky, N. 1966. *Language and Mind.* New York: Harcourt Brace Jovanovich.
Coslett, H. B. 2003. 'Body schema representation (patients and functional MRI)'. In *Behavioral Neurology: Issues in Cognitive Neuroscience,* 3FC 005–83–3FC. 005–96. American Academy of Neurology. 55th Annual Meeting, March 29–April 5.
Crick, F. and Mitchison, G.. 1983. 'The function of dream sleep'. *Nature* 304: 111–14.
Critchley, M. and Greenfield J. G. 1948. 'Olivo-ponto-cerebellar atrophy'. *Brain* 71(4): 343–64.
Damasio, A. R., Damasio, R., Rizzo, M., Varney, N., and Gersh, F. 1982. 'Aphasia with nonhemorrhegic lesions in the basal ganglia and internal capsule'. *Archives of Neurology* 39: 15–20.
Déjérine, J. and Thomas, A. 1900. 'L'atrophie olivo-ponto-cérébelleuse'. *Nouv. Iconogr. Salpèr* 13: 330–70.
de Saussure, F. 1959. *Cours de Linguistique Générale,* trans. Wade Baskin. New York: McGraw-Hill.
de la Torre, J. 2002. 'Alzheimer's disease is a vascular disorder: Nosological evidence'. *Stroke* 33: 1–11.
Everett, N. B. 1971. *Functional Neuroanatomy.* Sixth Edition, Philadelphia: Lea & Febriger.
Fraser, C. 1966. 'Discussion of D. McNeill's "The creation of language by children"'. In John Lyons and R. J. Wales (eds), *Psycholinguistics Papers.* Edinburgh: Edinburgh University Press.
Freeman, W. J. 1991. 'The physiology of perception'. *Scientific American* 78–85, February.
Frith 2004. 'Unravelling the mysteries of Schizophrenia'. *The Japan Times,* 2 October.
Gallagher, S. 1995. 'Body schema and intentionality'. In J. L. Bermudez, A. Marcel, and N. Eilan (eds), *The Body and the Self.* Cambridge, MA: MIT Press.
Gazzaniga, M. S. 1970. *The Bisected Brain.* New York: Appleton-Century-Crofts.
Gazzaniga, M. S. and LeDoux, J. E. 1978. *The Integrated Mind.* New York: Plenum Press.
Gesell, A. 1941. *Wolf Child and Human Child..* trans. Masako Ikutsuki from the English, 1972. Tokyo: Kasei Kyoiku Sha.
Gitelman, D. R. 2003. 'Cognitive neuroimaging of aging: focus on attention, language and working memory'. *Behavioral Neurology: Issues in Cognitive Neuroscience, Educational Program Syllabus,* 3FC 005. American Academy of Neuro-logy, 55th Annual Meeting, March 29–April 5.
Goldman-Rakic, P. S. 1992. 'Working memory and the mind'. *Scientific American* 111–17. September.
Hachinski, V. and Munso, D. 2002. 'Vascular factors in cognitive impairment: where are we now?' In R. N. Kalaria and P. Ince (eds), *Vascular Factors in Alzheimer's Disease.* Annals of the New York Academy of Sciences. Vol. 903. pp. 1–5.
Hall, E. 1959. *The Silent Language.* New York: Doubleday.

Hall, E. 1966. *The Hidden Dimension.* New York: Doubleday.
Halle, M. 1959a. *Sound Patterns of Russian.* The Hague: Mouton.
Halle, M. 1959b. 'Questions of linguistics'. *Nuovo Cimento* 13: 494–517.
Halle, M. 1961. 'On the role of the simplicity in linguistic description'. In R. Jakobson (ed.), *Structure of Language and Its Mathematical Aspects.* Proceedings of the Twelfth Symposium in Applied Mathematics, 89–94. Providence: American Mathematical Society.
Halle, M. 1962. 'Phonology in generative grammar'. *Word* 18: 72.
Halle, M. 1964. On the bases of phonology. In J. A. Fodor and J. J. Katz (eds),*The Structure of Language: Readings in the Philosophy of Language.* Englewood, NJ: Prentice-Hall.
Harnad, S. R., Steklis, H. D., and Lancaster, J. (eds). 1976. *Origins and Evolution of Language and Speech.* New York: The New York Academy of Sciences.
Hebb, D. O. 1949. *Organization of Behaviour.* New York: Wiley.
Hews, G. 1974. *Bibliograph of Works Relating to the Origin of Language.* The Hague: Mouton.
Hockett, C. F. 1958. *A Course in Modern Linguistics.* New York: Macmillan.
Hockett, C. F. 1986. 'Grammar for hearers' . In G. MacGregor (ed.), *Language for Hearers.* Oxford: Pergamon Press.
Honjo, I. 1999. *Language Viewed from the Brain.* Basel: Karger.
Hopkins, J. 1993. *Clinical Neurology: A Modern Approach.* Oxford: Oxford University Press.
Howard, D., Patterson, K. Wise, R., *et al.* 1992. 'The cortical localization of the lexicons'. *Brain* 115: 1769–82.
Hughes, J. R. 1982. *EEG in Clinical Practice,* Boston: Butterworth.
Itard, J. M-G. 1894. *Rapports et memoires sur Le Sauvage de L'Aveyron,* trans. Yasho Kotake from the French, 1970. Tokyo: Maki Shoten.
James, W. 1890. *The Principles of Psychology.* New York: Macmillan.
Jankowsky, K. R. 1972. *The Neogrammarians: A Re-evaluaton of their Place in the Development of Linguistic Science,* 1968. The Hague: Moton.
Kappers, C. U. A., Huber, G. C. and Crosby, E. C. 1936. *The Comparative Anatomy of the Nervous System of Vertebrates, Including Man.* New York: The Macmillan Company.
Katz, T. and Melzack, R. 1990 'Pain "memories" in phantom limbs: review and clinical observations'. *Pain* 43: 319–36.
Keidel, W. R. 1972. 'The D-C potential in the human cortical evoked response: a new contribution to the objective audiometry'. *Journal Français d'Otorhinolaryngologie* 121: 153–58.
Kennedy, M. and Murdoch, B. E. 1989. 'Speech and language disorders subsequent to subcortical vascular lesions. *Aphasiology* 3: 221–47.
Kimura, D. 1961. 'Cerebral dominance and the perception of verbal stimuli'. *Candian Journal of Psychology* 15: 166–71.
Kimura, D. 1964. 'Left-right differences in the perception of melodies'. *Quarterly Journal of Experimental Psychology* 16: 355–8.
Lamb, Sydney 1999. *Pathways of the Brain.* Amsterdam: John Benjamins.
Lees, R. B. 1953. 'The basis of glottochronology'. *Language* 29:113–27.
Lehmann, W. P. 1973. *Historical Linguistics: An Introduction.* New York: Holt, Rinehart & Winston, Inc.
Lester, M. (ed.) 1970. *Readings in Applied Transformational Grammar.* New York: Holt, Rinehart & Winston, Inc.

Lichtheim, L. 1885 'On aphasia'. *Brain* 7: 433–84.
Linton, R. 1945. 'The scope and aims of anthropology'. In Ralph Linton (ed.), *The Science of Man in the World Crisis.* New York: Columbia University Press, pp. 3–18.
Livingston, M. and Hubel, D. 1988. 'Segregation of form, color, movement and depth: anatomy, physiology, and perception'. *Science* 240: 740–49.
Llinás, R. R. 1975. 'The cortex of the cerebellum'. *Scientific American.* 56. 71.
Love, R. J. and Webb, W. G.. 1996. *Neurology for the Speech-Language Pathologist.* Third Edition. Oxford: Butterworth-Heinemann.
Lyons, J. 1971. *Introduction to Theoretical Linguistics.* Cambridge: Cambridge University Press.
Maher, J. P. 1980. 'The transformational-generative paradigm: a silver anniversary polemic'. *Forum Linguisticum* 5: 1–35, August.
Mandybur, T. I. and Chuirazzi, C. C. transformaional-generative 1990. 'Astrocytes and the plaques of Alzheimer's disease'. *Neurology* 40: 635–9.
Marange, M. 2001. *The Misunderstood Gene.* trans. Matthew Cobb from the French. Cambridge, MA: Harvard University Press.
Margolis, S. and Rabins, P. 1998. *Memory.* The Johns Hopkins White Papers. Baltimore: The John Hopkins Medical Institutions.
McGregor, G. (ed.) 1986. *Language for Hearers.* 1986. Oxford: Pergamon Press.
McKhann, G., Drachman, D., Folstein, M., Katzman, R., Price, D., and Stadlan, E. M. 1984. 'Clinical Diagnosis of Alzheimer's disease: Report of the NINCDS-ADRDA Work Group under the auspices of Department of Health and Human Services Task Force on Alzheimer's Disease'. *Neurology* 34: 939–44.
Melzack, R. 1992. 'Phantom limbs'. *Scientific American* 120–26.
Milner, B. 1962. 'Laterality effects in audition'. In V. B. Mountcastle (ed.), *Interhemispheric Relations and Cerebral Dominance.* Baltimore: The Johns Hopkins Press.
Mink J. 1996. 'The basal ganglia: Focused selection and inhibition of competing motor programs'. *Progress in Neurobiology* 50: 381–425.
Morange, M. 2001. *The Misunderstood Gene.* trans. from the French by M. Cobb. Cambridge, MA: Harvard University Press.
Murdock, B. E. 1987. 'Aphasia following right thalamic hemorrhage in a destral'. *Journal of Communication Disorders* 20: 459–69.
Myers, R. E. and Sperry, R. W. 1953. 'Interocular transfer of a visual form discrimination habit in cats after section of the optic chiasms and corpus callosum'. *Anatomical Record* 175: 351–2.
Nature Genetics 2001. 'Mutation of PVRL1 is associated with sporatic, non-syndromic cleft lip/palate in northern Venezuela'. 29: 141–2.
Nauta, W. J. H. and Feirtag, M. 1979. 'The organization of the brain'. *Scientic American* 241: 66–111.
Nida, E. A. 1949. *Morphology: The Descriptive Analysis of Words.* Ann Arbor, Mich: University of Michigan Press, 1949. Reprinted in 1976.
Nida, E. A. 1961 *Bible Translating: An Analysis of Principles and Procedures, with Specific Reference to Aboriginal Languages.* London: United Bible Societies.
Niedermeyer, E. and DaSilva, F. L. 1999. *Electroencephalography: Basic Principles, Clinical Applications, and Related Fields,* Baltimore: Williams and Wilkins.
Nora, J. J. and Fraser, F. C. 1974. *Medical Genetics: Principles and Practice.* Philadelphia: Lea and Febiger.
Ojemann, G.. Ojemann, J. *et al.* 1989. 'Cortical language localization in left dominant hemisphere'. *Journal of Neurosurgery* 71: 316–26.

Parret, H. 1984. 'Peirce and Hjelmslev: the two semiotics'. *Language Sciences* 6(2): 217–27.
Penfield, W. and Rasmussen, T. 1950. *The Cerebral Cortex of Man: A Clinical Study of Localization of Function*. New York: The Macmillan Company.
Peng, F. C. C. 1969. 'Review article of *Aspects of the Theory of Syntax*'. *Linguistics* 49: 91–128.
Peng, F. C. C. 1970. 'On the notions of accidental and systematic gaps'. In M. Estellie Smith (ed.), *Studies in Linguistics: In Honor of George L. Trager*. Greenwood Press, 81–86.
Peng, F. C. C. 1974. 'The place of generative phonology in the history of linguistics'. In Adam Makkai and Valerie Becker Makkai (eds),*The First LACUS Forum*, Columbia, South Carolina: Hornbeam Press, Inc, 81–119.
Peng, F. C. C. 1975a. 'The deaf and their acquisition of the various systems of communication: speculation against innatims'. In James Macris and Walburga von Raffler-Engel (eds), *Child Language, Word* 27 (1, 2, & 3): 225–46.
Peng, F. C. C. 1975b. 'On the fallacy of language innatism'. *Language Sciences* 37: 13–16.
Peng, F. C. C. 1976. 'A new explanation of language change: The sociolinguistic approach'. *Forum Linguisticum* 1(1): 67–94.
Peng, F. C. C. (ed.). 1978. *Sign Language and Language Acquisition in Man and Ape: New Dimensioins in Comparative Pedolinguistics*. AAAS Selected Symposium No. 16. Boulder: Westview Press.
Peng, F. C. C. 1979. 'Sound change and language change: a sociolinguistic interpretation'. *Language Sciences* 1: 94–123.
Peng, F. C. C. 1981. 'On the differences in the distribution of gray and white matter in human cerebral hemispheres. In Fred C. C. Peng (ed.), *Current Issues in Neurolinguistics: A Japanese Contribution*. The ICU Language Sciences Summer Institute, pp. 211–22.
Peng, F. C. C (ed.) 1984. *Language in A Semiotic Frame. Language Sciences* 6 (2).
Peng, F. C. C. 1992a. 'Review article of *Studies in Systemic Phonology*'. *Language Sciences* 14(4): 659–81.
Peng, F. C. C. 1992b. 'On de Saussure's theoretical construct of *le signe*: A neurolinguistics view'. *Journal of Neurolinguistics* 7: 1–10.
Peng, F. C. C. 1992c. 'Review article of *Agrammatic Aphasia*'. *Journal of Neurolinguistics* 7.4: 451–74.
Peng, F. C. C. 1994. 'Language disorders and brain functions'. *Acta Neurologica Sinica* 3: 103–30.
Peng, F. C. C. 1995. 'Language impairment in epileptics'. *Acta Neurologica Sinica*. 4: 1–21.
Peng, F. C. C. 2000. 'Review Article of *Re-reading Saussure. Lingua Posnaniensis*'. 42: 175–98.
Peng, F. C. C. 2001. 'Lexis and the dysfunctions of memory in the language behaviour of people with temporal lobe epilepsy'. *Lingua Posnaniensis* 43: 125–40.
Peng, F. C. C. 2003a. 'The anthropology of language disorders: a first approximation'. *Lingua Posnaniensis* 45: 39–62.
Peng, F. C. C. 2003b. 'Is dementia a disease?' *Gerontology* 49(6): 384–91.
Peng, F. C. C. 2004. 'A brief history of linguistics: what went wrong?' *Lingua Posnaniensis* 46: 46–72.

Peng, F. C. C. 2005. 'Dementia as a form of language disorder'. *Lingua Posnaniensis* 47: 101–9.

Peng, F. C. C. 2006. 'Review article of *Brain, Mind, and the Signifying Body*'. *Lingua Posnaniensis* (forthcoming).

Peng, F. C. C. and Huang, S. Y. 1996. 'Language disorders in Parkinson's disease'. *Acta Neurologica Taiwanica* 5: 175–89.

Peng, F. C. C., Chia, L. G. and Huang, S. Y. 1992a. 'Degrees of agrammatism and the recovery of aphasia'. *Journal of Neurolinguistics* 7: 363–78.

Peng, F. C. C., Chia, Y. W., Wang, Y. C. and Shih, C. J. 1986. 'Agrammatism of Chinese transcortical aphasics'. *Journal of Neurolinguistics* 2: 233–60.

Peng, F. C. C., Huang, S. Y. and Chen, Y. Y. and Chia, L. G.. 1992b. 'Parkinson's disease and degenerative language disorders'. *Journal of Neurolinguistics* 7: 439–50.

Peng, F. C. C., Shih, Y. H., Yiu, C. H, and Liu, R. S. 2002. 'A neurolinguistic account of the effect of ictal and interictal discharges on the results from surgical outcome of temporal lobe epilepsy'. *Lingua Posnaniensis* 44: 96–103.

Piction, T. W, and Hink, R. F. 1974. 'Evoked potentials: How? What? and Why? *American Journal Of EEG Technology* 14: 9–44.

Pike, K. L. 1947. *Phonemics: A Technique for Reducing Languages to Writing.* Ann Arbor, MI: University of Michigan Press.

Pollack, R. 2001. 'The misunderstood geneticist'. *Nature Genetics* 29: 115, October.

Pula, R. P. 2001. 'General semantics and semiotics: similarities and differences. *Lingua Posnaniensis* 43: 141–71.

Robins, R.1979. *A Short History of Linguistics.* London: Longman.

Sapir, E. 1921. *Language.* New York: Harcourt, Brace and Company.

Sapir, E. 1929. 'The status of linguistics as a science'. *Language* 5: 207–14.

Schmahmann, J. D. 2003. 'The cerebellum and cognition'. In *Education Program Syllabus.* American Academy of Neurology, 55th Annual Meeting, March 29–April 5, Honolulu, Hawaii.

Science. 2001. 'Nicaraguan sign language'. 1758–59, September 7.

Science. 2004. 'Evolution of Language'. Special Issue, February 27.

Scientific American. 2004. *New Look at 'Human Evolution'*. Special Edition.

Sebeok, T. A. 1972. *Perspectives in Zoosemiotics.* The Hague: Mouton.

Shepherd, G. M. (ed.). 1998. *The Synaptic Organization of the Brain.* Fourth Edition. Oxford: Oxford University Press.

Shock, N. W. 1962. 'The physiology of aging'. *Scientific American* 206: 100–10.

Siegal, J. M. 2003. 'Why we sleep'. *Scientific American* 289(5): 92–7, November.

Silveri, M. C. 1998. 'Verbal short-term store-rehearsal system and the cerebellum: evidence from a patient wth the right cerebellar lesion'. *Brain* 121: 2175–87.

Silveri, M. C. and Leggion, M. G.. 'The cerebellum contributes to linguistic production: A case of agrammatic speech following a right cerebellar lesion'. *Neurology* 44: 2047–50.

Skardo, A. and Freeman, W. J. 1987. 'How brains make chaos in order to make sense of the world'. *Behavioural and Brain Sciences* 10: 161–95.

Smalley, W. A. 1983. *Mannual of Articulatory Phonetics.* Pasadena, CA: William Carey Library.

Snider, M. C. 1976. 'Cerebellar contributions to the Papez Circuit'. *Journal of Neuroscience Research* 2: 133–46.

Snider, R. S. 1958. 'The cerebellum'. *Scientific American.* 84–9.

Snow, C. 1978. 'The conversational context of language learning'. In R. N.

Campbell and P. T. Smith (eds) *Recent Advances in the Psychology of Language: Language Development and Mother-Child Interaction.* New York: Plenum Press, 253–69

Snowdon, D. A., Greiner, L. H. and Markesbery, W. R. 2000. 'Linguistic ability in early life and neuropathology of Alzheimer's disease and cerebrovascular disease: findings from the Nun Study'. In R. N. Kalaria and P. Ince (eds),*Vascular Factors in Alzheimer's Disease.* Annals of the New York Academy of Sciences, 903: 34–8.

Squire, L. R. 1987. *Memory and Brain.* New York: Oxford University Press.

Starosta, S. 'Review of *Modern Linguistics: The Results of Chomsky's Revolution*'. *Language Sciences* 2: 339–42.

Stevens, C, F. 1994. 'CREB and memory consolidation: minireview'. *Neuron* 12: 769–70.

Stross, B. 1976. *The Origin and Evolution of Language.* Dubuque, IO: Wm. C. Brown Company.

The Diagram Group. 1982. *The Brain: A User's Manual.* New York: G. P. Putnam's Sons.

Thibault, P. J. 1997. *Re-reading Saussure: The Dynamics of Signs in Social Life.* London: Routledge.

Thibault, P. J. 2004a. *Brain, Mind, and the Signifying Body.* London: Continuum.

Thibault, P. J. 2004b. *Agency and Consciousness in Discourse.* London: Continuum.

Trager, G. L. and Smith, H. L, Jr. 1951. *An Outline of English Structure.* Studies in Linguistics Occasional Papers 3.

Tsukahara, N., Bando, T. and Kiyohara, T. 1973. 'The properties of the reverberating circuit in the brain'. In K. Yagi and S. Yoshida (eds), *Neuroendocrine Control.* K. Tokyo: Tokyo University Press.

Tsukahara, N., Bando, T., Kitai, S. T. and Kiyohara, T. 1971. 'Cerebello-pontine reverberatng circuit'. *Brain Research* 35: 233–6.

Twaddell, W. F. 1969–70. 'Remarks read at the 1966 Northeast Conference'. *Studies in Linguistics* 21: 101–3.

Voegelin, C. F. 1951. 'Culture, language and the human organism'. *Southwestern Journal of Anthropology* 7: 357–73.

Wilbur, R. B. and Petersen, L. 1998. 'Modality interactions of speech and signing in simultaneous communication'. *Journal of Speech, Language, and Hearing Research* 41: 200–12.

Wilkerson, B. W. 1989. *The Language Teacher.* XIII, April.

Williams, G.. and Lukin, A. (eds) 2004. *The Development of Language: Functional Perspectives on Species and Individuals.* London: Continuum.

Wise, R., Chollet, F., Hadar, U. *et al.* 1991. 'Distribution of cortical neural networks involved in word comprehension and word retrieval'. *Brain* 114: 1803–817.

Yngve ,V. 1986. 'To be a scientist'. In I. Fleming (ed.), *The Thirteen LACUS Forum.* Lake Bluff, IL: LACUS, 5–25.

Zeviani, M. and Klopstock, T. 2001. 'Mitochondrial disorders'. *Current Opinions in Neurology* 14: 538–60.

Name Index

Subject Index

www.ingramcontent.com/pod-product-compliance
Ingram Content Group UK Ltd.
Pitfield, Milton Keynes, MK11 3LW, UK
UKHW020133290926
15471UKWH00003B/464

9 780826 438843